# Case Studies
## for use with
# Computers in the Medical Office

### Ninth Edition

## Susan M. Sanderson, CPEHR

Mc
Graw
Hill
Education

CASE STUDIES FOR USE WITH COMPUTERS IN THE MEDICAL OFFICE, NINTH EDITION

Published by McGraw-Hill Education, 2 Penn Plaza, New York, NY 10121. Copyright © 2016 by McGraw-Hill Education. All rights reserved. Printed in the United States of America. Previous editions © 2013, 2011, and 2009. No part of this publication may be reproduced or distributed in any form or by any means, or stored in a database or retrieval system, without the prior written consent of McGraw-Hill Education, including, but not limited to, in any network or other electronic storage or transmission, or broadcast for distance learning.

Some ancillaries, including electronic and print components, may not be available to customers outside the United States.

This book is printed on acid-free paper.

1 2 3 4 5 6 7 8 9 0 RMN/RMN 1 0 9 8 7 6 5

ISBN    978-0-07-811759-6
MHID    0-07-811759-3

Senior Vice President, Products & Markets: *Kurt L. Strand*
Vice President, General Manager, Products & Markets: *Marty Lange*
Vice President, Content Design & Delivery: *Kimberly Meriwether David*
Managing Director: *Chad Grall*
Executive Brand Manager: *William R. Lawrensen*
Director, Product Development: *Rose Koos*
Senior Product Developer: *Michelle L. Flomenhoft*
Executive Marketing Manager: *Roxan Kinsey*
Market Development Manager: *Kimberly Bauer*
Digital Product Analyst: *Katherine Ward*

Director, Content Design & Delivery: *Linda Avenarius*
Program Manager: *Angela R. FitzPatrick*
Content Project Managers: *Vicki Krug / Brent dela Cruz*
Buyer: *Laura M. Fuller*
Senior Design: *Srdjan Savanovic*
Content Licensing Specialists: *Lori Hancock / Lorraine Buczek*
Cover Image: ©*Magnilion / Getty images*
Compositor: *Lumina Datamatics, Inc.*
Printer: *R. R. Donnelley*

All credits appearing on page or at the end of the book are considered to be an extension of the copyright page.

Design Element
Puppet on Monitor: ©frentusha/Getty RF.
CiMO logo: ©Magnilion / Getty images

Medisoft® is a registered trademark of McKesson Corporation and/or one of its subsidiaries. Screenshots and material pertaining to Medisoft® Software used with permission of McKesson Corporation. © 2013 McKesson Corporation and/or one of its subsidiaries. All Rights Reserved.

The Medidata (student data file), illustrations, instructions, and exercises in Computers in the Medical Office are compatible with the Medisoft Advanced Version 19 Patient Accounting software available at the time of publication. Note that Medisoft Advanced Version 19 Patient Accounting software must be available to access the Medidata. It can be obtained by contacting your McGraw-Hill sales representative.

All brand or product names are trademarks or registered trademarks of their respective companies.

CPT five-digit codes, nomenclature, and other data are © 2015 American Medical Association. All Rights Reserved. No fee schedules, basic units relative values, or related listings are included in CPT. The AMA assumes no liability for the data contained herein.

CPT codes are based on CPT 2015.
ICD-10-CM codes are based on ICD-10-CM 2015.

All names, situations, and anecdotes are fictitious. They do not represent any person, event, or medical record.

Library of Congress Cataloging-in-Publication Data

Sanderson, Susan M.
    Case studies for use with computers in the medical office / Susan M. Sanderson, CPEHR.—Ninth edition.
        pages cm
    Includes index.
    ISBN 978-0-07-811759-6 (alk. paper)
    1.  Medical assistants—Case studies.    2.  Medical offices—Case studies.
    3.  Medical fees—Computer programs—Case studies.    I.  Title.
R728.8.S258 2016

651'.9610285—dc23
                                                                    2015010801

The Internet addresses listed in the text were accurate at the time of publication. The inclusion of a website does not indicate an endorsement by the authors or McGraw-Hill Education, and McGraw-Hill Education does not guarantee the accuracy of the information presented at these sites.

# Table of Contents

## PART 3

## On the Job   95

# PART 4

## Source Documents   179

# Preface

## CiMO™: The Step-by-Step, Hands-On Approach…Case Studies: The Next Application of the Hands-On Approach

Welcome to the ninth edition of *Case Studies for use with Computers in the Medical Office!* This product reinforces the concepts and skills your students will need for a successful career in medical office billing, building on what they learned in *Computers in the Medical Office (CiMO),* 9e. It presents a capstone billing simulation, providing your students with hands-on practice with realistic source documents. Just like with *CiMO, Case Studies* gives not only the step-by-step instructions your students need to learn but also the "why" behind those steps.

*Case Studies* provides students with enhanced learning opportunities that lead to superior qualifications for employment in medical offices. The product contains a realistic and extensive simulation covering two weeks of billing work in a medical office. Students use Medisoft® Advanced Version 19, a widely distributed medical office administrative software program, to complete the simulation. In addition to practicing and reinforcing their Medisoft skills, *Case Studies* introduces fourteen new Medisoft training topics that expand their knowledge. Students must exhibit critical thinking and problem solving to pull together the resources they will need to handle their daily assignments.

The prerequisite for successful completion of *Case Studies* is a basic knowledge of Medisoft Advanced Version 19, which can be gained by studying *CiMO,* 9e (0077836383, 9780077836382).

Here's what you and your students can expect from *Case Studies:*

- Coverage of Medisoft Advanced Version 19 patient billing software, a full-featured software program, including screen captures showing how the concepts described in the book actually look in the medical billing software.

- Both a tutorial and a simulation of Medisoft, using a medical office setting, Polaris Medical Group, and related patient data.

- A program that builds important skills for handling computerized billing tasks in medical offices.

- A chance to perform various jobs during the simulation, reinforcing essential skills such as inputting patient information, scheduling appointments, and handling billing, reports, and insurance claims.

- An opportunity for students to exhibit the ability to research facts, think through priorities, and analyze problems.

- Realistic exercises, completed using Medisoft, that cover what students will see working in actual medical practices, no matter what software those practices might use.

- An understanding of the medical billing cycle and how completing the related tasks will positively affect the financial well-being of a medical practice.

## Organization of *Case Studies,* 9e

*Case Studies* is divided into four parts:

| Part | Coverage |
|------|----------|
| 1: Introduction to Polaris Medical Group | Sets the stage for the rest of the book. Based on the idea that Polaris Medical Group (PMG) has recently hired you. PMG is a general practice with a complex environment of patient cases, insurance affiliations, and schedule demands. Introduces the practice's staff, describes the guidelines for working with medical office records, and details the role of the patient services specialist, which the students will perform in the simulation. |
| 2: Polaris Medical Group Policy and Procedure Manual | Covers PMG's general policies and employment procedures. Has detailed guidelines on processing new patient registration and referrals, scheduling appointments, and billing. Also contains detailed information sheets on the insurance carriers with which the practice interacts. |
| 3: On the Job *This section requires the use of Medisoft Advanced Version 19. | Requires students to perform a series of assignments using Medisoft. Each day of the ten-day assignment at PMG contains applications of the knowledge required in a medical office. Medisoft training topics are introduced in the text at the points students need the knowledge to complete the specific tasks. Special tips are provided in Part 3. Health Plan Information Pages at the end of Part 2 give details about the insurance coverage percentages for the health plans used in Part 3. At the end of each day's jobs in Part 3, a daily worksheet is provided to help verify that the work was completed correctly. |
| 4: Source Documents | Provides the patient data needed to complete the daily tasks in Part 3. The variety of completed forms, similar to those used in medical offices, includes patient information forms, encounter forms, coding notes, chart notes, remittance advices, and audit/edit reports. |

## New to the Ninth Edition

As the ninth edition of *Case Studies* is published, the healthcare field continues to undergo major changes. More Americans than ever before have health insurance, which means more office visits for physician practices. At the same time, patients are responsible for a greater share of their healthcare expenses than in the past. Collecting from patients at the time of the visit and monitoring overdue accounts is essential to the financial well-being of the practice. The role of the billing specialist has never been more important!

In order to prepare students for the transition to ICD-10-CM, we introduced students to ICD-10-CM codes in the previous edition of *Case Studies*. However, due to a limitation in Medisoft at that time, we were not able to also include ICD-9-CM codes. In this edition we are adding back ICD-9-CM codes for those instructors who would like students to experience both sets of codes. An ICD mapping utility is also available in Medisoft Version 19, which is used in this new edition!

Key changes in the ninth edition include:

- Software
  - —Medisoft Version 19 is used for all databases and illustrations (screen captures).
  - —ICD-9-CM and ICD-10-CM codes are included in the diagnosis code database.
- Part 1
  - —Updated content includes changes in HIPAA brought about by the Health Information Technology for Economic and Clinical Health (HITECH) Act, the Affordable Care Act, and the HIPAA Omnibus Rule.
  - —Updated content on HIPAA enforcement and breaches.
- Part 3
  - —New Medisoft Training Topic: Changing an Insurance Carrier Code Set from ICD-9-CM to ICD-10-CM.
  - —New End-of-Month and Follow-Up Jobs focused on collections activities.

For a detailed transition guide between the eighth and ninth editions of *Case Studies*, go to the Instructor Resources under the Library Tab in Connect for *Computers in the Medical Office, 9e*.

## To the Instructor

McGraw-Hill knows how much effort it takes to prepare for a new course. Through focus groups, symposia, reviews, and conversations with instructors like you, we have gathered information about what materials you need in order to facilitate successful courses. We are committed to providing you with high-quality, accurate instructor support.

## Using Medisoft Advanced Version 19 with Case Studies

**medisoft**® *Case Studies* features Medisoft Advanced Version 19 patient accounting software. Students who complete *Case Studies* find that the concepts and activities in the textbook are general enough to cover most administrative software used by healthcare providers. McGraw-Hill has partnered with Medisoft from the very beginning, going back twenty years to when the software was DOS-based! The support you receive when you are using a McGraw-Hill text with Medisoft is second to none.

Your students will need the following:

- Minimum System Requirements
  - Pentium 4
  - 1.0 GHz (minimum) or higher processor
  - 500 MB available hard disk space
  - 1 GB RAM
  - 32-bit color display (minimum screen display of 1024 × 768)
  - Windows 7 Professional or Ultimate 32- or 64-bit
  - Windows 8 Professional 32- or 64-bit
- External storage device, such as a USB flash drive, for storing backup copies of the working database
- Medisoft Advanced Version 19 patient billing software
- Student Data Files, available for download from the website, www.mhhe.com/medisoft

**Instructor's Software:** Medisoft Advanced Version 19 CD-ROM

Instructors who use McGraw-Hill Medisoft-compatible titles in their courses receive a fully working version of Medisoft Advanced Version 19 software, which allows a school to place the live software on the laboratory or classroom computers. Only one copy is needed per campus location. Your McGraw-Hill sales representative will help you obtain Medisoft for your campus.

Another option is the Student At-Home Medisoft Advanced Version 19 CD (1259671747, 9781259671746); a great option for online courses or students who wish to practice at home. Available individually or packaged with the textbook—it's up to you!

Much more information on how to work with each of the Medisoft options can be found in the *McGraw-Hill Guide to Success for CiMO,* 9e at www.mhhe.com/medisoft. The guide covers the following topics: software installation procedures for both the Instructor Edition and the Student At-Home Edition of Medisoft, Student Data File installation procedures, use of flash drives, backup and restore processes, tips and frequently asked questions, instructor resources, and technical support.

## Instructors' Resources

You can rely on the following materials to help you and your students work through the material in the book, all of which are available in Connect Instructor Resources under the Library tab for any *CiMO* course.

| Supplement | Features |
|---|---|
| Instructor's Manual (organized by Learning Outcomes) | -Answer keys for all exercises<br>-Documentation of steps and screenshots for Medisoft exercises |
| PowerPoint Presentations (organized by Learning Outcomes) | -Key terms<br>-Key concepts |
| Tools to Plan Course | -Correlations of the Learning Outcomes to accrediting bodies such as CAHIIM, ABHES, and CAAHEP<br>-Sample syllabi and lesson plans<br>-Conversion guide for *Case Studies*, 8e to *Case Studies*, 9e |
| *Medisoft* Advanced Version 19 Tools | -*McGraw-Hill Guide to Success for CiMO*, 9e<br>-Technical support information<br>-Installation directions<br>-Student Data File<br>-Backup and restore directions and files for Medisoft use. (The Medisoft backup files are an important resource if a student makes mistakes with his or her data and you want the student to have the correct data to start the next chapter.)<br>-Instructions on how to load Student Data File for two books at the same time (i.e., *CiMO* and *Case Studies*) |

Need help? Contact McGraw-Hill's Customer Experience Group (CXG). Visit the CXG website at www.mhhe.com/support. Browse our FAQs (Frequently Asked Questions), browse the product documentation, and/or contact a CXG representative.

Want to learn more about this product? Attend one of our online webinars. To learn more about the webinars, please contact your McGraw-Hill sales representative. To find your McGraw-Hill representative, go to shop.mheducation.com and click "Find Your Learning Technology Representative" on the "CONTACT US" page.

## To the Student

## Make Sure Medisoft Version 19 Is Installed on Your School's Computer

Before you can complete the jobs in Part 3 of this text, you must make sure that Medisoft Version 19 (the actual software program) is installed on your school's computer. It is possible that Medisoft Version 19 has already been installed on the computer you are using. If this is the case, you do not need to install it again.

***Be sure to download a copy of the* McGraw-Hill Guide to Success *from www.mhhe .com/medisoft for much more detail on the items mentioned in this section.***

With this 9th edition of *Case Studies*, there are two options to access Medisoft. Students, please be sure to check with your instructor for the option you will use in your class.

*Install the Medisoft program from a CD and Download the Student Data File*

The Student Data File contains the medical practice, physicians, and patients required to complete the exercises in Part 3.

1. **If you are using a computer at your school [Instructor Edition CD]**

   Medisoft will most likely already be installed on the computer, in which case you don't need to install the program. You do still need to download and install the Student Data File (see below).

2. **If you are working on your own computer [Student At-Home Edition CD]**

   You will need to purchase the Student At-Home Medisoft CD and install the program on your computer. You also need to download and install the Student Data File (see page xiii).

*Instructions*

1. **If you are using a computer at your school [Instructor Edition CD]**

   **Step 1:** Determine whether Medisoft Advanced Version 19 is installed on your school's computer. (If it is already installed, skip to step 3.) To find out if it is installed:

   a. Click the Start button, select All Programs, and look for the Medisoft folder. If you find a Medisoft folder, click Medisoft Advanced to launch the program. Once the program is open, determine which version of Medisoft is installed. Click Help on the menu bar and then click About Medisoft. Look in the window that appears, which lists the version number of the program.

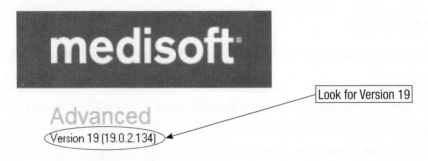

   b. If you see Version 19, skip to step 3.

   **Step 2:** Install *Medisoft Version* 19 if it is not already on your school computer. ***Students, please check with your instructor before proceeding.***

   a. To install the software from the CD, go to the "Guide" for instructions.

**Step 3:** Check to see if the CSMO9e Student Data File is installed. To find out if it is installed:

    a. Start Medisoft Advanced Version 19 by double-clicking the desktop icon. Look at the title bar that contains the words "Medisoft Advanced 19." If the CSMO9e Student Data File has already been installed, you should see "CSMO9e" to the right of "Medisoft Advanced 19".

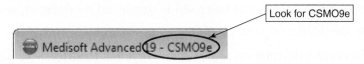

    b. If you see CSMO9e, close the program and you will be ready for Part 3! If not, proceed to step 4.

**Step 4:** Install the CSMO9e Student Data File if your computer does not have it.

    a. Go to www.mhhe.com/medisoft and click on the Case Studies link.

    b. Then you will find the installation file needed.

    c. Read the *McGraw-Hill Guide to Success*, which will walk you through downloading to your computer the zip file with the Student Data File installer.

    d. **Warning:** Make sure you do not have the Medisoft program open on your computer when you install the Student Data File.

**2. If you are working on your own computer [Student At-Home Edition CD]**

*To purchase a copy of this optional version, check with your instructor first.*

**Step 1:** To install the software from the CD, go to the "Guide" for instructions.

**Step 2:** To install the CSMO9e Student Data File, refer back to step 4 above.

Need help? Contact McGraw-Hill's Customer Experience Group (CXG). Visit the CXG website at www.mhhe.com/support. Browse our FAQs (Frequently Asked Questions), browse the product documentation, and/or contact a CXG representative.

## Backing Up Data in Medisoft

If you are in a school environment, it is important to make a backup copy of your work after each Medisoft session. This ensures that you can restore your work during the next session and be able to use your own data even if another student uses the computer after you or if, for any reason, the files on the school computer are changed or corrupted. This section provides instructions on backing up data in Medisoft.

**1.** You can use the Backup option on the File menu to back up your data at any time. However, by default, Medisoft also gives you the opportunity to back up your data each time you exit the program. Click the Exit option on the File menu to exit Medisoft.

2. The Backup Reminder dialog box appears. You will back up your data to the folder where you are storing your work for this course, for example, C:\...\My Documents\CaseStudies, and you will name the backup file according to the day of the simulation you are working on in the text. Click the Back Up Data Now button.

3. The Medisoft Backup dialog box appears. If the Destination File Path and Name box at the top of the dialog box does not show the folder where you will be storing your work (whichever folder was last used is displayed by default), use the Find button to locate this folder on your computer.

4. Once the correct destination folder is displayed in the Medisoft Backup dialog box, you are ready to key in the backup file name at the end of the path name. The backup file must end with the .mbk extension (which stands for Medisoft backup data). All Medisoft backup files end with the extension *.mbk.*

Using the End key or the right arrow key on the keyboard, move the cursor to the end of the path name. Depending on whether a backup file already exists in the destination folder, the end of the path may or may not display a file with the .mbk extension. If no file with the .mbk extension appears, simply key in the new file name, **Week1Day1.mbk** (for the first day of the simulation), at the end of the path name. If a backup file is already displayed, use the backspace key to delete the old file name and key in the new one. The end of the path should now read: \Week1Day1 .mbk, as shown in the following example. (*Note:* If you are sharing a computer, you may want to add your initials to the beginning of the file name.)

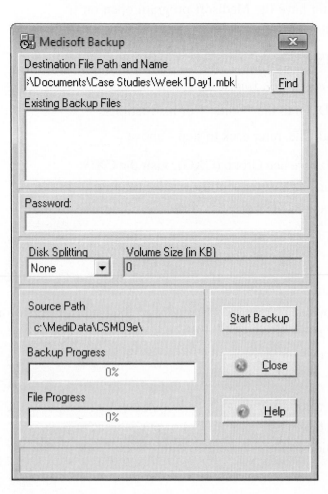

5. After the correct file name has been entered in the Destination File Path and Name box, click the Start Backup button to begin the backup.

6. Medisoft backs up the data under the new name and displays an Information box indicating that the backup is complete. Click the OK button to close the Information box.

7. Click the Close button to close the Medisoft Backup dialog box. Then exit the Medisoft program.

8. For safekeeping, copy your new backup file from the current drive on the computer to an external storage device, such as a flash drive. A separate backup copy

prevents you from losing your work if the current drive fails or if you or someone else accidentally deletes data on the computer.

## Restoring Data in Medisoft

If you are sharing a computer with other students in a school environment, you will need to perform a restore before a new Medisoft session to be certain you are working with your own data. If necessary, follow these steps to restore your latest backup file.

To restore the file *Week1Day1.mbk* to c:\MediData\CSMO9e:

1. Copy your backup file from your external storage device to the assigned location on the computer you are using. (Ask your instructor if you are not sure which folder this is.)

2. Start Medisoft.

3. Check the program's title bar at the top of the screen to make sure CSMO9e is displayed as the active data set. (If it is not, use the Open Practice option on the File menu to select it.)

4. Open the File menu, and click Restore Data.

5. When the Warning box appears, click OK. The Restore dialog box appears.

6. Use the Find button to locate your assigned storage folder (the folder used in step 1 above). Locate *Week1Day1.mbk* in the list of existing backup files displayed for that folder, and click on it to attach it to the Backup File Path and Name at the top of the dialog box. (The end of the path name should read \…\Week1Day1.mbk.)

7. The Destination Path at the bottom of the box will automatically display c:\MediData\CSMO9e. Your screen should look like the one shown here.

8. Click the Start Restore button.

9. When the Confirm box appears, click OK.

10. An Information dialog box appears indicating that the restore is complete. You have successfully restored the *Week1Day1.mbk* file for use with Medisoft for the next session. Click OK to continue and then click the Close button to close the Restore dialog box.

11. The Restore dialog box closes. You are ready to begin working.

# About the Author

Susan M. Sanderson has authored all Windows-based editions of *Computers in the Medical Office*. She has also written *Case Studies for use with Computers in the Medical Office, Electronic Health Records for Allied Health Careers,* and *Practice Management and EHR: A Total Patient Encounter for Medisoft® Clinical.*

In her more than fifteen years' experience with Medisoft, Susan has participated in alpha and beta testing, worked with instructors to site-test materials, and provided technical support to McGraw-Hill customers.

In 2009, Susan earned her CPEHR certification (Certified Professional in Electronic Health Records). In addition, she is a member of the Healthcare Information and Management Systems Society (HIMSS) and the eLearning Guild. Susan is a graduate of Drew University with further study at Columbia University.

# Acknowledgments

Thanks to the instructors and reviewers who have provided feedback on the ninth edition. Special thanks are due to the people listed below for accuracy checking the exercises.

- Dr. Tammie Bolling, CHTS, CBCS, CMA, CBCS, MOS-Master, CHI, MBA/HCM, Pellissippi State Community College

- Barbara Marchelletta, CMA ( AAMA ), RHIT, CPC, CPT, AHI, Beal College

- Suzanne Mays, BS, MSH, MSIT, University of Phoenix

- Tina M. Mazuch, MS, RHIA, Northeast Community College

A full list of reviewers can be found in the Acknowledgments section of *Computers in the Medical Office,* 9e.

# Introduction to Polaris Medical Group

## LEARNING OUTCOMES

*After successfully completing Part 1, you will be able to define the key terms and:*

1.1 Name the eight positions held by members of the Polaris Medical Group patient services team.

1.2 List eight facts that are documented in all medical records at Polaris Medical Group.

1.3 Identify the four parts of a SOAP note.

1.4 Describe how the HIPAA legislation sets standards for privacy and the electronic transmission of data.

1.5 Describe the qualities of an effective patient services specialist.

1.6 Identify ten tasks that a patient services specialist at Polaris Medical Group performs during a typical day.

## KEY TERMS

| | |
|---|---|
| audit trail | HIPAA Privacy Rule |
| continuity of care | HIPAA Security Rule |
| documentation | HITECH Act |
| electronic health record (EHR) | internist |
| electronic protected health information (ePHI) | medical record |
| family practitioner | National Provider Identifier (NPI) |
| Health Insurance Portability and Accountability Act of 1996 (HIPAA) | NSF (nonsufficient funds) check |
| | primary care physician |
| HIPAA Electronic Health Care Transactions and Code Sets (TCS) | protected health information (PHI) |
| | SOAP format |

This section is your introduction to Polaris Medical Group. You will learn about the purpose, the people, and the structure of the practice. In addition, you will be introduced to the topics of medical records and patient privacy. All staff members at Polaris Medical Group must understand the proper use and disclosure of patient health information.

Part 1 also provides information about the types of tasks you will complete in Part 3, On the Job. You will learn about your role and your specific responsibilities at Polaris Medical Group, including activities such as scheduling, billing, and responding to patient inquiries.

## CiMO 1.1 THE PMG PATIENT SERVICES TEAM

The physicians and staff of Polaris Medical Group (PMG) welcome you as a new member of our healthcare team. We are committed to providing each of our patients with the highest quality of healthcare. We hired you because we are confident that you can contribute to that goal. We are also committed to creating and maintaining a positive work environment for our employees.

At PMG, we work as a patient services team. The physicians, assistants, and medical office staff members work together, sharing information and resources to accomplish our common goals. We treat all patients and staff members with courtesy and patience. The caring environment we create is one reason that patients return to the clinic. A caring environment also makes the workplace a pleasant one for staff members. At PMG, we believe in treating others as we would like to be treated.

### Statement of Purpose

Polaris Medical Group provides medical care and services to individuals and families regardless of age, race, color, creed, national origin, gender, or disability. As a family practice, we respond to a broad range of patient needs. Our primary function is to treat illness, disease, injury, and disability through evaluation, examination, and the use of medical procedures. We also educate individuals and families regarding preventive care. Our goal is to help all patients achieve their maximum potential within their capabilities and to accelerate convalescence and reduce the length of the patient's recovery.

### Organization and Staff

The organization chart for PMG is illustrated in Figure 1-1. There are two physicians in the practice: Robin C. Crebore, M.D., F.A.A.F.P. (Fellow, American Academy of Family Physicians), and Michael P. Mahabir, M.D., F.A.C.P.

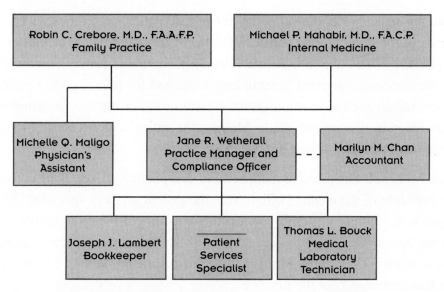

**FIGURE 1-1** Organization Chart of Polaris Medical Group

(Fellow, American College of Physicians). Dr. Crebore, a *family practitioner,* has a general practice and treats patients of all ages. Dr. Mahabir, as an *internist,* specializes in the care of adults.

*The physicians' backgrounds are as follows:*

**Robin C. Crebore, M.D., F.A.A.F.P.**

**Specialty:** Family Practice
**University:** Fairfield University, CT
**Medical School:** Tufts University School of Medicine, MA, 1996
**Internship:** Presbyterian University of Pennsylvania Medical Center, 1997
**Residency:** St. Elizabeth's Hospital, MA, 1999
**Board Certification Dates:**
    1999, Family Practice
    2015, Recertified Family Practice
    2016, Certificate of Added Qualifications in Geriatrics
**Memberships:** Fellow, American Academy of Family Practitioners; American Geriatrics Society

**Michael P. Mahabir, M.D., F.A.C.P.**

**Specialty:** Internal Medicine
**University:** University of Colorado
**Medical School:** East Virginia Medical School, VA, 2002
**Internship:** Medical Center Hospital of Vermont, 2003
**Residency:** Medical Center Hospital of Vermont, 2005
**Board Certification Date:** 2005, Internal Medicine
**Memberships:** American Society of Internal Medicine; Fellow, American College of Physicians; Diplomat, American Board of Internal Medicine

**family practitioner**
a physician who treats patients of all ages and does not specialize in one area of medicine.

**internist** a physician who specializes in the care of adults.

Both physicians offer consultations for private patients, and they accept assignment for Medicare and Medicaid. Both are also identified as **primary care physicians** in a number of managed care plans. In this role, they are responsible for overseeing patients' overall healthcare and for referring their patients to specialists, such as cardiologists for cardiovascular disease or dermatologists for skin disease. Michelle Maligo, the office's physician's assistant, works with both physicians.

**primary care physician** a physician in a managed care plan who directs all aspects of a patient's care, including routine services, referrals to specialists, and supervision of hospital admission.

Jane Wetherall, our practice manager and compliance officer, is responsible for oversight of the medical office. You, the patient services specialist (PSS), report to her, as does Thomas Bouck, the part-time medical laboratory technician. Accounting functions are handled by a bookkeeper, Joseph Lambert, whose work is checked by Marilyn Chan, an outside accountant who reviews the financial aspects of the practice.

Polaris Medical Group is located in a modern medical office building in Columbus, Ohio, three blocks from St. Mary's Hospital. Our offices have a patient reception area and a front office where the business transactions of the medical practice take place. Your desk is located in a glassed-in section of the front office. There is also a separate lunchroom.

Each doctor has a separate office. In addition, there are three examining rooms for the evaluation and treatment of patients and an office laboratory for analyzing blood and urine samples. PMG also contracts with an outside laboratory for other types of lab work. Specimens are picked up from the practice and processed on a daily basis.

## CiMO 1.2 MEDICAL RECORDS

Patients' records are a critical component of all services and treatments we provide at PMG. **Medical records** contain all information pertaining to a patient's health history. They also contain all communications with and about each patient. The medical record begins with a patient's first contact with the practice and continues through all treatments and services. These records provide continuity and communication among physicians and other healthcare professionals who are involved in a patient's care.

**medical record** a file that includes the patient information form, the patient's medical history, record of care, progress notes, insurance correspondence, and other pertinent documents.

**electronic health record (EHR)** patient medical record created using a computer.

In our practice, patient medical records are created on computers, rather than written by hand. In addition to physicians' notes, a patient's **electronic health record (EHR)** includes digital files of X-ray images, lab test results, medical history, and a picture of the patient. Electronic health records offer significant advantages over paper records. For example, a patient who is away from home or in an accident can authorize a local physician to access the record to locate needed history. In addition, large amounts of information gathered over many years about a patient's chronic condition can be organized for quick review.

## Information in the Medical Record

Information recorded in the patient's medical record is known as ***documentation.*** Accurate, complete documentation provides the physician with a detailed summary of each of the patient's visits, including information about treatments, progress, and outcomes.

The medical record originates when a patient visits the office for the first time. Using the information on the patient information form (see Figure 1-2), a patient chart is created. After that, the medical record is updated each time the patient visits the physician. PMG includes the following eight items in every medical record:

1. Patient's name.
2. Encounter date and reason.
3. Appropriate history and physical examination.
4. Review of all tests that were ordered.
5. Diagnosis.
6. Plan of care, or notes on procedures or treatments that were given.
7. Instructions or recommendations that were given to the patient.
8. Signature of the provider who saw the patient.

In addition, a patient's medical record contains

- Biographical and personal information, including the patient's full name, Social Security number, date of birth, full address and phone numbers, marital status, employer information as applicable, insurance information, and chart number.
- Copies of prescriptions and instructions given to the patient, including refills.
- A list of the patient's known allergies, created and updated as needed.
- A list of medications the patient is taking, created and updated as needed.
- Immunization records.
- Previous and current diagnoses, test results, health risks, and progress notes.
- Copies of all communications with the patient, including letters, telephone calls, faxes, and e-mail messages; the patient's responses; and a note of the time, date, topic, and physician's response to each communication.

## PATIENT INFORMATION FORM

### THIS SECTION REFERS TO PATIENT ONLY

| | | | | |
|---|---|---|---|---|
| Name: | Sex: | Marital Status: ☐ S ☐ M ☐ D ☐ W | Birth Date: | |

Address: | SS#:

City: | State: | Zip: | Employer: | Phone:

Home Phone: | Employer's Address:

Work Phone: | City: | State: | Zip:

Race:
___American Indian or Alaska Native
___Asian                    ___Other
___Black or African American    ___Native Hawaiian or Other Pacific Islander
___White                    ___Declined

Ethnicity:              Language:
___Hispanic or Latino
___Non-Hispanic or Latino
___Declined

Spouse's Name: | Spouse's Employer:

Emergency Contact: | Relationship: | Phone #:

### FILL IN IF PATIENT IS A MINOR

Parent/Guardian's Name: | Sex: | Marital Status: ☐ S ☐ M ☐ D ☐ W | Birth Date:

Phone: | SS#:

Address: | Employer: | Phone:

City: | State: | Zip: | Employer's Address:

Student Status: | City: | State: | Zip:

### INSURANCE INFORMATION

Primary Insurance Company: | Secondary Insurance Company:

Subscriber's Name: | Birth Date: | Subscriber's Name: | Birth Date:

Plan: | SS#: | Plan:

Policy #: | Group #: | Policy #: | Group #:

Copayment/Deductible: | Price Code:

### OTHER INFORMATION

Reason for visit: | Allergy to Medication (list):

Name of referring physician: | If auto accident, list date and state in which it occurred:

I authorize treatment and agree to pay all fees and charges for the person named above. I agree to pay all charges shown by statements, promptly upon their presentation, unless credit arrangements are agreed upon in writing.
I authorize payment directly to POLARIS MEDICAL GROUP of insurance benefits otherwise payable to me. I hereby authorize the release of any medical information necessary in order to process a claim for payment in my behalf.

_____        _____
(Patient's Signature/Parent or Guardian's Signature)                    (Date)

I plan to make payment of my medical expenses as follows (check one or more):

_____Insurance (as above)    _____Cash/Check/Credit/Debit Card    _____Medicare    _____Medicaid    _____Workers' Comp.

**FIGURE 1-2**   Patient Information Form

- Requests for information about the patient (from a health plan or an attorney, for example), and a detailed log indicating to whom information was released.

- Copies of referral or consultation letters.

- Original documents that the patient has signed, such as an authorization to release information and an advance directive.

The medical record allows healthcare professionals involved in the patient's care to provide continuity of care to individual patients. *Continuity of care* refers to coordination of care received by a patient over time and across multiple healthcare providers.

**continuity of care** coordination of care received by a patient over time and across multiple healthcare providers.

## Standards

Information in all patient medical records is recorded in a consistent manner. Without standardization, physicians and other medical office personnel would find locating the information they need difficult and time-consuming. To ensure that medical records are well organized and easy to use, the following standards are followed at PMG:

- *Records must be clear:* Medical records should be complete and accurate. If the records are handwritten, the entries should be legible to others, made in ink (not pencil), and dated.

- *Entries must be signed and dated:* Whether digitally entered by the provider, handwritten, or transcribed, each entry must have the signature or initials and title of the responsible provider and the date.

- *Changes must be clearly made:* An incorrect entry is marked with a single line through the words to be changed; the correct information is entered after it, so that the previous copy can be read. Corrections are also dated and signed by the person making the change. No part of a record should be otherwise altered or removed, deleted, or destroyed.

# 1.3 SOAP FORMAT

The Polaris Medical Group uses *problem-oriented medical records* (POMRs) to organize patient information. The problem-oriented medical record contains a general section with data from the initial patient examination and assessment. When the patient returns for subsequent visits, the reasons for those encounters are listed separately and have their own notes. A problem-oriented medical record contains SOAP notes. In the *SOAP format* (see Figure 1-3), a patient's encounter documentation is grouped into four parts: *s*ubjective, *o*bjective, *a*ssessment, and *p*lan:

**SOAP format** the documentation of medical records according to *s*ubjective data, *o*bjective data, *a*ssessment, and *p*lan of treatment.

*S:* The *subjective* information is based on the patient's descriptions of symptoms along with other comments.

*O:* The *objective* information (also called signs) includes the physician's descriptions of the presenting problem and data from examinations and tests.

*A:* The *assessment,* also called the impression or conclusion, is the physician's diagnosis, or interpretation of the subjective and objective information.

*P:* The *plan,* also called treatment, advice, or recommendations, includes the necessary patient monitoring, follow-up, procedures, and instructions to the patient.

Name: David Weatherly                     Telephone: 999-555-6798

Date of Birth:    8/12/59


3/5/18    **PROBLEM 1:** Tonsillitis
          **CHIEF COMPLAINT:** Sore throat x2 days.

          **S:**  Sore throat, fever, difficulty swallowing.
          **O:**  Temperature 101°, pharyngitis with exudative tonsils.
          **A:**  Tonsillitis.
          **P:**  1.    Throat culture.
                  2.    1.2 units CR Bicillin.
                  3.    Recheck in 10 days.

                                          Robin Crebore, M.D.


3/15/18 **PROBLEM 1:** Recheck

          **S:**  Feels better.
          **O:**  Temperature, normal.
          **A:**  Problem 1 resolved.
          **P:**  Saline gargles, if necessary.

                                          Robin Crebore, M.D.

**FIGURE 1-3**   SOAP Format

This format provides an orderly system for recording clinical information about a patient encounter.

## 1.4  HIPAA/HITECH AND PATIENT PRIVACY

Medical records are legal documents. Patients have rights to the information in their medical records. They also control the amount and type of information that is released from their records, except for the use of the data to treat them or conduct the normal business transactions of the practice.

Patient services specialists often handle requests for information from patients' medical records, and they must know what information can be released and under what circumstances. Staff members who work with a medical record are responsible for guarding the patient's privacy and confidentiality. Patient confidentiality is the basis of the physician-patient relationship. A violation of this understanding is not only a breach of trust; it may also violate federal law. The *Health Insurance Portability and Accountability Act of 1996,* known as *HIPAA,* is a federal law governing many aspects of healthcare, such as

**Health Insurance Portability and Accountability Act of 1996 (HIPAA)** a federal law governing many aspects of healthcare, such as standards for the electronic transmission of information and the security of healthcare records.

standards for the electronic transmission of information and the security of healthcare records.

When the legislation was passed in 1996, most physicians were recording patient information on paper. A decade later, the impact of the information technology revolution was being felt in hospitals and physician practices. Some healthcare providers were recording and storing patients' health records on computers. The information in the records could be transmitted electronically over a computer network from one provider to another, or from a provider to an insurance company.

Recognizing that the existing HIPAA legislation would not adequately safeguard health information in this new electronic environment, the *Health Information Technology for Economic and Clinical Health (HITECH) Act*, part of the American Recovery and Reinvestment Act of 2009, and the Affordable Care Act of 2010 contain updated rules to protect patients' healthcare information. The HIPAA Omnibus Rule of 2013 also made a number of significant changes to the privacy, security, and enforcement provisions of the original HIPAA legislation.

The original 1996 HIPAA law is divided into different sections that address unique aspects of healthcare reform.

HIPAA's Administrative Simplification provisions contain three rules that are important at PMG and in all medical offices:

1. Privacy Rule—provides privacy rights and protections for patients' health information.
2. Security Rule—the administrative, technical, and physical safeguards that are required to protect patients' health information.
3. Electronic Health Care Transactions and Code Sets—require every provider who does business electronically to use the same healthcare transactions, code sets, and identifiers.

## HIPAA Privacy Rule

The *HIPAA Privacy Rule* is the first comprehensive federal protection for the privacy of health information. These national standards protect individuals' medical records and other personal health information. The Privacy Rule must be followed by all health plans, healthcare clearinghouses, and healthcare providers and their business associates. The rules mandate that a provider or other group must

- Adopt a set of privacy practices that are appropriate for its healthcare services.
- Notify patients about their privacy rights and how their information can be used or disclosed.

**HITECH Act** the Health Information Technology for Economic and Clinical Health Act, part of the American Recovery and Reinvestment Act of 2009, that provides financial incentives to physicians and hospitals to adopt EHRs and strengthens HIPAA privacy and security regulations.

**HIPAA Privacy Rule** national standards that protect individuals' medical records and other personal health information.

- Train employees so that they understand the privacy practices.
- Appoint a staff member to be the privacy official responsible for seeing that the privacy practices are adopted and followed.
- Secure patient records containing individually identifiable health information so that they are not readily available to those who do not need them.

### Protected Health Information

The HIPAA Privacy Rule covers the use and disclosure of patients' *protected health information (PHI)*. PHI is defined as individually identifiable health information that is transmitted or maintained in any form or medium. *Electronic protected health information (ePHI)* is any protected health information (PHI) that is created, stored, transmitted, or received electronically.

Protected information includes the information below when it is used in connection with health information, such as a diagnosis or condition:

- Name
- Address (including street address, city, county, ZIP code)
- Names of relatives and employers
- Birth date
- Telephone numbers
- Fax number
- E-mail address
- Social Security number
- Medical record number
- Health plan beneficiary number
- Account number
- Certificate or license number
- Serial number of any vehicle or other device
- Website address
- Fingerprints or voiceprints
- Photographic images

Except for treatment, payment, and healthcare operations, the Privacy Rule limits the release of protected health information without the patient's authorization. *Treatment* means providing and coordinating the patient's medical care; *payment* refers to the exchange of information with health plans; and healthcare *operations* are the general business management functions. When using or disclosing protected health information at PMG, staff members must try to limit the information shared to the minimum amount necessary to accomplish the intended purpose.

## Notice of Privacy Practices

Under the HIPAA Privacy Rule, physician practices must provide patients with a Notice of Privacy Practices at their first contact or encounter. This document describes the medical office's practices regarding the use and disclosure of PHI. It also establishes the office's privacy complaint procedures, explains that disclosure is limited to the minimum necessary information that is required, and discusses how consent for other types of information release is obtained. Medical practices are required to display the Notice of Privacy Practices in a prominent place in the office. To satisfy this requirement, Polaris Medical Group gives patients a copy of a Notice of Privacy Practices (see Figure 1-4)

---

**POLARIS MEDICAL GROUP**
**NOTICE OF PRIVACY PRACTICES**

**THIS NOTICE DESCRIBES HOW MEDICAL INFORMATION ABOUT YOU MAY BE USED AND DISCLOSED AND HOW YOU CAN GET ACCESS TO THIS INFORMATION.**

**PLEASE REVIEW IT CAREFULLY.**

**YOUR RIGHTS**

When it comes to your health information, you have certain rights. This section explains your rights and some of our responsibilities to help you.

**GET AN ELECTRONIC OR PAPER COPY OF YOUR MEDICAL RECORD**

- You can ask to see or get an electronic or paper copy of your medical record and other health information we have about you. Ask us how to do this.
- We will provide a copy or a summary of your health information, usually within 30 days of your request. We may charge a reasonable, cost-based fee.

**ASK US TO CORRECT YOUR MEDICAL RECORD**

- You can ask us to correct health information about you that you think is incorrect or incomplete. Ask us how to do this.
- We may say "no" to your request, but we'll tell you why in writing within 60 days.

**REQUEST CONFIDENTIAL COMMUNICATIONS**

- You can ask us to contact you in a specific way (for example, home or office phone) or to send mail to a different address.
- We will say "yes" to all reasonable requests.

**ASK US TO LIMIT WHAT WE USE OR SHARE**

- You can ask us not to use or share certain health information for treatment, payment, or our operations. We are not required to agree to your request, and we may say "no" if it would affect your care.
- If you pay for a service or health care item out-of-pocket in full, you can ask us not to share that information for the purpose of payment or our operations with your health insurer. We will say "yes" unless a law requires us to share that information.

**GET A LIST OF THOSE WITH WHOM WE'VE SHARED INFORMATION**

- You can ask for a list (accounting) of the times we've shared your health information for six years prior to the date you ask, who we shared it with, and why.
- We will include all the disclosures except for those about treatment, payment, and health care operations, and certain other disclosures (such as any you asked us to make). We'll provide one accounting a year for free but will charge a reasonable, cost-based fee if you ask for another one within 12 months.

**GET A COPY OF THIS PRIVACY NOTICE**

- You can ask for a paper copy of this notice at any time, even if you have agreed to receive the notice electronically. We will provide you with a paper copy promptly.

**CHOOSE SOMEONE TO ACT FOR YOU**

- If you have given someone medical power of attorney or if someone is your legal guardian, that person can exercise your rights and make choices about your health information. We will make sure the person has this authority and can act for you before we take any action.

**FILE A COMPLAINT IF YOU FEEL YOUR RIGHTS ARE VIOLATED**

- You can complain if you feel we have violated your rights by contacting us using the information in this notice.

Page 1 of 4

---

**FIGURE 1-4**   Page from a Notice of Privacy Practices Booklet

<u>ACKNOWLEDGMENT OF RECEIPT OF NOTICE OF PRIVACY PRACTICES</u>

**Polaris Medical Group**
2100 Grace Avenue
Columbus, OH 43214-1111

I hereby acknowledge that I received or was provided the opportunity to receive a copy of Polaris Medical Group's Notice of Privacy Practices.

PATIENT INFORMATION

Print Name: _____

Signature : _____

Date: _____

Telephone : _____

PERSONAL REPRESENTATIVE INFORMATION (IF APPLICABLE)

Print Name: _____

Nature of Relationship: _____
(i.e.,– Parent, Guardian, Personal Representative, etc.)

Signature : _____

Date: _____

_For Office Use Only :_

___ Signed form received.
___ Acknowledgment not obtained.
___ Patient refused.
___ Emergency.
___ Other _____

Print Staff Member's Name: _____

Staff Member's Signature : _____

Date: _____

**FIGURE 1-5**   Acknowledgment of Receipt of Notice of Privacy Practices Form

and asks patients to sign an Acknowledgment of Receipt of Notice of Privacy Practices, illustrated in Figure 1-5.

## Authorizations

For use or disclosure other than for treatment, payment, or operations, the practice must have the patient sign an authorization to release the information. For example, information about alcohol and drug abuse may not be released without a specific authorization from the patient. The authorization document must be in plain language and include the following:

- A description of the information to be used or disclosed.
- The name or other specific identification of each person authorized to use or disclose the information.
- The name of the person or group of people to whom the covered entity may make the use or disclosure.
- A description of each purpose of the requested use or disclosure.
- An expiration date.
- Signature of the individual (or authorized representative) and date.

In addition, a valid authorization must include

- A statement of the individual's right to revoke the authorization in writing.
- A statement about whether the covered entity is able to base treatment, payment, enrollment, or eligibility for benefits on the authorization.
- A statement that information used or disclosed after the authorization may be disclosed again by the recipient and may no longer be protected by the rule.

A sample authorization form is shown in Figure 1-6.

## HIPAA Security Rule

The **HIPAA Security Rule** outlines safeguards required to protect the confidentiality, integrity, and availability of health information that is stored on a computer system or that is transmitted across computer networks, including the Internet. While the HIPAA Privacy Rule applies to all forms of patients' protected health information, whether electronic, paper, or oral, the Security Rule specifically covers PHI that is created, received, maintained, or transmitted in electronic form.

> HIPAA Security Rule national standards that outline the minimum administrative, technical, and physical safeguards required to prevent unauthorized access to protected healthcare information.

The security standards are divided into three categories of safeguards: administrative, physical, and technical.

*Administrative safeguards* are administrative policies and procedures designed to protect electronic health information. The management of security is assigned to one individual, who conducts an assessment of the current level of data security. Once that assessment is complete, security policies and procedures are developed or modified to meet current needs. Security training is provided to educate staff members on the policies and to raise awareness of security and privacy issues.

MRN_____

## Authorization for Release of Patient Information

Patient Name_____ Date of Birth_____

I hereby authorize _____
                  Name              Address              City        State      Zip
Telephone Number_____

to disclose the above named individual's health information as described below:

Date(s) of Service Requested (if known) or Provider: _____

Description of information to be released: (check all that apply)
___Immunization record                  ___Most recent history and physical
___Laboratory reports                    ___Consultations
___Radiology/Imaging reports          ___Progress notes
___Radiology films                       ___Entire medical record
___Other_____

I understand that the information in my health record may include information relating to communicable disease, Acquired Immunodeficiency Syndrome ("AIDS"), or Human Immunodeficiency Virus ("HIV"), behavioral or mental health, alcohol/drug (substance) abuse or any such related information.

This information may be disclosed to and used by the following individual or organization:

_____
Name                  Address                  City        State      Zip

Telephone Number_____

Description of the purpose of the use and/or disclosure:

___Continuing care        ___Second opinion          ___Social Security/Disability
___Consultation            ___Insurance
___Legal purposes        ___Personal use
___Other: Please describe: _____

I understand that this authorization is voluntary and I may refuse to sign this authorization. I further understand that my healthcare and the payment of my healthcare will not be affected if I do not sign this form. I understand I may inspect or copy the information to be used or disclosed. I understand that information used or disclosed pursuant to the authorization may be subject to redisclosure by the recipient and may no longer be protected by federal and state privacy regulations. I understand Polaris Medical Group may charge a processing fee for this service. I understand that this authorization will expire by law 180 days from the date of this authorization unless I otherwise specify. This authorization will be in effect until _____ (date or event).

I understand I may revoke this authorization at any time by notifying the Polaris Medical Group. I understand that if I revoke this authorization, I must do so in writing and the written revocation must be signed and dated with a date that is later than the date on this authorization. The revocation will not affect any actions taken before the receipt of the written revocation.

_____        _____
Signature of Patient or Patient's Representative      Date

_____
Printed name of Patient or Patient's Representative

_____        _____
Relationship to Patient           or      Legal Authority (attach supporting documentation)

**FIGURE 1-6** Sample Information Release Authorization Form

*Physical safeguards* are the mechanisms required to protect electronic systems, equipment, and data from threats, environmental hazards, and unauthorized intrusion. Unauthorized intrusion refers to access by individuals who do not have a need to know. For example, individuals who are not working with confidential patient information should not be able to view this type of information displayed on an office computer monitor. To prevent intrusion, PMG limits physical access to computers. A security measure can be as simple as a lock on the door or as advanced as an electronic device that requires fingerprint authentication to gain access.

*Technical safeguards* are the automated processes used to protect data and control access to data. Access to information is granted on an as-needed basis. For example, the individual responsible for scheduling may not need access to billing data. Examples of technical safeguards include computer passwords, antivirus and firewall software, and secure transmission systems for sending patient data from one computer to another.

Another type of technical safeguard is an **audit trail**—an electronic log that works in the background of a computer, tracing who has accessed information and when. When new information is entered or existing data are changed, the log records the time and date of the entry as well as the name of the computer operator. The practice manager reviews the log on a regular basis to detect any irregularities or errors.

## HIPAA Enforcement and Breaches

The HIPAA Security Rule and the HIPAA Privacy Rule are enforced by the Office for Civil Rights (OCR). The acquisition, access, use, or disclosure of unsecured PHI in a manner not permitted under the HIPAA Privacy Rule is known as a breach. Examples of a breach include stolen or improperly accessed PHI, unauthorized viewing of PHI, and PHI sent to the wrong provider. PHI is considered "unsecured" if it is not encrypted to government standards.

Under the HIPAA Omnibus Rule, the definition of breach has been expanded, and as a result, more unauthorized uses and disclosures of protected health information (PHI) must be reported. Previously, an incident was considered a breach only when it was found that the incident resulted in significant risk of harm to the individual. The updated definition presumes that any use or disclosure of PHI not allowed by HIPAA will harm an individual and is considered a breach, unless proven otherwise. The HIPAA Breach Notification Rule requires notification following a breach of unsecured protected health information. Notification must be provided to individuals, the Secretary of Health and Human Services, and if more than 500 individuals are affected, the media must be notified.

## HIPAA Electronic Health Care Transactions and Code Sets

The **HIPAA Electronic Health Care Transactions and Code Sets (TCS)** standards are rules that make it possible for physicians and health plans to exchange electronic data using the standard format and standard codes. Under this rule, three types of standards have been set:

1. Electronic formats
2. Code sets
3. Identifiers

**audit trail** a technical safeguard on a computer that keeps track of who has accessed information and when, which is regularly checked by a manager for errors or irregularities in data entry.

**HIPAA Electronic Health Care Transactions and Code Sets (TCS)** the HIPAA rule governing the electronic exchange of health information.

*Electronic Formats*

The HIPAA transactions standards apply to the data that are regularly sent back and forth between providers and health plans. HIPAA-covered transactions include electronic documents such as healthcare claims sent by physicians and hospitals to insurance companies, payments sent by the insurance companies in response, and employee enrollment information sent by employers to their insurance companies. Each standard is labeled with both a number and a name. Either the number (such as "the 837," which is the insurance claim form) or the name (such as the "HIPAA Claim") may be used to refer to the particular electronic document format.

*Code Sets*

There are also standard sets of codes for diseases; treatments and procedures; and supplies or other items used to perform these actions. These standards are listed in Table 1-1.

On October 1, 2015, two new code sets went into effect: the ICD-10-CM and the ICD-10-PCS. The ICD-10-CM replaced the original HIPAA standards for use in reporting diagnoses (ICD-9-CM, Volumes 1 and 2), and the ICD-10-PCS replaced the original standards for reporting inpatient hospital procedures (ICD-9-CM, Volume 3). The new ICD-10 code sets are greatly expanded.

*Identifiers*

*Identifiers* are numbers of predetermined length and structure, such as a person's Social Security number. They are important for billing because the

### TABLE 1-1

## HIPAA Standard Code Sets for Diagnoses and Procedures

| Purpose | Standard |
|---|---|
| Codes for diseases, injuries, impairments, and other health-related problems | *International Classification of Diseases*, Tenth Revision, *Clinical Modification* (ICD-10-CM) |
| Codes for procedures or other actions taken to prevent, diagnose, treat, or manage diseases, injuries, and impairments | Physicians' services: Current Procedural Terminology (CPT®)<br><br>Inpatient hospital services: *International Classification of Diseases*, Tenth Revision, *Procedure Coding System* (ICD-10-PCS) |
| Codes for other medical services | Healthcare Common Procedure Coding System (HCPCS) |

unique numbers can be used in electronic transactions. Two identifiers—for employers and for providers—have been set up by the federal government, and two—for patients and for health plans—are to be established in the future.

- The employer identifier is used to identify the patient's employer on claims. The Employer Identification Number (EIN) issued by the Internal Revenue Service is the HIPAA standard.

- The *National Provider Identifier (NPI)* is the standard unique health identifier for healthcare providers to use in filing healthcare claims and other transactions. The NPI is ten positions long, with nine numbers and a check digit.

- The *Health Plan Identifier (HPID)* has not yet been implemented.

### Polaris Medical Group HIPAA Compliance Program

Polaris Medical Group has established a special HIPAA compliance program to help its staff members comply with HIPAA legislation. This is part of the practice's overall compliance program, which includes adherence to all government regulations, including OSHA work-safety guidelines and fair labor laws.

The practice manager, Jane Wetherall, is the compliance officer for PMG. She is responsible for

- Training employees and new hires in all aspects of compliance.
- Monitoring adherence to current policies and procedures.
- Modifying policies and procedures to conform to changes in the HIPAA law.

The compliance officer also establishes the procedures for employees to follow when problems are identified. Every employee is required to sign, initial, and date a compliance form at the onset of employment, to make a record for chart identification purposes in case of legal issues.

**National Provider Identifier (NPI)** a unique identifier assigned to a healthcare provider that is used in standard transactions, such as healthcare claims. Polaris Medical Group HIPAA Compliance Program

## 1.5 QUALITIES AND ATTITUDES OF THE PATIENT SERVICES SPECIALIST

CiMO

Success as a PSS is not just about following procedures. It is also about the qualities you bring to the job and your attitude. The medical office has many things in common with other offices, but it also has unique environmental characteristics. For example, working in a medical office can be more stressful than working in other office environments because of people's reactions to illness. Some patients who come in for appointments are coping with serious illnesses or disabilities. New patients may be nervous when they see the doctor for the first time. Patients may experience a variety of emotions, ranging from fear to anger. Although the transactions you engage in (such as accepting payment from a patient) may be routine, the emotions you encounter may not be.

In the medical office, patience and enthusiasm are important qualities. It is important to appear calm in a crisis or when frustrations mount. Noise and confusion in the office create unnecessary stress for patients. To complete many of the tasks in the medical office, attention to detail is necessary. Information must be recorded with extreme accuracy. Finally, sincerity and helpfulness are always important. Be willing to assist other staff members not only when asked but also whenever the opportunity arises.

### General Responsibilities

Polaris Medical Group has identified the general responsibilities that are expected of every employee regardless of position.

All staff members must

- Arrive at the office on time and stay until the end of the shift.
- Return from breaks and meals on time.
- Follow office procedures and report issues concerning safety, infection control, and exposure control.
- Observe and follow all office policies, especially those related to confidentiality.
- Dress in a neat and appropriate style, with their identification tags visible at all times.
- Demonstrate effective verbal and written communication skills.
- Demonstrate their willingness to work cooperatively with all patients and coworkers.
- Interact with patients without prejudice with regard to age, gender, race, creed, and disability.
- Organize and prioritize their workloads in an efficient manner.
- Follow verbal and written instructions from supervisors, managers, and physicians.
- Maintain neat and legible records and documentation.
- Seek the advice of a supervisor when the proper or correct course of action is not clear.
- Adapt quickly to changes in the work environment or schedule.
- Learn new concepts and procedures as necessary.
- Juggle more than one task at a time when necessary.
- Complete work assignments within a reasonable time frame.

In this text-workbook, you are the PSS at PMG. In this role, you are responsible for a variety of tasks. This section provides an overview of the types of tasks you will complete later in Part 3, On the Job.

Like most medical practices, PMG has a Policy and Procedure Manual (PPM), located in Part 2 of this text. The PPM lists the procedures that should be followed when completing the tasks in Part 3. The PPM also contains detailed information on PMG's policies. Following the guidelines in the PPM ensures that all staff members use standard methods to complete tasks.

Polaris Medical Group also maintains a set of PPMs of the insurance carriers and managed care organizations with which the practice has contracts. For your convenience, summaries of these policies and procedures can also be found in PMG's PPM.

Each day, you will perform a variety of tasks. For example, you will interact with patients on the telephone and in the office. You will work on the office computer network to complete scheduling and billing tasks. You will look up information in medical records or in the PPM when necessary. The following sections describe the specific responsibilities of your position.

***Scheduling Patients for Appointments***   Patients call the office to schedule new appointments or reschedule existing appointments. Scheduling tasks include

- Scheduling, rescheduling, and canceling appointments.
- Adding patients to the recall list as appropriate.
- Maintaining computerized office schedules for physicians, including patient appointments, professional obligations, and personal time off.
- Printing copies of the day's schedule as soon as you arrive in the office in the morning; distributing copies to physicians and staff members; and maintaining an up-to-date schedule on the computer.
- On a weekly basis, generating a patient recall list.
- On a daily basis, calling patients on the recall list to schedule appointments.

***Recording and Maintaining Patient Information***   When a patient comes to PMG for the first time, information is collected and recorded in the medical record and in the computer. Similarly, patient records are updated each time the patient phones or visits the office. The patient information tasks include

- Gathering and recording information from a new patient over the telephone at the time the appointment is made.

- Asking new patients to fill out the patient information form (PIF) and reviewing it for completeness, paying particular attention to the insurance section.

- Distributing the Notice of Privacy Practices form to each patient and asking the patient to sign, date, and return the Acknowledgment of Receipt of Notice of Privacy Practices form.

- Asking to see the patient's insurance identification card, photocopying or scanning the front and back of the card, and filing the copy in the patient's electronic health record.

- Inputting data from the PIF and the insurance card (if appropriate) into the computer.

- Asking a patient whose information (such as employer, insurance, or address) has changed since his or her last visit to complete a new PIF, and recording changes in the computer the same day, before new charges are entered.

- Recording information gathered during patient phone calls regarding changes in address, employment, insurance carrier, marital status, and so on.

- Reading and storing e-mail messages.

***Maintaining Third-Party Payer Information***   Information is recorded and updated regarding each patient's insurance carrier or managed care organization. Information about each specific health plan is also recorded. Summary information about the major insurance plans in which PMG participates is listed in the PPM. To produce accurate claims, you must be familiar with the requirements of each third-party payer. Tasks include

- Looking up payer information for each patient as needed.

- Verifying each patient's insurance eligibility online or over the phone.

- Collecting a copayment from the patient at the time of the visit if the patient's insurance plan has a copayment requirement.

- Checking with patients who are participants in managed care plans to see if they need referrals before they can be seen by one of the physicians at PMG; if a referral is needed, checking for a proper referral or contacting the office of the patient's primary care physician for the necessary information.

- Checking for proper preauthorization; if preauthorization is required, contacting the health plan to obtain a preauthorization number.

- Recording referral information in the computer.

- Recording preauthorization numbers in the computer.

***Educating Patients and Responding to Patient Inquiries***   Educating patients often includes informing them about charges and the payment process in general. Some patients do not understand the fees. If the planned services are expected to be costly and are not covered by the patient's insurance, it is PMG's policy to discuss these charges with the patient before the services are provided. In addition, patients sometimes call or stop by the office to inquire about the status of a particular insurance claim or to ask about an account balance. You are responsible for researching the account and responding to the patient's question in a timely manner. This involves

- Researching and resolving patient inquiries regarding services, billing, or charges.
- Using relevant information to determine the validity of the inquiry and the source of the error, if there is one.
- Contacting the patient to communicate the resolution of the problem.

***Recording Charges, Payments, and Adjustments at the Time of an Encounter***   Every time a PMG physician sees a patient at the office, hospital, or nursing home, a service is performed and a charge needs to be recorded. Similarly, any payments received from patients must be recorded. Adjustments are required when there is a difference between the amount charged and the amount that is accepted as payment.

A new billing tool for collecting payment at the time of service is known as *real-time claims adjudication (RTCA)*. With RTCA, a billing assistant submits claims at the time the patient checks out. Once a claim is submitted, assuming the payer has RTCA capabilities, the payer's computer system adjudicates the claim within minutes and sends back a remittance advice (RA). The billing assistant then discusses the payer's decision with the patient in person, and the patient pays any balance due before leaving. If there is a problem with the claim, such as missing information, the billing assistant can work with the patient to resolve the problem and resubmit the claim. The only follow-up for the medical office is to verify that the payer's portion of the payment is received. Payment usually follows within twenty-four hours.

Regardless of whether a medical office uses RTCA or some other form of collecting payments at the time of an encounter, the billing tasks include

- Preparing encounter forms at the beginning of each day for all patients with appointments.
- At the conclusion of an office visit:
  — Reviewing charges with the patient.

— Recording charges on the encounter form and then entering them in the computer.

— Estimating the patient's financial responsibility.

— Collecting payments as appropriate—for example, deductibles, payments for noncovered services, or balances due. (*Note:* Depending on the particular health plan, some patients do not make payments at the time of office visits but are instead billed for the balance after the remittance advice from the plan has arrived.)

— Recording the amount of payment and type of payment (such as check or credit card) on the encounter form, entering the information in the computer, and applying the payment to the proper charge(s).

— Thanking patients for their payments and generating walkout receipts at the time payment is received or upon request.

***Generating Healthcare Claims*** Timely submission of claims helps solidify the finances of the practice. The sooner claims are created and submitted, the sooner payment arrives. It is your responsibility to prepare healthcare claims. If a claim is rejected, you must discover whether an error was made and, if so, resubmit the claim as soon as possible. Claim tasks include

- Generating healthcare claims and checking all claims for accuracy before submission, including

  — Diagnosis and procedure code compliance.

  — Correct linkage of diagnoses and procedures.

  — Medical necessity of procedures.

  — Billing compliance—making sure the charges are billable according to the payer's conditions.

- Reviewing claim acknowledgments to verify that claims have been received.

- Preparing claim status reports on a weekly basis.

***Monitoring Payments from Third-Party Payers*** Once a third-party payer makes a decision on a claim, you are responsible for checking the results. This includes

- Comparing the information on the RA with the expected payment.

- If a claim is denied, reduced, or overpaid, researching the reason and resolving any discrepancies regarding services or billing, analyzing relevant information to determine the validity of the payer's decision or the source of an error, if there is one, and contacting the payer to resolve the problem.

- Appealing denied or rejected claims as necessary.
- Posting payments to patients' accounts.
- Contacting the payer if a claim is not paid within thirty days; following up on and/or resubmitting the claim as necessary.

***Generating Patient Statements and Financial Reports***   The PSS prepares and prints patient statements regularly for billing. Depending on the insurance plan, the patient is billed for any remaining amount after all payers have paid on a claim. A patient who does not have insurance is billed for any amount that was not collected at the time of service.

When a patient makes a payment by check but does not have adequate funds in his or her checking account to cover the check, the check is not honored by the bank. Such a check is referred to as an ***NSF (nonsufficient funds) check,*** commonly called a "bounced" check. When the practice receives an NSF notice from a bank, the PSS posts a negative adjustment to the patient's account, since the patient now owes the practice the amount of the check. The PSS also posts a fee for the returned check to the patient's account. The maximum amount of the fee is governed by state laws. At PMG, the fee for a returned check is $35. These new amounts are reflected on the patient's next statement.

NSF (nonsufficient funds) check   a check that is not honored by a bank because the account it was written on does not have sufficient funds to cover it.

In addition, the financial transactions of the medical practice must also be reported daily, weekly, and monthly. Patient day sheets summarize the number of patients seen by the physicians on a given day, the procedures performed, the charges and payments for the day, and other information. Reports that are generated on a weekly or monthly basis include patient and insurance aging reports.

***Collecting Overdue Payments from Patients***   An unpaid account with a balance that is thirty days past due is considered overdue. It is usually the job of the PSS to collect payments on patients' overdue accounts. Each week, the PSS generates an aging report showing which patients' accounts are overdue ("aged") and by how many days. The report indicates whether the account is thirty, sixty, or ninety days past due. Generally, if the account is thirty days past due, the PSS sends out a reminder notice or a second statement or phones the patient about the payment.

In some cases, or for large amounts, the office may decide to extend credit to a patient by setting up a payment plan. Usually the agreement is to divide the bill over a period of months, with the patient making regular monthly payments. Finance charges may or may not be applied. In the case of Polaris Medical Group, finance charges are not applied to the payment plan.

At Polaris Medical Group, when an account is ninety days overdue, the PSS generates a collection letter. If a patient does not respond, additional collection letters are sent. Ultimately, if the office's collection procedures fail, an office may hire an outside collection agency to pursue the matter. If the agency is able to collect money from the patient, the agency retains a portion, for example, 30 percent, as payment for its services. When the remaining amount is sent to the practice, the PSS posts it to the patient's account using the appropriate billing code.

The office may also decide that the account is uncollectible and write off the uncollected amount as a bad debt. Future services for patients with such accounts are usually on a cash-only basis. It is the job of the PSS to keep track of where an account is in the collection process and to follow up on collections on a weekly basis.

***Updating CPT and ICD-10-CM Codes in the Database*** The Current Procedural Terminology (CPT) and *International Classification of Diseases* (ICD-10-CM) codes are updated annually. New codes are added; existing codes are modified; and old codes are marked inactive. When the practice manager requests it, these changes must be made by the PSS to PMG's computer database.

## PART SUMMARY

| | |
|---|---|
| **1.1** Name the eight positions held by members of the Polaris Medical Group patient services team. | 1. Family practitioner<br>2. Internist<br>3. Physician's assistant<br>4. Practice manager/compliance officer<br>5. Accountant<br>6. Bookkeeper<br>7. Patient services specialist (PSS)<br>8. Medical laboratory technician |
| **1.2** List eight facts that are documented in all medical records at Polaris Medical Group. | 1. Patient's name<br>2. Encounter date and reason<br>3. Appropriate history and physical examination<br>4. Review of all tests that were ordered<br>5. Diagnosis<br>6. Plan of care, or notes on procedures or treatments that were given<br>7. Instructions or recommendations that were given to the patient<br>8. Signature of the provider who saw the patient |
| **1.3** Identify the four parts of a SOAP note. | A SOAP note, or SOAP format, groups the clinical information for a patient's encounter into four parts:<br><br>*S:* The *subjective* information is based on the patient's descriptions of symptoms along with other comments.<br><br>*O:* The *objective* information includes the physician's descriptions of the presenting problem and data from examinations and tests.<br><br>*A:* The *assessment*, also called the impression or conclusion, is the physician's diagnosis, or interpretation of the subjective and objective information.<br><br>*P:* The *plan*, also called treatment, advice, or recommendations, includes the necessary patient monitoring, follow-up, procedures, and instructions to the patient. |

| | |
|---|---|
| **1.4** Describe how HIPAA legislation sets standards for privacy and the electronic transmission of data. | 1. The HIPAA Privacy Rule: The privacy requirements cover patients' health information.<br><br>2. The HIPAA Security Rule: The security requirements state the administrative, technical, and physical safeguards that are required to protect patients' health information.<br><br>3. The HIPAA Electronic Health Care Transactions and Code Sets: These standards require every provider who does business electronically to use the same healthcare transactions, code sets, and identifiers. |
| **1.5** Describe the qualities of an effective patient services specialist. | An effective patient services specialist is patient, enthusiastic, accurate in attention to detail, sincere, and helpful in dealing with the often stressful environment of a medical office. |
| **1.6** Identify ten tasks that a patient services specialist at Polaris Medical Group performs during a typical day. | 1. Schedules patients for appointments<br>2. Records and maintains patient information<br>3. Maintains third-party payer information<br>4. Educates patients and responds to patient inquiries<br>5. Records charges, payments, and adjustments at the time of an encounter<br>6. Generates healthcare claims<br>7. Monitors payments from third-party payers<br>8. Generates patient statements and financial reports<br>9. Collects overdue payments from patients<br>10. Updates CPT and ICD codes in the database as needed |

*For questions 1 through 15, write the letter that corresponds to the correct answer in the space provided.*

_____ **1.** *[LO 1.1]* An internist specializes in treating:
    **a.** patients of all ages
    **b.** adults
    **c.** diseases of the organs
    **d.** families

_____ **2.** *[LO 1.1]* Physicians responsible for overseeing patients' overall healthcare and for referring patients to specialists are known as:
    **a.** family practitioners
    **b.** primary care physicians
    **c.** internists
    **d.** family care physicians

_____ **3.** *[LO 1.2]* Which of the following is generally not part of a patient's medical record?
    **a.** insurance correspondence
    **b.** chart notes
    **c.** patient information form
    **d.** remittance advice (RA)

_____ **4.** *[LO 1.4]* The HIPAA security standards are divided into which three categories:
    **a.** electronic, paper, and oral
    **b.** Internet, PHI, and networks
    **c.** confidentiality, integrity, and availability
    **d.** administrative, physical, and technical

_____ **5.** *[LO 1.3]* The *O* in SOAP refers to:
    **a.** obstetrical
    **b.** observation
    **c.** objective
    **d.** ordinary

_____ **6.** *[LO 1.5, 1.6]* Which of the following is not considered a general responsibility of all employees at PMG?
    **a.** Organize and prioritize their workloads in an efficient manner.
    **b.** Seek the advice of a supervisor when the correct course of action is not clear.
    **c.** Update diagnosis and procedure codes in the practice's database.
    **d.** Maintain neat and legible records and documentation.

7. *[LO 1.2]* The coordination of care received by a patient over time, and across several providers, is known as:
   a. electronic health records
   b. medical records
   c. documentation
   d. continuity of care

8. *[LO 1.3]* The patient's diagnosis is contained in the _____ section of a SOAP note.
   a. subjective
   b. objective
   c. assessment
   d. plan

9. *[LO 1.2]* If an error is made in a patient's medical record, the incorrect information should be:
   a. deleted
   b. marked with a single line through the words to be changed
   c. placed inside parentheses
   d. marked with yellow highlighting

10. *[LO 1.4]* The _____ is the first comprehensive federal protection for the privacy of health information.
    a. HITECH Privacy Act
    b. American Recovery and Reinvestment Act
    c. HIPAA Privacy Rule
    d. Meaningful Use Act

11. *[LO 1.4]* A patient's health information can be released without the patient's authorization when it is for treatment, payment, and:
    a. disclosure to family members
    b. marketing
    c. operations
    d. disclosure to pharmaceutical companies

12. *[LO 1.4]* An audit trail is an example of a(n) _____.
    a. code set
    b. technical safeguard
    c. identifier
    d. electronic format

13. *[LO 1.6]* The Polaris Medical Group sends collection letters to patients when their account is _____ days past due.
    a. 30
    b. 45
    c. 60
    d. 90

_____ **14.** *[LO 1.6]* The Polaris Medical Group generates a patient recall list once a _____.

    **a.** day

    **b.** week

    **c.** month

    **d.** year

_____ **15.** *[LO 1.4]* The HITECH Act, the Affordable Care Act, and the _____ made updates to the HIPAA privacy, security, and enforcement rules.

    **a.** HIPAA Technology Rule

    **b.** HIPAA Omnibus Rule

    **c.** Electronic Health Records and Standards Act

    **d.** Centers for Medicare and Medicaid Electronic Health Information Act

## Critical Thinking Questions

*Answer the questions below in the space provided.*

16. *[LO 1.2]* This year, Sam Donovan's primary care physician and his cardiologist began using an electronic health record (EHR) to document Sam's encounters, including related lab work, diagnostic tests, and prescriptions. Each office uses a different software program. The first time Sam's health information was transmitted between the two programs, data in certain fields were lost or truncated. Why is it essential for EHR programs to be compatible? Why is compatibility difficult to ensure?

_____

_____

_____

17. *[LO 1.4 ]* A medical office has hired Jamaica Townsend to work for one week in the summer to scan patients' paper records. After she is finished, the scanned files will be input into an EHR. Because she has been hired for a very short time and is not an official staff member, Jamaica has not been required to sign a confidentiality agreement. Do you think this policy is in keeping with HIPAA rules? Why?

_____

_____

_____

18. *[LO 1.1, 1.5]* In your role as a patient services specialist at a large medical practice, you notice that two of the physicians in the group are documenting procedures they have not actually performed. Because you are responsible for preparing and following up on their claims, you notice that both physicians are receiving payments regularly for these procedures. What should you do about this problem?

_____

_____

_____

19. *[LO 1.4]* A physician consults by e-mail with another physician about a patient's condition. Has the HIPAA Privacy Rule been followed? Explain your answer.

_____

_____

_____

20. *[LO 1.4]* A medical assistant at a small medical practice took an office laptop home to do some work. The laptop contained clinical and billing information for the practice. The assistant stopped at a coffee shop on the way home and left the laptop on the table while getting a refill. While she was gone, it was stolen. Both the clinical data and the billing database were protected by passwords. An encryption program was also used to protect the data. What types of safeguards do these represent? Do you think these security methods will be enough to block a breach in the patient information? Do you think it was a good idea for the medical assistant to take the laptop home?

_____

_____

_____

# Part 2

# Polaris Medical Group Policy and Procedure Manual

The Policy and Procedure Manual (PPM) provides staff members with information about the practice's general policies. It also covers the specific procedures that you are expected to follow while employed as a patient services specialist at Polaris Medical Group. The PPM contains detailed guidelines on the way the practice processes new patient registration, insurance verification, appointment scheduling, billing, and payments.

Read the PPM before proceeding with your work in Part 3. After you have read the PPM, sign in the box at the bottom of page 32. Then, as you work through the daily assignments in Part 3, refer to the PPM as needed.

## LEARNING OUTCOMES

*After successfully completing Part 2, you will be able to define the key terms and:*

2.1 List the types of outside entities for which PMG stores contact information in the PPM.

2.2 Describe the steps a PMG employee follows when he or she has a grievance.

2.3 Explain the difference between the resignation, termination, and discharge of an employee.

2.4 Summarize the main personnel conduct issues addressed in the PPM.

2.5 Provide examples of excused and unexcused absences according to PMG's attendance policy.

2.6 Describe the steps used to screen routine and emergency telephone calls.

2.7 Describe the PMG guidelines for the protection of patients' PHI in general, and when using information technology in particular.

2.8 List five tasks the PSS performs during each patient visit.

2.9 Describe how the PSS uses Medisoft, the practice's billing program, in processing payments.

2.10 List the required daily reports.

2.11 Describe the different populations that Medicare, Medicaid, and workers' compensation plans serve.

2.12 Explain the purpose of the health plan information pages in the PPM.

## KEY TERMS

| | |
|---|---|
| COBRA | Medi-Medi beneficiary |
| ethics | preauthorization |
| grievance | Universal Precautions |
| medical necessity | workers' compensation insurance |
| Medigap insurance | |

### Reading Acknowledgment

The PPM is not an employment contract. Polaris Medical Group makes every attempt to offer secure employment and rewarding careers to its employees. However, PMG makes no guarantee of length of employment or possible advancement. Length of employment and pace of advancement are related to a number of factors, including your adherence to the standards of performance and conduct contained in this PPM. Thus, all employees of PMG are employed for an unspecified length of time, and employment may be terminated at any time at the will of either the employee or the practice.

Polaris Medical Group reserves the right to alter or deviate from these policies and procedures from time to time as is necessary.

---

I have read and understood Polaris Medical Group's Policy and Procedure Manual. (Sign after reading entire PPM.)

_____

Employee's Signature                                    Date

---

# CONTENTS

The first section of the PPM provides contact information about the practice, the physicians and staff, its accounting firm and referring physician, the hospital and nursing home with which the practice is affiliated, and the laboratory service it uses. It also contains the practice's equal employment opportunity, nondiscrimination, and affirmative action statements, and it describes the various full-time and part-time employment levels available.

### Polaris Medical Group

**Address:** 2100 Grace Avenue, Columbus, OH 43214-1111
**Phone:** 999-555-9800
**Fax:** 999-555-9801
**Office Hours:** 9:00 a.m. to 5:00 p.m., Monday through Friday
6:00 p.m. to 9:00 p.m., Thursday, for evening walk-in appointments

### Personnel

**Physician:** Robin C. Crebore, M.D., F.A.A.F.P., NPI 1145678922
**Beeper Number:** 999-666-9436

**Physician:** Michael P. Mahabir, M.D., F.A.C.P., NPI 2167891336
**Beeper Number:** 999-666-9756

**Practice Manager:** Jane Wetherall
**Physician's Assistant:** Michelle Maligo
**Medical Laboratory Technician:** Thomas Bouck
**Bookkeeper:** Joseph Lambert
**Patient Services Specialist:** _____ (your name)

### Accounting Firm

**Name:** Marilyn M. Chan, Chan and Grimwald
**Address:** 9000 South Street, Cincinnati, OH 43214
**Phone:** 999-555-6060
**Fax:** 999-555-6061

### Referring Physician

**Name:** Rachel P. Innanni, M.D., F.A.A.F.P., NPI 5211361139
**Facility:** Rennsit Clinic
**Address:** 98 Broadway, Columbus, OH 43214
**Phone:** 800-555-1920
**Fax:** 800-555-1212
**Medicare Participating:** Yes

### Hospital Affiliation

**Name:** St. Mary's
**Address:** 2500 Grace Avenue, Columbus, OH 43214

**Phone:** 999-555-0001
**Fax:** 999-555-0002

*Nursing Home Affiliation*
**Name:** Grandview Home
**Address:** 300 Center Street, Grandview, OH 46757
**Phone:** 999-555-1010
**Fax:** 999-555-1011
**Contact Person:** Louise Schroth
**Extension:** 325

*Laboratory Services*
**Name:** Medco
**Address:** 1415 Central Avenue, Columbus, OH 43214
**Phone:** 999-555-8989
**Fax:** 999-555-8990
**Contact Person:** John Witkowski
**Extension:** 1014
**Medicare Participating:** Yes

*Emergency Phone Numbers*
**Local Emergency Police/Fire/Ambulance:** 911
**Local Poison Control Center:** 999-777-0000

## Equal Employment Opportunity, Nondiscrimination, and Affirmative Action Statements

Polaris Medical Group does not discriminate on the basis of race, color, age, sex, national origin, religion, creed, or disability in the admission or access to, or treatment or employment of, its programs and activities. The practice manager has been designated as the Human Resource Coordinator to coordinate all efforts to comply with section 504 of the Rehabilitation Act of 1973 and its implementing regulation that prohibits discrimination on the basis of disability.

The clinic is an equal opportunity employer. All applicants for employment will be considered. All persons employed, including management staff, professionals, technicians, and others, will be treated without regard to age, race, color, religion, sex, national origin, handicap, or disability. Such action includes, but is not limited to, the following:

- Employment, promotion, demotion, transfers, layoffs, and termination.
- Recruitment and recruitment advertising.

- Rates of pay and other forms of compensation.
- Training opportunities.
- Practice-sponsored social and recreational programs.

All employees are responsible for reporting perceived illegal discrimination to the practice manager.

## Employment Levels

PMG classifies employees in the following categories:

- *Regular full-time employee:* An employee who is regularly scheduled for at least forty hours a week and who has worked for more than three months. Eligible for benefits.

- *Probationary period full-time employee:* An employee who is regularly scheduled for a least forty hours a week and who has not yet worked for three months. Does not receive benefits.

- *Temporary full-time employee:* An employee who is regularly scheduled for at least forty hours a week and whose length of employment will be less than six months. Does not receive benefits.

- *Regular part-time employee:* An employee who is regularly scheduled for less than forty hours a week and who has worked for more than three months. Does not receive benefits.

- *Probationary period part-time employee:* An employee who is regularly scheduled for less than forty hours a week and who has not yet worked for three months. Does not receive benefits.

- *Temporary part-time employee:* An employee who is regularly scheduled to work less than forty hours a week and whose length of employment will be less than six months. Does not receive benefits.

## 2.2 WAGES AND COMPENSATION

Polaris Medical Group's policy is that wage compensation will be in accordance with the Fair Labor Standards Act (FLSA) and state law. Some employees and occupations are considered exempt from additional payment for working more than forty hours in a week. The practice manager determines which employees are exempt and which are nonexempt.

## Pay Rates

Polaris Medical Group compensates all employees with at least the federal minimum wage, or the state minimum wage if it is higher, for each hour of work performed voluntarily. Rates are based on

- Job performance
- Length of employment
- Additional qualifications, education, or certifications
- Prior salary history

## Overtime Compensation

All overtime must be approved by management before it is worked. If overtime is not preapproved, the employee may be disallowed those hours and not compensated. Employees who are considered nonexempt are entitled to overtime pay at the rate of not less than one and a half times their regular pay for any portion of hours worked in excess of forty hours in a single workweek.

If the forty-hour requirement has not yet been met, an employee will not be paid overtime for hours in excess of eight per day or for work on Saturdays, Sundays, holidays, or regular days of rest. Any overtime compensation earned during a specific pay cycle will be paid on the regular payday for the period in which that pay cycle ends.

## Pay Dates

Pay dates for the current year are posted on the bulletin board. Checks or electronic funds will be available at 9:00 a.m. on the dates listed. Employees who need to obtain their checks early must contact the practice manager at least three working days in advance.

## Employee Time Records

Nonexempt employees will be responsible for clocking in and out on a time card. The time card serves as a permanent record of the time worked. An error on the time card must be immediately reported and corrected in the same week in which the error occurred. At the end of the pay period, time cards are submitted to the practice manager. Falsification of a time card will be grounds for immediate dismissal.

Employees record their own starting and ending times on their own time cards. Clocking in or out for another employee will be grounds for progressive disciplinary action, beginning with verbal reprimand and progressing to written reprimand, suspension, and finally to termination.

All nonexempt employees are required to clock out for a one-hour lunch during shifts of five hours or more. Employees are not allowed to skip this lunch break without approval. Failure to clock out for lunch break will result in progressive disciplinary action.

An employee who needs to leave the clinic on personal business is required to clock out before leaving. Failure to do so will result in progressive disciplinary action.

Repeated failure to clock in or out at the beginning or end of a shift, when leaving for or returning from lunch, or when leaving for or returning from personal business, will result in progressive disciplinary action.

## Performance Evaluations

Performance evaluations are conducted at three months, twelve months, and each year thereafter, or more often if necessary. Reviews are held annually on the employee's anniversary date. The practice manager will prepare the evaluation and discuss it with the employee. The employee will be given an opportunity to ask questions and discuss matters of concern. The practice manager and the employee will sign the evaluation at the completion of the review. All evaluations become part of the employee's permanent personnel file.

A review of salary and wages may also occur during the performance evaluation. Pay increases are not automatic. If an increase is recommended, it will be in accordance with approved scheduled wages, unless otherwise authorized. Increases become effective the first pay period after the anniversary date.

## Employee Benefits

Below are some of the benefits offered by PMG to regular full-time employees. Employees are advised to consult with the practice manager for a comprehensive description of available benefits.

- Employee assistance program
- Health service program
- Medical/health insurance
- Professional liability insurance
- Workers' compensation insurance
- Unemployment insurance
- Paid holidays
- Credit union membership
- Investment, retirement, or pension plans
- Severance pay

- Short-term/long-term disability
- Personal time off/personal emergency leave
- Tuition reimbursement
- Paid continuing education/reimbursement for continuing education
- Paid time off for jury duty
- Military leave/time off for active reserve or National Guard duty
- Paid time off for death in immediate family/bereavement
- Maternity leave
- Paid vacation time
- Paid sick time
- Family leave
- Compensatory time off

## Employee Grievances

**grievance** a job-related problem that an employee feels should be corrected.

A *grievance* related to discrimination based on race, color, sex, age, creed, marital status, national origin, or disability is processed in accordance with the nondiscrimination grievance procedure described below.

A grievance procedure must be initiated within ten days of the incident. No employee is criticized or penalized in any way for using the grievance procedure; it is the means of resolving an employee problem when normal conversation between an employee and supervisor cannot resolve the problem. Employees and supervisors alike should consider this procedure as another part of PMG's management of open communication. All employee grievance discussions are strictly confidential.

In order to provide the employee with a means of expressing dissatisfaction relating to wages, hours of work, administration of personnel policies and procedures, and perceived unfair or inequitable treatment or discipline or other conditions of employment, PMG has adopted the following grievance procedure:

1. The employee should talk over the problem with the practice manager within ten working days of the date of the problem.
2. If the problem is not resolved informally, the employee must submit a written statement describing the situation, with dates and signatures, to the practice manager.
3. Within five working days, the practice manager, the employee, and one of the physicians will meet to discuss, and attempt to resolve, the situation. The physician's decision will be final and binding.

## 2.3 RESIGNATION, TERMINATION, DISCHARGE, AND COBRA BENEFITS

Polaris Medical Group has specific written policies regarding resignation, termination, discharge, and COBRA benefits. This section of the manual provides an overview of these policies. For a complete copy of the policies, ask the practice manager.

### Resignation

When an employee decides to end employment with PMG, advance notice of one month is requested from all managers, supervisors, and registered/licensed personnel. All other employees are requested to give two weeks' notice. Once a resignation notice from an employee is received, management reserves the right to allow the employee to continue employment to the resignation date or to accept the date of notice as the employee's last date of employment. All resignations are to be submitted in writing to the practice manager.

### Termination

In some instances, termination may be initiated by management for nondisciplinary reasons including, but not limited to, the following:

- Work assignment completed (temporary employee).
- Workforce reduction.
- Position abolished; employee cannot be transferred to another position.
- Workload decreased or work assignments changed.

### Discharge

Discharge is immediate dismissal for misconduct. No advance notice is given, and terminal pay covers only the time actually worked prior to discharge.

### COBRA Benefits

The Consolidated Omnibus Reconciliation Act of 1986 *(COBRA),* also known as Public Law 99-272, states that an employer is required to provide continuation of group plan health insurance to terminated employees and other qualified beneficiaries for a period of up to eighteen months. Any employee eligible for PMG benefits is also eligible for COBRA benefits. Beneficiaries are generally required to pay the entire premium for the coverage.

COBRA federal legislation requiring an employer with twenty or more employees that sponsors a group health benefit plan to continue health insurance coverage of terminated employees and other qualified beneficiaries for a period of up to eighteen months.

Polaris Medical Group has developed guidelines for employee conduct while on the job. The following section of the PPM provides an overview of these guidelines.

## Contributions and Solicitations

Solicitations or distribution of printed material by employees and/or visitors for purposes other than an officially approved program is prohibited. Such unapproved action by an employee will be considered grounds for progressive disciplinary action.

## Identification Badges

In order to readily identify all staff members to our patients and visitors, identification (ID) badges must be worn at all times during working hours. This creates an atmosphere of professionalism, courtesy, and efficiency. The employee ID badge is clinic property and must be turned in to the practice manager upon resignation or termination. The final paycheck will not be given to the employee until the badge is received.

## Inclement Weather

Polaris Medical Group does not close during adverse weather conditions. Each employee should determine whether it is safe to travel to work. Employees are expected to make an attempt to report to work. Notify the practice if you are unable to arrive at work at the normal time. Those who are unable to report to work will not be paid unless they substitute vacation or other paid time off for the time missed.

## Sexual Harassment

Sexual harassment is a form of discrimination prohibited by Title VII of the Civil Rights Act of 1964. It is defined by the Equal Employment Opportunity Commission as "unwelcome sexual advances, requests for sexual favors, and other verbal or physical conduct of a sexual nature when submission to the conduct enters into employment decisions and/or the conduct unreasonably interferes with an individual's work performance or creates an intimidating, hostile, or offensive working environment."

Polaris Medical Group does not tolerate verbal or physical conduct by any employee that harasses, disrupts, or interferes with another employee's work performance or that creates an intimidating, offensive, or hostile environment. Prohibited behavior includes

- Sexual flirtations, touching, advances, or propositions.
- Verbal abuse of a sexual nature.
- Graphic or suggestive comments about an individual's dress or body.
- The use of sexually degrading words to describe an individual.
- The display in the workplace of sexually suggestive objects or pictures.

Any employee who believes that the actions or words of a supervisor or employee constitute sexual harassment must immediately report the incident to the practice manager. The complaint will be taken seriously and investigated immediately. If an employee is not satisfied with the handling of a complaint or the action taken, the employee should bring the complaint to the attention of a physician. In all cases, the employee will be informed of the ongoing findings and conclusion.

Any employee, supervisor, or manager who is found to have engaged in the harassment of another individual, whether coworker, patient, vendor, or anyone else, will be subject to progressive disciplinary action, up to and including termination.

## Dress Code

Employees are expected to appear neat, clean, and well groomed at all times. It is important for employees to be aware that patients and visitors may judge the entire practice and the attention they receive on the basis of the personal appearance of an employee. Employees are expected to use good judgment and moderation in dress and grooming at all times while on the job. Employees whose appearance is not acceptable in a conservative, professional environment, or whose attire represents a safety hazard, are subject to progressive disciplinary action.

## Smoking and Tobacco Use

In order to promote the health and well-being of patients, visitors, and employees, no cigarettes or tobacco products of any kind are allowed inside the building, on the grounds, or in the parking lot. Personnel found smoking or using tobacco will be subject to progressive disciplinary action.

## Substance Abuse

It is the duty of PMG to provide a safe work environment in accordance with the Drug-Free Workplace Act of 1988. While the intention is not to intrude on the private lives of employees, the concern that chemical substance use that might affect job competence, public or employee safety, public trust, or the practice's reputation requires adherence to the following policy.

Illegal use or working under the influence of alcohol, illegal drugs, or prescription drugs (to the extent that work performance is affected) will not be tolerated. The purpose of any drug testing conducted is to ensure that public safety and the personal safety of employees and patients are not endangered as a result of drug use by employees and that all employees perform their jobs both efficiently and in a manner to promote public trust. Violations of this policy will result in disciplinary action up to and including termination and may also have legal consequences.

## Personal Telephone Calls and Visits

Personal telephone calls and visits to employees must be kept to a minimum and must not interfere with an employee's work. It is not appropriate for employees to receive personal visits while working. Personal visits should take place after work hours and away from the clinic.

Phone calls to arrange transportation and check on the safety of immediate family members, as well as other important outgoing calls, may be made. These calls should be local calls and should be made during breaks or lunch periods. Incoming calls should be kept to a minimum and restricted primarily to emergency messages. Employees whose work is frequently interrupted by personal calls or visits may be subject to progressive disciplinary action.

## Personal Use of Computers and E-mail

The Polaris Medical Group e-mail system belongs to the medical group. Staff members are permitted access to the computer system to assist them in the performance of their jobs. Personal use of the computer system is prohibited if the use interferes with the user's or any other employee's work performance; has a negative effect on the operation of the computer system; or violates any other provision of this policy or any other policy of the Polaris Medical Group.

The e-mail system may not be used for unlawful activities or for commercial purposes that are not directly related to the practice's business. Prohibited uses of e-mail include but are not limited to

- Sending commercial advertisements, solicitations, or promotions.
- Sending destructive programs such as computer viruses.
- Sending copies of documents in violation of copyright laws.

- Using e-mail to harass, intimidate, defame, or discriminate against others or to interfere with the ability of others to conduct business.

- Using e-mail for any purpose restricted or prohibited by laws or PMG policies.

- Constructing an e-mail communication so it appears to be from someone else.

- Accessing electronic mail without authorization, breaching security measures on any electronic mail system, or intercepting electronic mail transmissions without authorization.

## Cell Phones

Medical practices have a responsibility to protect the confidentiality of their patients as well as their professional reputation. In addition to having a negative effect on work productivity, cell phones with cameras and video recorders also create potential legal issues by compromising the integrity of protected health information and individual rights to privacy.

Personal cell phones are to be used only during breaks/lunch hours and must be kept on nonringing mode during business hours. When your cell phone is OFF and your voicemail is ON and a family emergency occurs, family members should be instructed to call the main number and ask that you be contacted in person immediately. The same applies to texting; this mode must also be OFF and can be turned ON only during breaks/lunch hours.

Texting to arrange transportation and check on the safety of immediate family members, as well as sending other important messages, is acceptable.

No photos or videos may be taken inside the workplace that could capture documents, paperwork, patient charts, or other information protected by privacy law.

## Social Networking

Similarly, accessing social networking sites such as Twitter, Facebook, and Pinterest on the office network for non-work-related reasons is not permitted. Because of the negative effect on work productivity, employees who engage in this activity regularly may be subject to progressive disciplinary action.

## Universal Precautions

All employees are required to utilize the Centers for Disease Control and Prevention (CDC)–approved Universal Precaution techniques while performing patient care functions. *Universal Precautions* are specific techniques designed to prevent healthcare workers from exposing themselves and others to infection by pathogens, such as the human immunodeficiency virus (HIV).

Universal Precautions techniques issued by the Centers for Disease Control and Prevention (CDC) to protect healthcare workers from infection.

## Ethics

Medical *ethics* are standards of behavior requiring truthfulness, honesty, and integrity. Ethics guide the behavior of physicians, who have the training, the primary responsibility, and the legal right to diagnose and treat human illnesses and injuries. All medical office employees and those working in health-related professions share responsibility for observing the ethical code. In general, this code states that information about patients, other employees, and confidential business matters should not be discussed with anyone not directly concerned with them. Staff members at PMG work regularly with patients' medical records and with finances. It is essential to maintain the confidentiality of patient information and communications, as well as to act with integrity, when handling these tasks.

## CiMO 2.5 OFFICE HOURS AND ATTENDANCE

The normal hours of operation are 9:00 a.m. to 5:00 p.m., Monday through Friday, and 6:00 p.m. to 9:00 p.m., Thursday evenings, for walk-in appointments. Working additional hours outside the normal range will sometimes be necessary. This is not a common occurrence, but when it does become necessary, all employees are expected to be available to work.

During each workday, you are allowed two fifteen-minute breaks. These breaks are usually taken at regularly scheduled times. The practice manager will determine the schedule of breaks. A staff member who works a five-hour day or longer is required to take a one-hour lunch break.

Staff members who work on a part-time basis must clock in at the beginning of each shift and clock out at the end of each shift. In addition, they should not clock in more than fifteen minutes prior to their regular start time. When a part-time staff member works more than five hours, he or she should clock out for a one-hour lunch break. Part-time personnel should not exceed eight hours per day or forty hours per week. These regulations should be followed without deviation unless authorization is given by the practice manager. All overtime requires prior approval from the practice manager.

Employees are hired to perform certain duties in the medical office during a specified time period. For patients to receive quality care and for the practice to run efficiently, all staff members must be present. One employee's lateness or absence can disrupt the efficient functioning of the entire practice. For this reason, PMG has developed an attendance policy. While we recognize that everyone has an occasional emergency that prevents on-time arrival at the office (for example, an automobile breakdown or a family illness), we expect all employees to be at work when they are scheduled.

## Definitions of Absences

***Scheduled Absences***   Holidays, vacation days, and other days off, scheduled in advance and approved by the practice manager, are considered scheduled absences.

***Unscheduled Absences***   Failure to be present during scheduled working hours, during overtime hours, or at a required class or meeting is considered an unscheduled absence.

***Lateness/Leaving Early***   Employees are considered late if they arrive more than ten minutes after the scheduled start of their shift. Employees are considered to have left early if they leave the office before the scheduled end of their shift.

***Excused Absences***   The following are considered excused absences:

- Scheduled absences.
- Absences that have been preapproved by the practice manager.
- Absences or lateness on a day the practice has defined as a weather-related emergency.
- Absences for assigned jury duty.
- Absences due to the death of a family member.
- Other absences as defined by the practice manager.

***Unexcused Absences***   The following are considered unexcused absences:

- Unscheduled absences or lateness.
- Absences without proper notification (for example, having a friend or family member call in to report your absence).
- Late arrivals or early departures to and from work.
- Other absences as defined by the practice manager.

## Attendance Policy

The key elements of PMG's attendance policy are

- All employees are expected to be at the office during their assigned work hours.
- An employee who is not at work during the required period must have prior authorization from the practice manager.
- Employees are not permitted to leave the building except during their lunch breaks without prior approval from the practice manager.

- All employees should inform the practice manager as far in advance as possible of any known reasons for lateness or absence. It is not appropriate to have a family member or friend call in and speak to the practice manager. This discussion must take place between the employee and the practice manager.

- If advance notice is given and the practice manager does not approve the lateness or absence, and if the time is taken anyway, it will be considered an unexcused absence.

- The first incidence of an unexcused absence results in a written notation in the employee's personnel file. The second incidence of an unexcused absence results in immediate dismissal.

- Any absences that occur during an employee's ninety-day probationary period will not be paid except in the case of illness.

- An employee who is not at work for two consecutive days without informing the practice manager will be subject to immediate dismissal.

- An employee who is absent two or more consecutive days due to illness will be required to present a medical note from a physician upon returning to work. If such a document is not submitted, the employee will not be paid for the time.

## CiMO 2.6 TELEPHONE PROCEDURES

The voice on the other end of the telephone is often the first contact patients have with the practice. Callers form impressions about the office as a whole based on the nature of the phone call and the tone of voice of the person answering the phone. For this reason, it is very important to sound calm, friendly, and efficient when answering the phone. Even if you are having a stressful day, it is important to not sound that way on the telephone.

The patient services specialist is responsible for answering the telephone. As in all medical offices, the telephone should be answered promptly. There is always the possibility that a call is an emergency. The proper way to answer the phone is "Polaris Medical Group, this is _____ (your name). May I help you?"

### Documenting Telephone Calls

Physicians must keep records of all telephone conversations with patients. These notes are stored in the patients' medical records. The patient services specialist must also document telephone calls with patients that involve requests for appointments or complaints.

## Screening Telephone Calls

The practice receives a variety of telephone calls throughout the day. Common types of calls relate to

- Appointments.
- Billing questions.
- Insurance questions.
- General office questions, such as office hours.
- Requests for prescription renewals.
- Reports from outside labs or X-ray sites.
- Reports from a hospital concerning a patient's condition.
- Reports from a patient concerning his or her condition.
- Referral requests.

All calls must be screened before they are transferred within the office. To determine whether the call should be transferred and who should receive it, certain information should first be obtained from the caller:

1. Determine who the caller is (patient, family member of patient, physician, pharmacist, insurance claim specialist, and so on).

2. Determine what the call is about (billing question, lab report, referral, and so on). (See step 4 below and pages 50–52 for information concerning what to do in the case of an emergency call.)

3. Decide whether to transfer the call. Using the information obtained in steps 1 and 2, review Table 2-1 and make a decision about whether to put the call through to the appropriate person.

4. Put emergency calls through to a physician immediately. If neither physician is available, seek the advice of your manager. You may need to suggest that the patient go to the emergency room or to another physician's office.

## Taking Telephone Messages

Sometimes you will need to take a message rather than transfer the call. This usually happens when the call is for a staff member who is unable to take the call at that time. When taking a telephone message, write down the following information:

- Name of person calling.
- Patient's name.
- Date and time of the call.
- The caller's phone number.

## TABLE 2-1

# Polaris Medical Group
# Telephone Routing Chart

| Type of Call | Transfer to Physician | Take Message for Physician | Route to Personnel Listed |
|---|---|---|---|
| Emergency | X | | |
| Other physician | if possible | | |
| Appointments | | | PSS |
| Patient billing or insurance inquiry | | | PSS |
| Patient progress report | | X | |
| Patient request for test results | | X | |
| Prescription renewals | | X | |
| Patient questions about medication | | X | |
| Office business | | | Practice manager |
| Personal calls for physicians | | X | |
| Business calls | | | Practice manager |
| Personal call for others | | | Appropriate personnel |

- Reason for the call.
- Name of person who took the call.
- How urgent the call is—that is, whether the call needs to be returned, is for someone's information only, and so on.

## Handling Emergency Telephone Calls

During the course of the day, patients may call the office with emergencies. The following procedures must be followed when an emergency call is taken:

1. Remain calm. You will be better able to assist the patient if you remain calm and focused on the problem.
2. Obtain the following information:
   - Phone number and exact address where the patient is located.
   - Name of the caller.
   - Caller's relationship to the patient (if the caller is not the patient).
   - Patient's name.
   - Patient's age.

- Patient's detailed symptoms or complaints and the duration of those symptoms.
- If the call is about an accident or injury, a description of how the accident or injury occurred.
- Patient's reaction to the situation.
- Description of any treatment that has been given.

3. Summarize the information and speak it back to the caller to confirm that you have heard and understood the situation.

4. Refer to PMG's list of symptoms and complaints that require emergency attention to determine whether this situation requires immediate action.

5. If the situation is a medical emergency, immediately transfer the call to a physician. If neither of the physicians is available, put the caller on hold and discuss the situation with the practice manager.

6. If the situation is not a medical emergency, schedule the patient for an appointment as soon as possible.

*Symptoms/Complaints Considered Emergencies*   The following symptoms and complaints are handled as emergency calls:

- Loss of consciousness.
- Lack of breathing or difficulty breathing.
- Symptoms of a heart attack, including severe chest pain or pressure; pain radiating from the chest to the arm, neck, shoulder, jaw, back, or abdomen; nausea or vomiting; shortness of breath; weakness; pale skin color.
- Symptoms of a stroke, including severe headache, slurred speech, dizziness.
- Symptoms of shock, including feeling faint; sweating; pale skin color; weakness; rapid pulse; cold, moist skin; drowsiness or confusion.
- Severe bleeding.
- Pain or pressure in the abdomen that does not cease.
- Severe vomiting.
- Bloody stools.
- Severe swelling/edema of extremities.
- Poisoning.
- Electrical shock.
- Drowning.
- Snake bites.
- Injuries from an automobile accident.
- Back, head, or neck injuries.
- Broken bones.

- Allergic reactions to foods or insect bites or stings.

- Chemicals or foreign objects in the eye.

- Severe burns or injuries from an explosion.

- Deep bites from humans or animals.

- Symptoms of sunstroke, including loss of consciousness or confusion; strong, rapid pulse; flushed skin that is hot and dry.

- Symptoms of hypothermia, including slurred speech; becoming increasingly clumsy, irritable, confused, unreasonable, and tired; being in a coma with slow, weak breathing and heartbeat.

## CiMO 2.7 PATIENT PRIVACY AND CONFIDENTIALITY PROCEDURES

You are required to maintain a patient's privacy and to safeguard the protected health information (PHI) of anyone who receives services at PMG. Patient information should be provided only on a need-to-know basis to individuals or organizations that use the information to provide treatment, obtain payment, or perform other related healthcare operations. This includes all patient information regardless of the format in which it occurs—verbal, written, or electronic.

If, in the course of doing your job, you accidentally see or hear patient information that you do not need to know, remember that this information is confidential and that you are not permitted to repeat it to or share it with others. This is the case even when you no longer work for PMG.

Polaris Medical Group's HIPAA compliance officer has developed policies to ensure compliance with the HIPAA rules for protecting patients' PHI. Every employee is responsible for complying with these policies and protecting patient privacy. You must read and understand the policies related to your job function.

### Polaris Medical Group Patient Privacy Guidelines—General

*Oral Communication*

Oral communication is a common source of confidentiality breaches because others in the office may have the opportunity to overhear a discussion. The following actions should be taken to ensure patient privacy:

- Consider who may overhear your conversation.

- Tell confidential information only to those who have a need to know.

- Speak in an appropriate tone of voice.

- Move the discussion to an area where others will not be able to hear.

If you overhear others discussing confidential information:

- Let them know they can be overheard.
- Keep the information to yourself.

### Physical Security

Simple measures can be taken to keep an unauthorized person from gaining access to information:

- Accompany visitors and repair/maintenance personnel to and from their destinations.
- Question individuals whom you do not recognize if they are near areas that contain confidential information.
- Lock all file cabinets, desk drawers, and the like when you walk away.

### Using Photocopy Machines

The following guidelines apply to the use of photocopy machines:

- Never leave a photocopier unattended when making copies of confidential information.
- Make sure you have removed all papers from the copy machine before leaving it. Check all areas of the copier—the top of the glass surface as well as all output and input trays.
- Do not allow others to see the information you are copying.

### Using Fax Machines

The following guidelines should be followed when operating fax machines:

- Use a cover sheet that shows your contact information and contains a confidentiality disclaimer.
- Confirm the recipient's contact information, including fax and telephone numbers.
- Advise the recipient prior to faxing confidential information, so that he or she may immediately retrieve it from the fax machine.
- Follow up with the recipient to verify that he or she received the fax.
- Immediately remove confidential information from the fax machine.

### Disposing of Confidential Information

Never discard paper that contains patient information in a trash can. Doing so makes the information vulnerable to unauthorized personnel and may lead to identity theft. Always shred or dispose of confidential information in a designated container.

## Polaris Medical Group Patient Privacy Guidelines—Information Technology

To protect patient privacy and to comply with HIPAA regulations, Polaris Medical Group adopted the following guidelines related to passwords, computer viruses, printers, e-mail messages, laptop computers, cell phones and smartphones, tablets, and social networking sites.

### Protecting Your Password

You are responsible for all actions performed under your user name and password. Treat your password as you would treat any personal and confidential information by taking measures to keep it confidential. The best way to ensure that your password remains confidential is to use one that is difficult to guess and to change the password as often as every ninety days.

Don't write your password where it can be seen, and don't share your password with anyone, not even the practice manager. If someone asks for your password or if you believe that another person has learned it, report this to the practice manager. If you forget your password or need assistance changing it, contact the practice manager. Remember, you are accountable for any transactions made under your user name and password.

### Protecting Your Computer from Computer Viruses

A virus is a computer program that performs unexpected or unauthorized actions. A virus can render a system unavailable and corrupt information contained in a system. To help protect your computer from becoming infected with a virus, never open an unsolicited e-mail attachment or download a file from a source you don't trust. Use antivirus software to scan all e-mail messages and downloads. If you believe that your computer may be infected with a virus, contact the practice manager.

### Using Printers

Printers are shared by staff members, which makes it necessary to take measures to protect confidential information when printing:

- Notice the name and location of the printer to which you are sending a file.
- Immediately remove confidential items from the printer output tray.
- Deliver or dispose of confidential information found on a printer.

### Using Electronic Mail (E-mail)

Electronic mail (e-mail) is provided for the purpose of conducting PMG business and providing service to our customers. Appropriate use of e-mail can prevent the accidental disclosure of confidential information and the disruption of computer services.

Before communicating directly with a patient through e-mail, you should add the following disclaimer to the bottom of all e-mail communications:

> "By communicating with PMG staff through e-mail, you agree to comply with the e-mail terms and conditions found at www.pmg.com/emailterms. Should you decide that you do not want to comply with these terms, it is your obligation to (1) reply to the PMG staff member with whom you are corresponding, indicating that you do not agree to comply with these terms, and (2) cease further communication with PMG by e-mail."

The following guidelines should be followed when using e-mail:

- Use e-mail only for official PMG business. Don't forward humor, stories, chain letters, or the like.
- Do not send an e-mail message that may be interpreted as disruptive, offensive, or harmful to others.
- When transmitting confidential information, double-check the e-mail addresses of intended recipients.
- Tell the recipient that the information being conveyed is sensitive in nature and should be protected. You can do this by adding the following disclaimer:

  > "This e-mail may contain confidential information of Polaris Medical Group. Any unauthorized or improper disclosure, copying, distribution, or use of the contents of this e-mail and attached document(s) is prohibited. The information contained in this e-mail and attached document(s) is intended only for the personal and confidential use of the recipient(s) named above. If you have received this communication in error, please notify the sender immediately by e-mail, and delete the original e-mail and attached document(s)."

- Use available security methods to encrypt messages.

### Using Laptop Computers, Tablets, and Smartphones

Laptops, tablets, and smartphones often contain confidential information. Steps must be taken to secure the information contained on these devices.

- Physically secure the device with a locking mechanism.
- Require a password for access.
- Do not leave a laptop or other device unattended in a public place.

### Using Social Networking Sites

Current policies regarding patient privacy and the protection of PHI apply to activities on personal social networking sites. Sharing any PHI, including photographs of, conversations with, or comments about patients socially, whether on a personal device or on a computer in the office, is a violation of the HIPAA Privacy Rule and may have serious legal consequences.

### Using Personal Computers

Computers are an access point to confidential information. To protect confidential information:

- *Restrict the view or access of others:* If possible, position your computer screen so that others cannot view it. This will prevent someone from seeing confidential information. Set your screen saver to automatically activate, and hide confidential information when your computer is not in use.

- *Follow appropriate log-on and sign-off procedures:* Never use someone else's user name and password or allow another person to use yours. Prevent others from using your log-on by locking your computer workstation when leaving it unattended. Protect the log-ons of others by always looking away when someone types his or her password.

- *Store files properly:* Do not store confidential information on a local computer workstation unless you are authorized to do so. Instead, store information on your network's shared drive. Delete files that are no longer needed. Secure removable media such as CDs and flash drives from unauthorized access by keeping them in a locked drawer or cabinet.

- *Adhere to software installation and removal procedures:* Do not install software that is not approved for use on PMG computer workstations. This includes software downloaded from the Internet, such as screen savers and games, and personal software purchased for home use. PMG must own a valid software license for all software installed on its computers.

## Violations of PMG's Patient Privacy Guidelines

HIPAA calls for stiff penalties for privacy and security violations. The violation of regulations under HIPAA can result in civil and possibly criminal penalties. If you feel that a patient's privacy or confidentiality has been violated, report the incident to the HIPAA compliance officer. You may remain anonymous when making the report.

## CiMO  2.8  OFFICE VISIT PROCEDURES

When a patient is seen by one of the physicians in the office, employees must follow specific procedures. This section of the PPM describes PMG's office visit procedures.

## Receptioning

When patients arrive at the office, the patient services specialist greets them in a friendly manner. If the patient has an appointment, suggest that he or she have a seat and indicate the approximate waiting time to see the physician. If the patient does not have an appointment, ask, "How may I help you today?" If the situation is an emergency, calmly escort the patient to an examining room and immediately alert the practice manager.

If the situation is not an emergency, determine the reason for the visit. Inform the patient that the physician sees patients by appointment only, except in the case of an emergency, but that you will look at the schedule to see whether the patient can be accommodated. Once you have checked the schedule, tell the patient the approximate waiting time.

## Gathering Patient Information

The office requires that certain information be on file for each patient of the practice. Basic information is usually obtained over the telephone before the first appointment; more detailed information is gathered when the patient arrives at the office.

### Preregistration Information Obtained from New Patients over the Telephone

When a new patient calls to request an appointment, basic information is obtained during the telephone call. This information is used to determine whether the patient is appropriate for PMG (for example, ensuring that the condition is within the physicians' practice areas and determining insurance coverage) and to begin a medical record for the patient. The information must be entered in the computer before the patient can be scheduled for an appointment. The information to be obtained is as follows:

- Name of patient
- Phone number/alternate number
- Address
- Date of birth
- Gender
- Social Security number
- Name of insurance plan
- Reason for call/complaint

A new patient should be asked to fill out a patient information form at the time of the initial office visit. When an established patient comes in for an office visit, ask whether any information has changed since the last visit. If there are any changes, provide the patient with a patient update form to complete. The new information must then be entered in the office computer.

New patients must also be given a copy of the PMG Notice of Privacy Practices and must be asked to sign an Acknowledgment of Receipt of Notice of Privacy Practices form.

### *Information from Other Sources*

When a new patient visits the office, it is often necessary to request patient medical records from the patient's prior physician. The office has a special form, Authorization for Release of Medical Records (see Figure 2-1), that must be signed by the patient and then forwarded to the other physician.

AUTHORIZATION FOR USE OR DISCLOSURE OF MEDICAL RECORD INFORMATION

Patient Full Name: ______________________ Medical Record #: ______________________
Patient Address: ______________________ Date of Birth: ______________________
______________________ Home Phone: ______________________
Work Phone: ______________________

I HEREBY AUTHORIZE POLARIS MEDICAL GROUP (check one):
__ To release my Medical Record information to:
__ To speak about my Medical Record information with:
Other: ______________________
Name/Facility: ______________________
Attention: ______________________
Address: ______________________
______________________

INFORMATION NEEDED (Be specific; include provider name and dates of treatment, if applicable): ______________________
______________________

(Note: We do not provide copies of records Polaris received from another physician or institution. Please request those records directly from the original healthcare provider.)

FOR THE PURPOSE OF: ______________________
So that we can be sure that your Medical Record information is complete, did you have an appointment with or receive services from us today? If yes, please indicate with whom: ______________________

AUTHORIZATION FOR RELEASE OF SENSITIVE OR STATUTORILY PROTECTED INFORMATION.
IMPORTANT: If your Medical Records contain information in any of the following areas and you want this information to be included in your request, you need to indicate your authorization by initialing next to the corresponding category(ies). Otherwise, Polaris will not release the following categories, except as required by law.

| | YES Release | NO Do not Release | Initials | | YES Release | NO Do not Release | Initials |
|---|---|---|---|---|---|---|---|
| Abortion | | | | AIDS/ARC | | | |
| Alcohol Abuse | | | | HIV Tests or Related Information | | | |
| Substance Abuse | | | | Domestic/Sexual Assault | | | |
| Mental Health | | | | Sexually Transmitted Disease | | | |

Does your medical record contain any other information that you would like withheld under this release? If yes, please specify; include provider names and dates, as applicable. ______________________
______________________

______________________
Patient's Signature Date*

______________________
Parent/Legally Recognized Representative Signature** Date*

______________________
Witness Date

*This Authorization is valid for 90 days (30 days for alcohol/drug abuse treatment) unless you specify otherwise: __________. You may revoke this Authorization at any time by providing a written statement to the Health Information Management Department, except to the extent that Polaris has already completed action on it.

**By my signature, I attest that I am the legally recognized representative of the above-mentioned patient in accordance with the following:
______________________.

The information released pursuant to this Authorization may be redisclosed by the receiving institution or individual to other individuals or organizations that are not subject to privacy protection laws.

Polaris will not condition treatment or payment on the provision of this Authorization.

**FIGURE 2-1** Authorization for Release of Medical Records

## Verifying Insurance Coverage

A patient's insurance coverage should be verified before treatment is given, except in emergency situations. Insurance coverage changes under many circumstances, such as when patients change jobs, get divorced, or complete college (in the case of a dependent). Unless patients are seen on a frequent basis (monthly or more often), you should ask the patient whether there has been any change in insurance coverage. In cases in which there have been changes, insurance coverage should be verified before the patient receives treatment.

### *Guidelines*

- If the patient is new or the insurance has changed, photocopy or scan both sides of the insurance identification card (see Figure 2-2 for a sample insurance identification card). Insurance identification cards usually indicate the type of coverage, effective date, phone numbers to call, and other data. Verify that the identification number and/or group number matches the number(s) on the patient information form. Also check to make sure the policy is in effect as of the date of treatment. A patient may have a card for a policy that is not yet in effect or for one that has terminated.

- Obtain employment information from the patient, especially the length of time with the current employer. Many companies have thirty-, sixty-, or ninety-day waiting periods before insurance benefits are effective.

- Medicaid patients must provide proof of eligibility at the start of every office visit. If a patient's eligibility is not checked, benefits may not be paid to the physician, since Medicaid eligibility changes on a continuing basis.

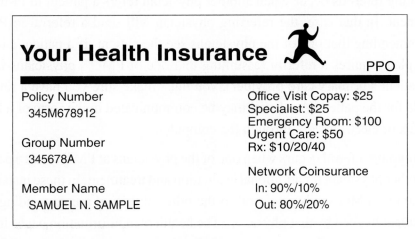

**FIGURE 2-2**   Sample Insurance Identification Card

- If a patient has an insurance plan that is not already on file in the office, call or e-mail the insurance carrier or go to the plan's website to request information. You will need to obtain the following terms of the plan:

  — Is there a deductible for this plan? If yes, how much? Has the deductible been met for this year?

  — Is there a copayment for this plan? If yes, how much is it?

  — What are the plan benefits for office visits? Outpatient hospitalization? Inpatient hospitalization? Preventive care?

  — What percentage do you reimburse?

  — Which services require preauthorization?

## Checking for Preauthorization Requirements

**preauthorization** prior approval from an insurance carrier that must be received before a procedure for a patient will be covered under the particular plan.

Many payers require preauthorization before they provide coverage for hospital admissions, surgeries, and certain procedures. ***Preauthorization*** refers to the process of obtaining permission, in the form of a preauthorization number, from the payer for a particular service before the care is provided. Since the office works with many different health plans, it is impossible to remember the requirements of each carrier. For this reason, PMG has the Policy and Procedure Manuals of all insurance carriers on file. The requirements of the major health plans are summarized at the end of this manual (see pages 77–87).

## Checking for Referral Requirements

A few managed care plans require referrals from a patient's primary care physician before services provided by another physician will be covered. A referral consists of two items—a referral number from the insurance carrier and a referring letter from the primary care physician.

Incoming referrals occur when another physician refers a patient to PMG for treatment. In that case, the referring physician will send a referral to PMG, recommending that one of the physicians see the patient. If a patient's insurance plan requires a referral (assuming that one of PMG's physicians is not the patient's primary care provider), you must make sure you have a referral on file for the patient. A referral may be communicated in the form of a letter or a fax or electronically through the computer.

An outgoing referral occurs when one of the physicians at PMG sends a patient to another physician for additional evaluation and treatment. In these instances, if required, PMG sends a referral to the other physician recommending that the patient be seen by that physician. The health plan information pages in this manual (pages 77–87) specify which plans require a patient to obtain a referral.

## Concluding the Patient's Visit

Before the patient leaves the office at the conclusion of an office visit, you need to perform certain tasks. If there is a payment or copayment due at this time, inform the patient of the charges, accept the payment, thank the patient, and provide a walkout receipt. If the patient has Medicare or another insurance carrier for which the practice accepts assignment, no payment is due at the time of service. If the physician has indicated that the patient needs a follow-up appointment, schedule the appointment before the patient leaves the office.

## Appointments

During the day, many telephone calls coming into the office are requests for appointments. Except on Thursday evenings, the physicians do not see patients without appointments.

### Scheduling Appointments

Scheduling is sometimes a balance between the clinical needs of patients and the productivity needs of the office. Ideally, patients should not have to wait to see the physician, and the physician should not have to wait for the next patient to arrive. In practice, to ensure that the physician is not kept waiting, multiple patients may be scheduled at the same time. This allows for variations that naturally occur each day—one patient arrives ten minutes early, another arrives fifteen minutes late.

### Patient Flow

All patients are scheduled according to their medical complaints. All new or established patients who require lab work, the completion of insurance forms, or the like are asked to report fifteen minutes before they are scheduled to see the physician so that the procedures or paperwork will be completed prior to the appointment time. When scheduling a patient, suggest several available time slots and allow the patient to choose the one that is most convenient.

If patients are worked into the daily schedule, inform them that they may have to wait a little longer than usual since they were not scheduled in advance. Informed patients are less likely to complain. If it is not an emergency, ask the patient to consider an appointment for another day or to come in during the Thursday evening walk-in hours.

In addition to patient appointments, the following activities are entered on a physician's appointment schedule:

- Regularly scheduled meetings
- Lunch hours

- Hospital rounds
- Days the physician is scheduled to be out of town
- Days the physician is scheduled to be off
- Surgical schedules
- Other outside activities

### Allotments

The office has a list of the different levels of office visits for new and established patients and the approximate time needed for each. The time needed is listed in the General tab of the Procedure/Payment/Adjustment dialog box in Medisoft. When a patient calls to request a first appointment, a follow-up appointment, or a comprehensive physical exam, for example, you will know approximately how much time is required. New patients should arrive fifteen minutes before the scheduled appointment to allow time to complete paperwork.

## CiMO  2.9  PAYMENT PROCESSING

Polaris Medical Group accepts insurance coverage from the major insurance carriers in the region. Both physicians accept assignment for Medicare, Medicaid, and TRICARE patients. Most of the insurance carriers are already entered in the Medisoft database. Occasionally, a new carrier must be added when the practice has established a contract with it.

At a patient's first visit, the patient signs a release form that assigns all insurance benefits to be paid directly to PMG. Should a claim be denied or a portion of the bill not paid by the insurance carrier, the patient may be responsible for the remaining amount. Polaris Medical Group accepts payment in the form of cash, personal check, or credit/debit card.

### The Collections Policy

The Polaris Medical Group policy regarding the collection of overdue payments is as follows:

- Patients are responsible for making arrangements to pay for services they receive.
- A patient is required to pay any outstanding balance within thirty days of the date of the service (unless an insurance claim is being resubmitted or appealed).
- If payment is not received within thirty days, a second statement or a notice will be sent reminding the patient that payment is overdue. The patient services specialist may also telephone the patient directly.

## ☐ Job 3

Cynthia Cashell, a cash patient, is examined by Dr. Crebore for a flare-up of psoriasis. Record the transaction using SD 51. Calculate the amount Cynthia owes and enter her payment. She pays in full with check 102. Print a walkout receipt.

## ☐ Job 4

Chantalle Usdan arrives for her sigmoidoscopy with Dr. Mahabir. Complete her patient information areas in Medisoft using SD 52. Create a new case. Since Chantalle is not a patient of Polaris Medical Group (she was referred by Dr. Rachel Imanni), a visit authorization number has been obtained by contacting her insurance carrier. Enter authorization number 321404 in Medisoft.

Enter today's transactions using SD 53. Note that her diagnosis has been omitted from the encounter form—it is "other specified examination." Look up the ICD code and enter the diagnosis in the Diagnosis tab of the Case folder. Enter Chantalle's copayment, which is made with check 409 (note that Dr. Mahabir is in the network). Print a walkout receipt.

## ☐ Internet Activity

Go to the website for CIGNA. Look up information on the different types of health plans offered. Explore the member and provider areas of the website.

## ☐ Job 5

A memo from the practice manager states that Jimmy LeConey's fever case and Roberta Yange-Sang's urinary tract infection case can now be closed. Close the cases.

## ☐ Job 6

Dr. Mahabir visits Rachel Atchely at Grandview Nursing Home. Rachel had cellulitis of the left foot and has been on a treatment regimen. Enter the transactions in Medisoft using SD 54. The copayment is paid with check 1078.

## ☐ Job 7

Mae Deysenrothe arrives at the office for a routine annual comprehensive physical examination with Dr. Mahabir. Create a new case. Record the transactions using SD 55. (Optional: Use the MultiLink feature to enter all the transactions except for the office visit code.) Payment is made with check 2043. Print a walkout receipt.

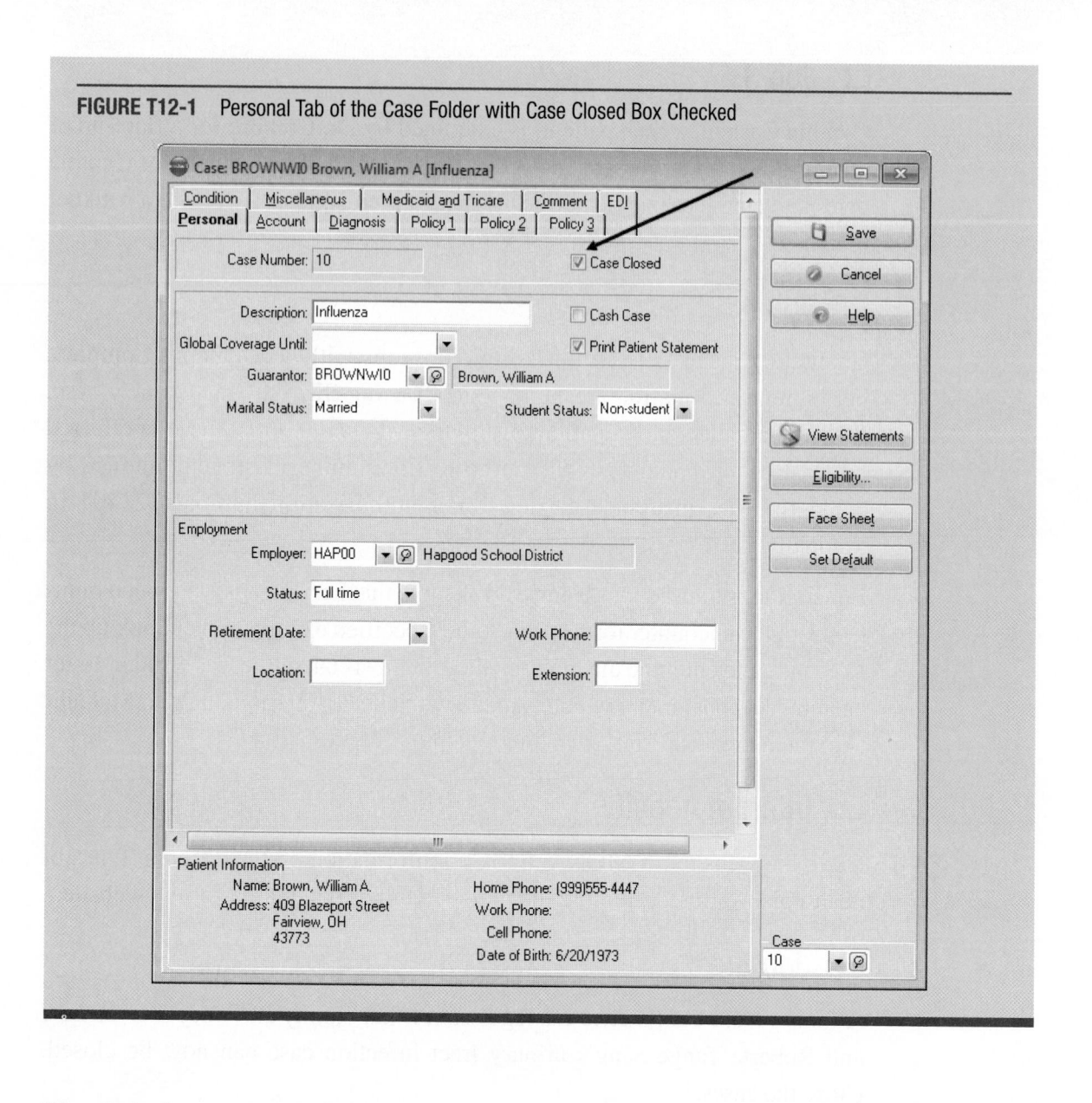

**FIGURE T12-1** Personal Tab of the Case Folder with Case Closed Box Checked

## ❏ Job 1

Change the Medisoft Program Date to June 20, 2018.

Print today's schedules for Dr. Crebore and Dr. Mahabir. Today is Wednesday, June 20, 2018.

## ❏ Job 2

Susan Jonas accompanies Felidia, her daughter, for an appointment with Dr. Crebore. Felidia has been successfully treated for impetigo and needs a release to attend summer camp. Record the transactions using SD 50. Susan pays with check 2349. Print a walkout receipt.

Figure T10-1). The provider referral is entered by selecting the physician from the list of choices in the Referring Provider drop-down list. A provider who is not listed in the Referring Provider drop-down list needs to be added to the database by selecting Referring Providers on the Lists menu and then clicking the New button.

In addition, some practices keep track of other types of referrals, such as the way a new patient found out about the practice. Many physicians like to have a record of referrals so they can review the sources of their referrals. This type of referral can be recorded by selecting the appropriate person or entity in the Referral Source drop-down list, also located in the Account tab (see Figure T10-1).

## MEDISOFT TRAINING TOPIC 11:

## Entering Visit Authorization Numbers

Visit authorization numbers are assigned by managed care insurance carriers, usually when a patient has a referral. In Medisoft, these authorization numbers are entered in the Visit Series Authorization Number box located in the Account tab of the Case folder (see Figure T10-1).

## MEDISOFT TRAINING TOPIC 12:

## Closing Cases

Medical practices have different policies regarding when a case may be closed. Cases are generally closed when (1) the patient is no longer receiving treatment for the condition specified in the case and (2) the case has a zero balance. For example, a patient's case for influenza may be closed once the physician indicates that the patient has fully recovered from the condition and when all payments have been received. Cases for chronic conditions, such as diabetes mellitus, may never be closed as long as the individual is a patient of the practice. When an individual is no longer a patient and the account has a zero balance, the case is usually closed.

Cases are closed in Medisoft by clicking the Case Closed box in the Personal tab of the patient's Case folder (see Figure T12-1). A check mark in the Case Closed box indicates that a case is closed.

# WEEK 2

## Day 3

*Study the Medisoft Training Topics, and complete the jobs listed for today.*

---

**MEDISOFT TRAINING TOPIC 10:**

### Entering Referrals

Some patients may be referred to the practice by other physicians. These physicians are called referring providers. For insurance billing purposes, these referrals must be recorded in Medisoft. Many managed care plans require patients to be referred by their primary care physician before being treated by another physician. In these situations, if there is no referral, the insurance carrier is not obligated to pay the claim. Often, as part of the referral, a visit authorization number is also required (see Training Topic 11 below).

---

**FIGURE T10-1**   Account Tab of the Case Folder

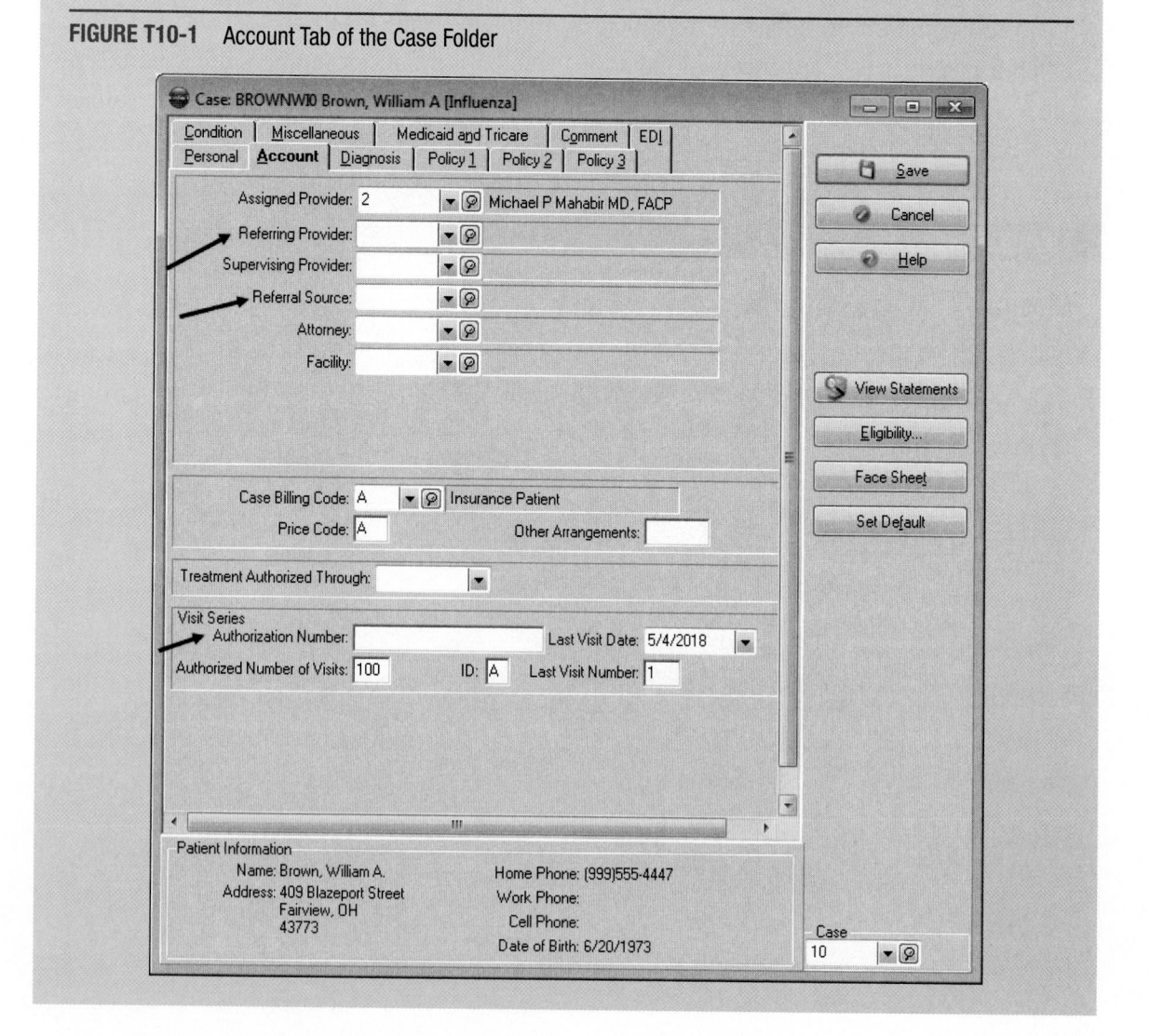

# Daily Worksheet

## WEEK 2

## Day 2

*After completing all the jobs for Week 2 Day 2, answer the following questions in the spaces provided.*

1. When diagnosis codes are listed by code number in the Diagnosis List dialog box, what diagnosis code comes right before L03.031, Cellulitis of right toe?

2. What is the charge for the procedure performed on Flora Torres-Gil on June 19?

3. Who is scheduled to see Dr. Crebore before Eugene Kadar on June 22?

4. What code is used for entering payments from Ohio Maxcare?

5. What is the balance on Diana O'Keefe's account as of June 19?

6. What is the net effect on accounts receivable for transactions on June 19?

7. How many insurance claims were created on June 19?

## ❏ Job 8

Diana O'Keefe comes in for her sedimentation rate test. Record the transaction using SD 49.

## ❏ Internet Activity

Go to the website for the Blue Cross and Blue Shield Association. Look up information about the different health plans offered. Explore areas of interest.

## ❏ Job 9

Print a patient day sheet for June 19, 2018.

## ❏ Job 10

Create insurance claims for June 19, 2018. Change the status of the claims.

- If full payment is not received within sixty days of the date of service, the patient's credit at PMG will be limited until arrangements are made to pay the outstanding balance.

- In some instances, patients may request a monthly payment plan. These requests are considered on a case-by-case basis by the practice manager.

- If full payment is not received within ninety days of the date of service, the patient services specialist sends a collection letter to the patient, requesting immediate payment.

- Depending on the amount in question, the office may hire an outside collection agency to pursue the matter if payment is not received after several collection letters are sent.

- Questions regarding the practice's collection policy are directed to the practice manager.

## The Billing Cycle

Polaris Medical Group uses a single set of fees for its procedures. The procedure codes and their corresponding fees are listed in the Amounts tab of the Procedure/Payment/Adjustment dialog box in Medisoft. For ease of reference, Polaris Medical Group's current fee schedule is also displayed on page 76 of this manual.

### Allowed Amounts

An allowed amount is the amount a given insurance carrier agrees to pay for a given procedure. In some cases, an allowed amount may be the same amount as the provider is charging, as in a fee-for-service plan. In other cases, the allowed amount will be less than the charge amount, as in a managed care plan or a government plan such as Medicare. In Medisoft, the allowed amounts for each procedure by each insurance carrier are stored in the Allowed Amounts tab of the Procedure/Payment/Adjustment dialog box (accessed through the Lists menu). The program uses the allowed amounts in this table to calculate the correct adjustment and to arrive at an estimate of how much the insurance carrier and/or the patient can be expected to pay for a procedure.

### Billing Codes, Patient Statements, and Place of Service Codes

The practice uses two billing codes—A and B—to indicate whether patients are insurance patients (Code A) or cash patients (Code B). Patient statements are mailed to patients on a monthly basis. Cash patients are billed at the end of the third and fourth weeks of the month, and insurance patients are billed at the end of the month.

The practice uses the following place of service (POS) codes when entering billing transactions in Medisoft:

| Code | Description |
|------|-------------|
| 11 | Office |
| 12 | Home |
| 21 | Inpatient hospital |
| 22 | Outpatient hospital |
| 23 | Emergency room—hospital |
| 24 | Ambulatory surgical center |
| 25 | Birthing center |
| 31 | Skilled nursing facility |
| 32 | Nursing facility |
| 33 | Custodial care facility |

## Insurance Claims

Insurance claims are generated on a daily basis. Information needed to generate the claims is gathered by the patient services specialist from data found on the encounter forms located in the patients' medical records. The encounter form lists the codes for the most common procedures and diagnoses. After the physician sees the patient, the applicable procedure and diagnosis codes are marked on the encounter form.

The information on the encounter form is then entered in Medisoft. If the patient is receiving treatment for an existing condition, locate the appropriate case in Medisoft. Verify that the diagnosis on the encounter form matches the diagnosis in the Medisoft case. If they match, go to the Transaction Entry dialog box, locate the appropriate case, and enter the procedure code and charges for the current visit. If the diagnosis is for a new condition, a new case must be created before the procedure code and charges are entered.

### Reviewing Linkage and Compliance

Before entering diagnosis and procedure codes, always check the data on the encounter form for errors. Make sure the diagnosis listed and the medical services received are logically connected so that the medical necessity of the charges will be clear to the insurance company.

*Medical necessity* refers to provisions set up by third-party payers requiring medical treatments to be appropriate and provided in accordance with generally accepted standards of medical practice. These standards require that the service or procedure

- Matches the diagnosis.

- Is not elective.

- Is not experimental.

- Has not been performed for the convenience of the patient or the patient's family.

- Has been provided at the appropriate level.

If the insurance company determines that the criteria have not been met—for example, that the procedure performed does not match or link up with the diagnosis listed for the patient—the company will issue a medical necessity denial and refuse to pay for the procedure.

## Billing Guidelines

To ensure that payment for services is received in a timely manner, the patient services specialist must follow these billing guidelines:

- Explain the practice's payment for services policy to all patients before services are provided. Discuss insurance coverage as well as patient responsibility.

- Verify insurance coverage before the patient receives services, including deductibles, copayments, limits, and preauthorization requirements.

- If a copayment is required at the time of service, collect the copayment before the patient leaves the office.

- If a patient is unable to pay the amount due at the time of service, ask for a commitment to a regular payment plan.

- Be familiar with currently used procedure and diagnosis codes; understand how to use the CPT and ICD-10-CM manuals to research information.

- Use Medisoft Advanced Patient Accounting to post charges, payments, and adjustments; generate and submit insurance claims; and generate patient statements.

- Follow up on all outstanding insurance claims on a weekly basis.

- Mail patient statements on a monthly basis.

- Provide clear, easy-to-understand statements that list the date the service was provided, the procedures performed, and the charges for those procedures.

- Help patients if they have questions about their bills.

- Follow up on all outstanding patient accounts on a monthly basis. Balances are aged as follows: current (0–30 days), past (31–60 days), past (61–90 days), and past (91 or more days).

- If a patient does not make a payment when requested and no payment plan has been discussed, speak to the practice manager about the situation.

- In the event of an overpayment by an insurance carrier or a patient, notify the company or person in writing, file a copy in the patient's insurance file, and issue a repayment if appropriate.

## Review of RAs

When a remittance advice (RA) arrives from an insurance carrier, it is important to compare the information on it with other information in the computer. (See Figure 2-3 for a sample RA.) The RA should be reviewed before payments or adjustments are entered in the computer, paying attention to the following items:

- Confirm that the charges for the services in Medisoft are the same as the charges listed on the RA.

- Confirm that the CPT codes listed in Medisoft match the codes on the RA.

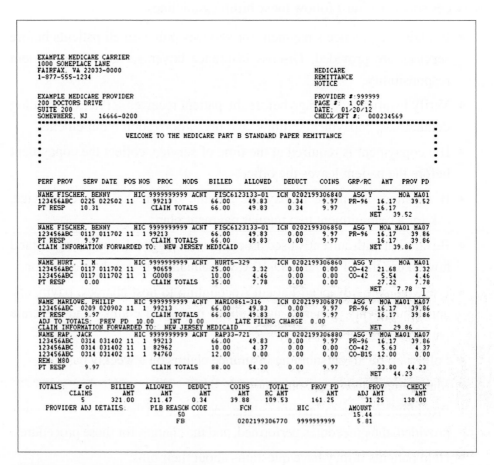

**FIGURE 2-3**  Sample Remittance Advice

- Confirm that the payment for each procedure is in line with the expected payment for that procedure. Depending on the type of insurance plan the patient has, the billed amount and the allowed amount will vary. For instance, if a patient is enrolled in a PPO that has arrangements with Polaris Medical Group for a discounted fee schedule, the billed amount will be more than the allowed amount, since the latter will reflect the discount. The patient services specialist must therefore be familiar with the different payment arrangements for each insurance plan when reviewing RAs.

- If the payment is less than expected, review the claim to make sure correct CPT and ICD-10-CM codes were used. If a coding mistake was made, resubmit the claim. If no coding mistake was found and you believe that the payment is not what it should be, file a request for review with the insurance carrier.

- If there are unpaid or denied claims, review the explanation provided and resubmit the claim if appropriate.

### Patient Billing Disputes

In the course of your employment with PMG, you may encounter patients who question the amount they were charged for services. If a patient disputes the charges, refer to the following guidelines:

- Remain calm and always treat patients with respect. Remember that they are questioning charges and services provided, not you as an individual. In addition, medical billing and insurance claims are complex; patients cannot be expected to be familiar with all aspects of billing.

- Gather and review the documents relevant to the amount in question (such as the encounter form).

- If, after reviewing the documents, you still believe PMG's figures to be correct, explain your reasoning to the patient in a logical, step-by-step manner. If the patient is not satisfied with your explanation, refer the problem to the practice manager. No matter how upset or irate the patient may be, you must remain calm.

- If you find an error on the part of PMG, apologize for the mistake and assure the patient that you will correct it today and provide corrected paperwork.

## 2.10 DAILY REPORTS

At the end of each day, several reports are generated that provide valuable information to the practice. These include the patient day sheet and the procedure day sheet. The patient day sheet (see Figure 2-4) provides a summary of patient activity on a given day. It lists the procedures for the day, grouped by

Polaris Medical Group
## Patient Day Sheet
Show all data where the Date From is between 6/11/2018, 6/11/2018

| Entry | Date | Document | POS | Description | | Provider | Code | Amount |
|---|---|---|---|---|---|---|---|---|
| **CONNODA0 Connolly, Daniel** | | | | | | | | |
| 378 | 06/11/2018 | 1806110000 | 11 | | | 2 | 99214 | 105.00 |
| | | | | Patient Charges | Patient Receipts | Adjustments | | Patient Balance |
| | | | | $105.00 | $0.00 | $0.00 | | $403.00 |
| **KAVANGR0 Kavanaugh, Gregory W** | | | | | | | | |
| 372 | 06/11/2018 | 1806110000 | 11 | | | 1 | 99212 | 54.00 |
| 373 | 06/11/2018 | 1806110000 | 11 | | | 1 | 36415 | 22.00 |
| 374 | 06/11/2018 | 1806110000 | 11 | | | 1 | 86360 | 263.00 |
| 375 | 06/11/2018 | 1806110000 | 11 | | | 1 | COPAYSTA | -15.00 |
| | | | | Patient Charges | Patient Receipts | Adjustments | | Patient Balance |
| | | | | $339.00 | -$15.00 | $0.00 | | $396.00 |
| **KOPELMA0 Kopelman, Mary Anne C** | | | | | | | | |
| 361 | 06/11/2018 | 1806110000 | 11 | | | 1 | 99202 | 88.00 |
| 362 | 06/11/2018 | 1806110000 | 11 | | | 1 | 36415 | 22.00 |
| 363 | 06/11/2018 | 1806110000 | 11 | | | 1 | 80050 | 143.00 |
| 365 | 06/11/2018 | 1806110000 | 11 | | | 1 | COPAYTRI | -10.00 |
| | | | | Patient Charges | Patient Receipts | Adjustments | | Patient Balance |
| | | | | $253.00 | -$10.00 | $0.00 | | $243.00 |
| **STEPHLY0 Stephanos, Lydia P** | | | | | | | | |
| 366 | 06/11/2018 | 1806110000 | | #3642987 Nationwide Medicare ( | | 2 | PAYMEDIC | 0.00 |
| 367 | 06/11/2018 | 1806110000 | | Adjustment | | 2 | ADJMEDIC | -37.00 |
| 368 | 06/11/2018 | 1806110000 | | #3642987 Nationwide Medicare ( | | 2 | PAYMEDIC | -23.20 |
| 369 | 06/11/2018 | 1806110000 | | Adjustment | | 2 | ADJMEDIC | -55.00 |
| 370 | 06/11/2018 | 1806110000 | 11 | | | 2 | 99213 | 72.00 |
| 371 | 06/11/2018 | 1806110000 | 11 | | | 2 | 10060 | 117.00 |
| | | | | Patient Charges | Patient Receipts | Adjustments | | Patient Balance |
| | | | | $189.00 | -$23.20 | -$92.00 | | $312.80 |
| **SZINOMA0 Szinovacz, Martin G** | | | | | | | | |
| 376 | 06/11/2018 | 1806110000 | | #267498 Standard Health Care, | | 1 | PAYSTAND | -47.00 |
| 377 | 06/11/2018 | 1806110000 | | Adjustment | | 1 | ADJSTAND | -10.00 |
| | | | | Patient Charges | Patient Receipts | Adjustments | | Patient Balance |
| | | | | $0.00 | -$47.00 | -$10.00 | | $434.00 |

Polaris Medical Group
## Patient Day Sheet
Show all data where the Date From is between 6/11/2018, 6/11/2018

| Entry | Date | Document | POS | Description | Provider | Code | Amount |
|---|---|---|---|---|---|---|---|
| | | | | Total # Patients | 5 | | |
| | | | | Total # Procedures | 9 | | |
| | | | | Total Procedure Charges | $886.00 | | |
| | | | | Total Product Charges | $0.00 | | |
| | | | | Total Inside Lab Charges | $0.00 | | |
| | | | | Total Outside Lab Charges | $0.00 | | |
| | | | | Total Billing Charges | $0.00 | | |
| | | | | Total Charges | $886.00 | | |
| | | | | Total Insurance Payments | -$70.20 | | |
| | | | | Total Cash Copayments | $0.00 | | |
| | | | | Total Check Copayments | -$25.00 | | |
| | | | | Total Credit Card Copayments | $0.00 | | |
| | | | | Total Patient Cash Payments | $0.00 | | |
| | | | | Total Patient Check Payments | $0.00 | | |
| | | | | Total Credit Card Payments | $0.00 | | |
| | | | | Total Receipts | -$95.20 | | |
| | | | | Total Credit Adjustments | $0.00 | | |
| | | | | Total Debit Adjustments | $0.00 | | |
| | | | | Total Insurance Debit Adjustments | $0.00 | | |
| | | | | Total Insurance Credit Adjustments | -$102.00 | | |
| | | | | Total Insurance Withholds | $0.00 | | |
| | | | | Total Adjustments | -$102.00 | | |
| | | | | Net Effect on Accounts Receivable | $688.80 | | |

**FIGURE 2-4** Patient Day Sheet

patient, in alphabetical order by chart number. Besides listing procedures performed for a patient or group of patients, it lists charges, receipts, adjustments, and balances for the patient or group of patients; and it displays a summary of a practice's charges, payments, and adjustments.

The procedure day sheet (see Figure 2-5) lists all procedures performed on a particular day and gives the dates, patients, document numbers, places of service, debits, and credits relating to these procedures. Procedures are listed in numerical order.

Polaris Medical Group
**Procedure Day Sheet**
Show all data where the Date From is between 6/11/2018, 6/11/2018

| Entry | Date | Chart | Name | Document | POS | Debits | Credits |
|---|---|---|---|---|---|---|---|
| **10060** | | | | | | | |
| 371 | 6/11/2018 | STEPHLY0 | Stephanos, Lydia P | 1806110000 | 11 | 117.00 | |
| | | | Total of 10060 | | Quantity: 1 | $117.00 | $0.00 |
| **36415** | | | | | | | |
| 373 | 6/11/2018 | KAVANGR0 | Kavanaugh, Gregory W | 1806110000 | 11 | 22.00 | |
| 362 | 6/11/2018 | KOPELMA0 | Kopelman, Mary Anne C | 1806110000 | 11 | 22.00 | |
| | | | Total of 36415 | | Quantity: 2 | $44.00 | $0.00 |
| **80050** | | | | | | | |
| 363 | 6/11/2018 | KOPELMA0 | Kopelman, Mary Anne C | 1806110000 | 11 | 143.00 | |
| | | | Total of 80050 | | Quantity: 1 | $143.00 | $0.00 |
| **86360** | | | | | | | |
| 374 | 6/11/2018 | KAVANGR0 | Kavanaugh, Gregory W | 1806110000 | 11 | 263.00 | |
| | | | Total of 86360 | | Quantity: 1 | $263.00 | $0.00 |
| **99202** | | | | | | | |
| 361 | 6/11/2018 | KOPELMA0 | Kopelman, Mary Anne C | 1806110000 | 11 | 88.00 | |
| | | | Total of 99202 | | Quantity: 1 | $88.00 | $0.00 |
| **99212** | | | | | | | |
| 372 | 6/11/2018 | KAVANGR0 | Kavanaugh, Gregory W | 1806110000 | 11 | 54.00 | |
| | | | Total of 99212 | | Quantity: 1 | $54.00 | $0.00 |
| **99213** | | | | | | | |
| 370 | 6/11/2018 | STEPHLY0 | Stephanos, Lydia P | 1806110000 | 11 | 72.00 | |
| | | | Total of 99213 | | Quantity: 1 | $72.00 | $0.00 |
| **99214** | | | | | | | |
| 378 | 6/11/2018 | CONNODA0 | Connolly, Daniel | 1806110000 | 11 | 105.00 | |
| | | | Total of 99214 | | Quantity: 1 | $105.00 | $0.00 |
| **ADJMEDIC** | | | | | | | |
| 367 | 6/11/2018 | STEPHLY0 | Stephanos, Lydia P | 1806110000 | | | -37.00 |
| 369 | 6/11/2018 | STEPHLY0 | Stephanos, Lydia P | 1806110000 | | | -55.00 |
| | | | Total of ADJMEDIC | | Quantity: 2 | $0.00 | -$92.00 |
| **ADJSTAND** | | | | | | | |
| 377 | 6/11/2018 | SZINOMA0 | Szinovacz, Martin G | 1806110000 | | | -10.00 |
| | | | Total of ADJSTAND | | Quantity: 1 | $0.00 | -$10.00 |
| **COPAYSTAND** | | | | | | | |
| 375 | 6/11/2018 | KAVANGR0 | Kavanaugh, Gregory W | 1806110000 | 11 | | -15.00 |
| | | | Total of COPAYSTAN | | Quantity: 1 | $0.00 | -$15.00 |
| **COPAYTRI** | | | | | | | |
| 365 | 6/11/2018 | KOPELMA0 | Kopelman, Mary Anne C | 1806110000 | 11 | | -10.00 |
| | | | Total of COPAYTRI | | Quantity: 1 | $0.00 | -$10.00 |

Printed on 06/11/2018  2:03 pm                                                                Page 1

**FIGURE 2-5**  Procedure Day Sheet (Page 1)

**Procedure Day Sheet**

Show all data where the Date From is between 6/11/2018, 6/11/2018

| Entry | Date | Chart | Name | Document | POS | Debits | Credits |
|-------|------|-------|------|----------|-----|--------|---------|
| **PAYMEDIC** | | | | | | | |
| 366 | 6/11/2018 | STEPHLY0 | Stephanos, Lydia P | 1806110000 | | | |
| 368 | 6/11/2018 | STEPHLY0 | Stephanos, Lydia P | 1806110000 | | | -23.20 |
| | | Total of PAYMEDIC | | | Quantity: 2 | $0.00 | -$23.20 |
| | | | | | | | |
| **PAYSTAND** | | | | | | | |
| 376 | 6/11/2018 | SZINOMA0 | Szinovacz, Martin G | 1806110000 | | | -47.00 |
| | | Total of PAYSTAND | | | Quantity: 1 | $0.00 | -$47.00 |
| | | | | | Total of Codes: | $886.00 | -$197.20 |
| | | | | | Balance: | $688.80 | |

**FIGURE 2-5** Concluded (Page 2)

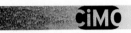

## 2.11 GUIDELINES FOR MEDICARE, MEDICAID, AND WORKERS' COMPENSATION

Some patients of PMG are insured by federal government programs such as Medicare and Medicaid. Individuals who are injured while on the job are covered by government workers' compensation programs. This section provides an overview of these different programs.

### Medicare

Medicare is the federal government's insurance program for individuals age sixty-five and older. Some individuals with disabilities and end-stage renal disease (ESRD) also receive Medicare benefits.

Medicare consists of two major parts, Part A and Part B. Part A covers inpatient hospital services, nursing home care, home healthcare, and hospice care. People who are eligible for Social Security benefits are automatically enrolled in Medicare Part A. No payments or insurance premiums are required. Those not eligible for Social Security benefits may enroll in Part A if they pay premiums.

Medicare Part B is optional. It helps pay for physician services, outpatient hospital services, durable medical equipment, and other services and supplies. Individuals who choose to enroll in Part B pay monthly premiums, coinsurance, and annual deductibles. Polaris Medical Group files Medicare Part B claims with Medicare for physician services, even physician services that are performed in a hospital. For some patients, Medicare is the secondary insurance carrier. In these cases, the primary insurance carrier is billed first, and then any remaining unpaid amount is billed to Medicare.

In 2006, Medicare began a prescription drug coverage program, known as Medicare Part D, to help beneficiaries pay for the medications they need. This help is available to all individuals with Medicare, although the program offers extra help to those most in need. Enrollment is voluntary; to receive help in paying for prescription drugs, beneficiaries must elect to enroll in the Medicare Part D program. An enrollee must also pay a premium for the coverage.

### Medically Unnecessary Services

Services that the Medicare program does not consider generally medically necessary are not covered unless certain conditions are met, such as the relation of the procedure, treatment, or service to the diagnoses. For example, a vitamin B12 injection is a covered service only for patients with certain diagnoses, such as pernicious anemia.

If a physician believes that a procedure will not be covered by Medicare because it will be deemed not reasonable and necessary, the patient must be notified before the treatment begins. PMG uses a standard *advance beneficiary notice of noncoverage (ABN)* in these cases (see Figure 2-6). The ABN form, which can be downloaded from the Centers for Medicare and Medicaid Services (CMS) website, is designed to

- Identify the service or item that Medicare is unlikely to pay for.
- State the reason Medicare is unlikely to pay.
- Estimate how much the service or item will cost the beneficiary if Medicare does not pay.

### Excluded Services

Some services are not covered under Medicare policies. Excluded services are those that are not covered under any circumstances, such as routine physical examinations and many screening tests. These services change each year. Participating providers, such as those at Polaris Medical Group, may bill patients for services that are not covered by the Medicare program. Giving a patient written notification that Medicare will not pay for a service before providing it is a good policy, although it is not required. When patients are notified ahead of time, they understand their financial responsibility to pay for the service. The ABN form may be used for this type of voluntary notification. In this case, the purpose of the ABN is to advise beneficiaries, before they receive services that are not Medicare benefits, that Medicare will not pay for them and to provide beneficiaries with an estimate of how much they may have to pay.

**Medigap insurance** an insurance plan offered by a federally approved private insurance carrier that is designed to supplement Medicare coverage.

### Medigap Insurance

Many Medicare patients purchase supplemental insurance plans known as **Medigap insurance**. Since Medicare does not cover all medical expenses,

| (A) Notifier(s): | | |
| (B) Patient Name: | | (C) Identification Number: |

## ADVANCE BENEFICIARY NOTICE OF NONCOVERAGE (ABN)

**NOTE:** If Medicare doesn't pay for **(D)**_____ below, you may have to pay.

Medicare does not pay for everything, even some care that you or your healthcare provider have good reason to think you need. We expect Medicare may not pay for the **(D)**_____ below.

| (D)_____ | (E) Reason Medicare May Not Pay: | (F) Estimated Cost: |
|---|---|---|
| | | |
| | | |

### WHAT YOU NEED TO DO NOW:

- Read this notice, so you can make an informed decision about your care.
- Ask us any questions that you may have after you finish reading.
- Choose an option below about whether to receive the **(D)**_____ listed above.
  **Note:** If you choose Option 1 or 2, we may help you to use any other insurance that you might have, but Medicare cannot require us to do this.

| **(G) OPTIONS:** | Check only one box. We cannot choose a box for you. |
|---|---|

❏ **OPTION 1.** I want the **(D)**_____ listed above. You may ask to be paid now, but I also want Medicare billed for an official decision on payment, which is sent to me on a Medicare Summary Notice (MSN). I understand that if Medicare doesn't pay, I am responsible for payment, but **I can appeal to Medicare** by following the directions on the MSN. If Medicare does pay, you will refund any payments I made to you, less co-pays or deductibles.

❏ **OPTION 2.** I want the **(D)**_____ listed above, but do not bill Medicare. You may ask to be paid now as I am responsible for payment. **I cannot appeal if Medicare is not billed.**

❏ **OPTION 3.** I don't want the **(D)**_____ listed above. I understand with this choice I am **not** responsible for payment, and **I cannot appeal to see if Medicare would pay.**

**(H) Additional Information:**

**This notice gives our opinion, not an official Medicare decision.** If you have other questions on this notice or Medicare billing, call **1-800-MEDICARE** (1-800-633-4227/**TTY**: 1-877-486-2048).
Signing below means that you have received and understand this notice. You also receive a copy.

| (I) Signature: | (J) Date: |
|---|---|

According to the Paperwork Reduction Act of 1995, no persons are required to respond to a collection of information unless it displays a valid OMB control number. The valid OMB control number for this information collection is 0938-0566. The time required to complete this information collection is estimated to average 7 minutes per response, including the time to review instructions, search existing data resources, gather the data needed, and complete and review the information collection. If you have comments concerning the accuracy of the time estimate or suggestions for improving this form, please write to: CMS, 7500 Security Boulevard, Attn: PRA Reports Clearance Officer, Baltimore, Maryland 21244-1850.

| Form CMS-R-131 (03/11) | Form Approved OMB No. 0938-0566 |
|---|---|

**FIGURE 2-6**  Advance Beneficiary Notice of Noncoverage (ABN)

Medigap insurance plans literally fill in the gaps in Medicare coverage. Medigap plans are regulated by federal and state laws. Most states have adopted the ten standard Medigap benefit plans that can be sold to individuals living in that state.

Some Medigap plans pay the patient's deductible and coinsurance. If a patient has a Medigap plan, it is the secondary payer; Medicare is the primary payer.

The claim is filed with Medicare first. Then, in many cases, the claim is automatically sent from Medicare to the secondary payer (this information is noted on the RA). If the claim is not automatically forwarded to the secondary payer, the office must submit the secondary claim.

### Medicare Managed Care Plans

Some Medicare patients choose to enroll in a managed care plan. Doing so eliminates the need for a Medigap policy. Medicare managed care plans, also known as Medicare Part C, often provide services not covered under Medicare at a small cost or no cost at all. However, there are drawbacks to Medicare managed care plans. Under most policies, services must be provided by a specific network of physicians, hospitals, and facilities.

All Medicare managed care plans must provide beneficiaries with coverage for Medicare Parts A and B, assuming that the beneficiary is covered by both parts. In addition to standard Medicare benefits, many managed care members do not have to pay deductibles or coinsurance. In addition, they may have policies that do not limit the number of days of medically necessary hospital stays. In contrast, Medicare Part A inpatient hospital care is paid during the first sixty days less any unmet amount of the annual deductible. After sixty days, the patient is responsible for paying a portion of the daily charges. Other benefits of many managed care plans include low-cost or no-cost preventive care, such as physical examinations and inoculations, and coverage for services such as prescription drugs, eyeglasses, hearing aids, dental care, and more.

Medicare pays the managed care plan a monthly premium to cover the services patients receive. Most plans charge policyholders monthly premiums, although some have no monthly premiums. In addition, many Medicare managed care plans require patients to pay small copayments at the time of each office visit. These copayments are usually between $10 and $25. Other than the monthly premiums and the copayments, there are typically no other charges, regardless of how many times the patient sees the physician or how many days he or she is in the hospital.

The following guidelines must be adhered to when providing care to a Medicare patient:

- Since PMG's physicians accept assignment for Medicare, the office must accept the amount allowed by Medicare as payment in full for services provided.
- The office is responsible for filing the insurance claims for all Medicare patients.

- If the annual deductible has not been met, the office can collect the charge for the service (up to the amount of the deductible that has not been met) at the time of service. For example, if the unmet deductible is $40 and the allowable amount for today's service is $30, the amount of the service ($30) can be collected from the patient. (This does not apply if the patient is covered by a Medicare managed care plan.)
- If the patient has a Medicare managed care plan with a copayment provision, collect the copayment at the time of the office visit.
- If the office has reason to believe that a service may not be covered by Medicare, the patient can be asked to sign an ABN form.

## Medicaid

Medicaid provides coverage for physician services, laboratory and X-ray services, prescription drugs, hospital services, skilled nursing and home health services, family planning, and periodic checkups and treatment for children. Medicaid-participating providers must accept Medicaid pricing for services. Typically, Medicaid recipients are individuals with low incomes who have children, are over age sixty-five, are blind, or have permanent disabilities. People applying for Medicaid benefits must meet minimum federal requirements and any additional requirements of the state in which they live. Medicaid eligibility varies on a month-to-month basis if the individual's income fluctuates. For this reason, it is essential to confirm a patient's eligibility at every office visit. A patient who was eligible for Medicaid last month may not be eligible this month.

If a patient who is eligible for Medicaid has additional healthcare coverage through an insurance plan or another government program such as workers' compensation, Medicaid is the secondary payer. When other coverage exists, Medicaid is always billed after that plan; for this reason, it is known as the *payer of last resort*. File the insurance claim with the other carrier first, and then file for Medicaid benefits after receiving the RA from the primary carrier.

### Medi-Medi Beneficiary

**Medi-Medi beneficiary**
person who is eligible for both Medicare and Medicaid benefits.

An individual who is eligible for both Medicaid and Medicare benefits is known as a **Medi-Medi beneficiary.** Medicare pays benefits for a Medi-Medi beneficiary first, followed by Medicaid.

## Workers' Compensation

When an individual is accidentally injured while performing his or her job or a job-related duty or becomes ill due to the employment environment, government plans called ***workers' compensation insurance*** pay for medical services. These plans also provide benefits for lost wages and permanent disabilities. When a patient is covered by workers' compensation insurance, other insurance plans such as long-term disability do not cover the charges until all workers' compensation benefits are exhausted.

Medical information about a patient who is being treated under workers' compensation insurance must be recorded in a separate case in Medisoft. In addition, a separate release form for the workers' compensation claim should be filed. At PMG, workers' compensation claims are submitted to Blue Cross and Blue Shield of Ohio.

**workers' compensation insurance** the government plan that covers medical care and other benefits for employees who suffer accidental injury or who become ill as a result of employment.

## POLARIS MEDICAL GROUP
Fee Schedule

### OFFICE VISITS - SYMPTOMATIC

**NEW**

| | | |
|---|---|---|
| 99201 | OF-New Patient Minimal | 66 |
| 99202 | OF-New Patient Low | 88 |
| 99203 | OF-New Patient Detailed | 120 |
| 99204 | OF-New Patient Moderate | 178 |
| 99205 | OF-New Patient High | 229 |

**ESTABLISHED**

| | | |
|---|---|---|
| 99211 | OF-Est. Patient Minimal | 36 |
| 99212 | OF-Est. Patient Low | 54 |
| 99213 | OF-Est. Patient Detailed | 72 |
| 99214 | OF-Est. Patient Moderate | 105 |
| 99215 | OF-Est. Patient High | 163 |

### PREVENTIVE VISITS

**NEW**

| | | |
|---|---|---|
| 99381 | Under 1 Year | 181 |
| 99382 | 1 - 4 Years | 189 |
| 99383 | 5 - 11 Years | 186 |
| 99384 | 12 - 17 Years | 231 |
| 99385 | 18 - 39 Years | 215 |
| 99386 | 40 - 64 Years | 233 |
| 99387 | 65 Years & Up | 259 |

**ESTABLISHED**

| | | |
|---|---|---|
| 99391 | Under 1 Year | 143 |
| 99392 | 1 - 4 Years | 161 |
| 99393 | 5 - 11 Years | 168 |
| 99394 | 12 - 17 Years | 194 |
| 99395 | 18 - 39 Years | 178 |
| 99396 | 40 - 64 Years | 194 |
| 99397 | 65 Years & Up | 155 |

### HOSPITAL/NURSING HOME VISITS

| | | |
|---|---|---|
| 99221 | Initial hospital care, det. | 185 |
| 99222 | Initial hospital care, comp. | 205 |
| 99223 | Initial hospital care, high | 250 |
| 99281 | ER visit, min. | 100 |
| 99282 | ER visit, low | 125 |
| 99283 | ER visit, det. | 150 |
| 99284 | ER visit, moderate | 175 |
| 99285 | ER visit, high | 200 |
| 99307 | Subseq. nursing facility care, pf. | 63 |

### PROCEDURES

| | | |
|---|---|---|
| 10060 | Incision/drainage, abscess | 117 |
| 20610 | Aspiration, bursa | 112 |
| 29505 | Splint, long leg | 130 |
| 29515 | Splint, short leg | 114 |
| 36415 | Routine venipuncture | 22 |
| 45330 | Sigmoidoscopy, flex | 276 |
| 46600 | Anoscopy, collection | 89 |
| 71030 | Chest x-ray, complete | 153 |
| 73610 | Radiology, ankle, complete | 113 |
| 93000 | Routine ECG | 84 |
| 93018 | Cardiovascular stress test | 202 |
| 99070 | Supplies and materials | ----- |

### LABORATORY

| | | |
|---|---|---|
| 80050 | General health panel | 143 |
| 81000 | Urinalysis, complete | 22 |
| 82270 | Blood, occult, feces screening | 19 |
| 82607 | Vitamin B-12 test | 90 |
| 82948 | Glucose, blood reagent | 18 |
| 85027 | CBC, automated | 34 |
| 85651 | Sedimentation rate test, manual | 24 |
| 86360 | Absolute CD4/CD8 ratio | 263 |
| 86592 | Syphilis test | 27 |
| 87070 | Throat culture | 48 |
| 87088 | Urine culture | 42 |
| 88150 | Cytopathology, cervical or vaginal | 35 |

### INJECTIONS

| | | |
|---|---|---|
| 90471 | Immunization administration | 18 |
| 90472 | Immunization administration, 2nd | 10 |
| 90658 | Influenza injection, ages >3 | 28 |
| 90702 | DT immunization, ages <7 | 32 |
| 90703 | Tetanus immunization | 29 |
| 90707 | MMR immunization | 90 |
| 96372 | Therapeutic injection | 27 |
| 90723 | DTaP - HepB - IPV | 81 |
| 90732 | Pneumococcal immunization | 38 |

# Standard Health Care, Inc.
## PPO

1500 Summit Avenue, Suite 500, Cincinnati, OH 45000

Phone Number .................................... 999-555-2900

Precertification Phone Number ...................... 999-555-5556

Fax .......................................... 999-555-8333

### CONTACT PERSON
**Gloria R. Saniszar**

### PLAN TYPE
**High-Deductible Health Plan (HDHP)**
Qualifies for use with a Health Savings Account (HSA)

### COVERAGE PROVIDED FOR:
Physician Services ................................ Yes

Comprehensive Physical Examinations ........................ Yes

Prescription Drugs ................................ Yes

### PRECERTIFICATION REQUIRED FOR:
Office Visits .................................... No

Surgery ...................................... Yes

Second Opinions ................................ No

Lab Services ................................... No

Referral to Specialist ............................. No

### DEDUCTIBLES/COPAYMENTS
Deductible Amount ............................... $1,000

Copayment Amount ............................... $15.00

Insurance Coverage Percents ......................... 100%

.......................... $5,000 maximum annual out-of-pocket cap

### MISCELLANEOUS
Accept Assignment ............................... Yes

Number of Days to File Claims ........................ 30

Diagnosis Code Set ............................... ICD-10

# Blue Cross and Blue Shield of Ohio
## Fee-for-Service Plan

5000 First Street, Worthington, OH 43085

Phone Number .......................................... 999-555-1414

Precertification Phone Number ....................... 999-555-1416

Fax .................................................... 999-555-1415

**CONTACT PERSON**

**Rosalyn C. Rimbord**

**PLAN TYPE**

**Indemnity**

**COVERAGE PROVIDED FOR:**

Physician Services ........................................ Yes

Comprehensive Physical Examinations ................... Yes

Prescription Drugs ...................................... Yes

**PRECERTIFICATION REQUIRED FOR:**

Office Visits ............................................. No

Surgery ................................................. Yes

Second Opinions ........................................ No

Lab Services ............................................ No

Referral to Specialist ................................... No

**DEDUCTIBLES/COPAYMENTS**

Deductible Amount ...................................... $500

Insurance Coverage Percents .......... Carrier 70%; policyholder 30%

........................................ $2,000 maximum annual coinsurance cap

**MISCELLANEOUS**

Accept Assignment ....................................... Yes

Number of Days to File Claims ........................... 30

Diagnosis Code Set ..................................... ICD-10

**CiMO**

## TRICARE

### HMO

PO Box 1000, Columbus, OH 43214

Phone Number . . . . . . . . . . . . . . . . . . . . . . . . . . . . . . . . . . . 999-555-0303

Precertification Phone Number . . . . . . . . . . . . . . . . . . . . . . 999-555-0304

Fax . . . . . . . . . . . . . . . . . . . . . . . . . . . . . . . . . . . . . . . . . . . . 999-555-0305

### CONTACT PERSON

**Lt. Regina Cotswold**

### PLAN TYPE

**HMO**

### COVERAGE PROVIDED FOR:

Physician Services . . . . . . . . . . . . . . . . . . . . . . . . . . . . . . . . . . Yes

Comprehensive Physical Examinations . . . . . . . . . . . . . . . . . . . . Yes

Prescription Drugs . . . . . . . . . . . . . . . . . . . . . . . . . . . . . . . . . . Yes

### PRECERTIFICATION REQUIRED FOR:

Office Visits . . . . . . . . . . . . . . . . . . . . . . . . . . . . . . . . . . . . . . . No

Surgery . . . . . . . . . . . . . . . . . . . . . . . . . . . . . . . . . . . . . . . . . . Yes

Second Opinions . . . . . . . . . . . . . . . . . . . . . . . . . . . . . . . . . . . No

Lab Services . . . . . . . . . . . . . . . . . . . . . . . . . . . . . . . . . . . . . . No

Referral to Specialist . . . . . . . . . . . . . . . . . . . . . . . . . . . . . . . . No

### DEDUCTIBLES/COPAYMENTS

Copayment Amount . . . . . . . . . . . . . . . . . . . . . . . . . . . . . . . $10.00

Insurance Coverage Percents . . . . . . . . . . . . . . . . . . . . . . . . . 100%

### MISCELLANEOUS

Accept Assignment . . . . . . . . . . . . . . . . . . . . . . . . . . . . . . . . . Yes

Number of Days to File Claims . . . . . . . . . . . . . . . . . . . . . . . . . 30

Diagnosis Code Set . . . . . . . . . . . . . . . . . . . . . . . . . . . . . . . ICD-10

# Columbus Medical Care
## PPO

3000 Arkady Street, Columbus, OH 43214

Phone Number ..................................... 999-555-7777

Precertification Phone Number ...................... 999-555-7779

Fax ............................................... 999-555-7778

### CONTACT PERSON
**George R. Coranelli**

### PLAN TYPE
**PPO**

### COVERAGE PROVIDED FOR:

Physician Services ................................... Yes

Comprehensive Physical Examinations ........................ Yes

Prescription Drugs ................................... Yes

### PRECERTIFICATION REQUIRED FOR:

Office Visits ...................................... No

Surgery ......................................... Yes

Second Opinions .................................... No

Lab Services ...................................... No

Referral to Specialist ................................ No

### DEDUCTIBLES/COPAYMENTS

Copayment Amount .................................. $12.00

Insurance Coverage Percents ............................ 100%

### MISCELLANEOUS

Accept Assignment .................................. Yes

Number of Days to File Claims .......................... 30

Diagnosis Code Set .................................. ICD-10

## Cigna Healthplan
## HMO

1200 Green Avenue, Cincinnati, OH 45000

Phone Number ....................................... 999-555-9000

Precertification Phone Number ....................... 999-555-9002

Fax ................................................. 999-555-9001

### CONTACT PERSON
**Ralph B. Granger**

### PLAN TYPE
**HMO, Capitated**

### COVERAGE PROVIDED FOR:

Physician Services ................................................. Yes

Comprehensive Physical Examinations ......................... Yes

Prescription Drugs ................................................ Yes

### PRECERTIFICATION REQUIRED FOR:

Office Visits ...................................................... No

Surgery .......................................................... Yes

Second Opinions ................................................. Yes

Lab Services ...................................................... No

Referral to Specialist ............................................ Yes

### DEDUCTIBLES/COPAYMENTS

Copayment Amount ........................... $18.00 (in network)

........................................ $25.00 (out of network)

Insurance Coverage Percents ................................ 100%

### MISCELLANEOUS

Accept Assignment ............................................. Yes

Number of Days to File Claims ................................. 30

Diagnosis Code Set .......................................... ICD-10

## Aetna Health Plans
## Ohio HMO—Network

5777 Royal Boulevard, Columbus, OH 43214

Phone Number  . . . . . . . . . . . . . . . . . . . . . . . . . . . . . . . . . . . . . .  999-555-1000

Precertification Phone Number  . . . . . . . . . . . . . . . . . . . . . . .  999-555-1002

Fax  . . . . . . . . . . . . . . . . . . . . . . . . . . . . . . . . . . . . . . . . . . . . .  999-555-1003

### CONTACT PERSON
**Elizabeth Kelley**

### PLAN TYPE
**HMO, Capitated**

### COVERAGE PROVIDED FOR:

Physician Services  . . . . . . . . . . . . . . . . . . . . . . . . . . . . . . . . . . . . . . . .  Yes

Comprehensive Physical Examinations  . . . . . . . . . . . . . . . . . . . . . . . .  Yes

Prescription Drugs  . . . . . . . . . . . . . . . . . . . . . . . . . . . . . . . . . . . . . . . .  Yes

### PRECERTIFICATION REQUIRED FOR:

Office Visits  . . . . . . . . . . . . . . . . . . . . . . . . . . . . . . . . . . . . . . . . . . . . .  No

Surgery  . . . . . . . . . . . . . . . . . . . . . . . . . . . . . . . . . . . . . . . . . . . . . . . . .  Yes

Second Opinions  . . . . . . . . . . . . . . . . . . . . . . . . . . . . . . . . . . . . . . . . . .  Yes

Lab Services  . . . . . . . . . . . . . . . . . . . . . . . . . . . . . . . . . . . . . . . . . . . . .  No

Referral to Specialist  . . . . . . . . . . . . . . . . . . . . . . . . . . . . . . . . . . . . . .  Yes

### DEDUCTIBLES/COPAYMENTS

Copayment Amount  . . . . . . . . . . . . . . . . . . . . . . . . . . . . . . . . . . . . .  $15.00

Insurance Coverage Percents  . . . . . . . . . . . . . . . . . . . . . . . . . . . . . .  100%

### MISCELLANEOUS

Accept Assignment  . . . . . . . . . . . . . . . . . . . . . . . . . . . . . . . . . . . . . . . .  Yes

Number of Days to File Claims  . . . . . . . . . . . . . . . . . . . . . . . . . . . . . . .  30

Diagnosis Code Set  . . . . . . . . . . . . . . . . . . . . . . . . . . . . . . . . . . . . .  ICD-10

## Ohio Insurance Company
## Fee-for-Service Plan

1600 Galleria Way, Cleveland, OH 44000

Phone Number ........................................999-555-5600

Precertification Phone Number ........................999-555-5602

Fax ...................................................999-555-5601

**CONTACT PERSON**

**Lynn Q. Farrell**

**PLAN TYPE**

**Indemnity**

**COVERAGE PROVIDED FOR:**

Physician Services ...................................... Yes

Comprehensive Physical Examinations ........................ Yes

Prescription Drugs ...................................... Yes

**PRECERTIFICATION REQUIRED FOR:**

Office Visits ........................................... No

Surgery ............................................... Yes

Second Opinions ....................................... No

Lab Services .......................................... No

Referral to Specialist ................................... No

**DEDUCTIBLES/COPAYMENTS**

Deductible Amount ....................................$100

Insurance Coverage Percents ............Carrier 90%; policyholder 10%

.........................$2,500 maximum annual coinsurance cap

**MISCELLANEOUS**

Accept Assignment ...................................... Yes

Number of Days to File Claims............................. 30

Diagnosis Code Set .................................... ICD-10

# Nationwide Medicare

## HMO

P.O. Box 7000, Columbus, OH 43214

Phone Number . . . . . . . . . . . . . . . . . . . . . . . . . . . . . . . . . . . . . . 999-555-8000

Precertification Phone Number . . . . . . . . . . . . . . . . . . . . . . . 999-555-8001

Fax . . . . . . . . . . . . . . . . . . . . . . . . . . . . . . . . . . . . . . . . . . . . . . 999-555-8002

### CONTACT PERSON

**Steve Delaplane**

### PLAN TYPE

**HMO**

### COVERAGE PROVIDED FOR:

Physician Services . . . . . . . . . . . . . . . . . . . . . . . . . . . . . . . . . . . . Yes

Comprehensive Physical Examinations . . . . . . . . . . . . . . . . . . . . . No

Prescription Drugs . . . . . . . . . . . . . . . . . . . . . . . . . . . . . . . . . . . . Yes*

*In some instances

### PRECERTIFICATION REQUIRED FOR:

Office Visits . . . . . . . . . . . . . . . . . . . . . . . . . . . . . . . . . . . . . . . . . No

Surgery . . . . . . . . . . . . . . . . . . . . . . . . . . . . . . . . . . . . . . . . . . . . Yes

Second Opinions . . . . . . . . . . . . . . . . . . . . . . . . . . . . . . . . . . . . . Yes

Lab Services . . . . . . . . . . . . . . . . . . . . . . . . . . . . . . . . . . . . . . . . No

Referral to Specialist . . . . . . . . . . . . . . . . . . . . . . . . . . . . . . . . . . Yes

### DEDUCTIBLES/COPAYMENTS

Copayment Amount . . . . . . . . . . . . . . . . . . . . . . . . . . . . . . . . . . $5.00

Insurance Coverage Percents . . . . . . . . . . . . . . . . . . . . . . . . . . . . 100%

### MISCELLANEOUS

Accept Assignment . . . . . . . . . . . . . . . . . . . . . . . . . . . . . . . . . . . Yes

Number of Days to File Claims . . . . . . . . . . . . . . . . . . . . . . . . . . . 30

Diagnosis Code Set . . . . . . . . . . . . . . . . . . . . . . . . . . . . . . . . . . ICD-10

**CiMO**

## Ohio Department of Human Services
## Medicaid

P.O. Box 4000, Columbus, OH 43214

| | |
|---|---|
| Phone Number | 999-555-3050 |
| Precertification Phone Number | 999-555-3051 |
| Fax | 999-555-3052 |

### CONTACT PERSON
**Carrie Repinski**

### PLAN TYPE
**HMO**

### COVERAGE PROVIDED FOR:

| | |
|---|---|
| Physician Services | Yes |
| Comprehensive Physical Examinations | No |
| Prescription Drugs | Yes |

### PRECERTIFICATION REQUIRED FOR:

| | |
|---|---|
| Office Visits | No |
| Surgery | Yes |
| Second Opinions | No |
| Lab Services | No |
| Referral to Specialist | Yes |

### DEDUCTIBLES/COPAYMENTS

| | |
|---|---|
| Copayment Amount | $8.25 |
| Insurance Coverage Percents | 100% |

### MISCELLANEOUS

| | |
|---|---|
| Accept Assignment | Yes |
| Number of Days to File Claims | 30 |
| Diagnosis Code Set | ICD-10 |

## Blue Cross and Blue Shield of Ohio
### Workers' Compensation

5000 First Street, Worthington, OH 43085

Phone Number . . . . . . . . . . . . . . . . . . . . . . . . . . . . . . . . . . . . . 999-555-1414

Precertification Phone Number . . . . . . . . . . . . . . . . . . . . . . . 999-555-1416

Fax . . . . . . . . . . . . . . . . . . . . . . . . . . . . . . . . . . . . . . . . . . . . . 999-555-1415

**CONTACT PERSON**

**Harley Burand**

**PLAN TYPE**

**Indemnity**

**COVERAGE PROVIDED FOR:**

Physician Services . . . . . . . . . . . . . . . . . . . . . . . . . . . . . . . . . . . Yes

Comprehensive Physical Examinations . . . . . . . . . . . . . . . . . . . No

Prescription Drugs . . . . . . . . . . . . . . . . . . . . . . . . . . . . . . . . . . Yes

**PRECERTIFICATION REQUIRED FOR:**

Office Visits . . . . . . . . . . . . . . . . . . . . . . . . . . . . . . . . . . . . . . . No

Surgery . . . . . . . . . . . . . . . . . . . . . . . . . . . . . . . . . . . . . . . . . . Yes

Second Opinions . . . . . . . . . . . . . . . . . . . . . . . . . . . . . . . . . . . No

Lab Services . . . . . . . . . . . . . . . . . . . . . . . . . . . . . . . . . . . . . . No

Referral to Specialist . . . . . . . . . . . . . . . . . . . . . . . . . . . . . . . . No

**DEDUCTIBLES/COPAYMENTS**

Insurance Coverage Percents . . . . . . . . . . . . . . . . . . . . . . . . . 100%

**MISCELLANEOUS**

Accept Assignment . . . . . . . . . . . . . . . . . . . . . . . . . . . . . . . . . Yes

Number of Days to File Claims . . . . . . . . . . . . . . . . . . . . . . . . . 30

Diagnosis Code Set . . . . . . . . . . . . . . . . . . . . . . . . . . . . . . . . ICD-9

**CiMC**

## Nationwide Medicare

### Parts A and B

P.O. Box 7000, Columbus, OH 43214

Phone Number .................................... 999-555-8000

Precertification Phone Number ..................... 999-555-8001

Fax ............................................. 999-555-8002

### CONTACT PERSON

**Steve Delaplane**

### PLAN TYPE

**Indemnity**

### COVERAGE PROVIDED FOR:

Physician Services .................................... Yes

Comprehensive Physical Examinations ................... No

Prescription Drugs .................................... Yes*

*In some instances

### PRECERTIFICATION REQUIRED FOR:

Office Visits ......................................... No

Surgery .............................................. No

Second Opinions ...................................... No

Lab Services ......................................... No

Referral to Specialist ................................ No

### DEDUCTIBLES/COPAYMENTS

Deductible Amount ................................... $110

Insurance Coverage Percents ........... Carrier 80%; policyholder 20%

### MISCELLANEOUS

Accept Assignment .................................... Yes

Number of Days to File Claims ......................... 30

Diagnosis Code Set ................................... ICD-10

# PART SUMMARY

| | |
|---|---|
| **2.1** List the types of outside entities for which PMG stores contact information in the PPM. | • Accounting firm<br>• Referring physician<br>• Affiliated hospital<br>• Affiliated nursing home<br>• Laboratory services |
| **2.2** Describe the steps a PMG employee follows when he or she has a grievance. | 1. The employee discusses the problem with the practice manager (PM) within ten working days.<br>2. If the problem is not resolved, the employee submits a written statement describing the situation, with dates and signatures, to the PM.<br>3. Within five working days, the PM, the employee, and one of the physicians meet to discuss the situation. The physician's decision is final and binding. |
| **2.3** Explain the difference between the resignation, termination, and discharge of an employee. | Employee *resignation* occurs when an employee decides to end employment with PMG, giving advance notification.<br><br>*Termination* is initiated by management for nondisciplinary reasons, such as workforce reduction.<br><br>*Discharge* is immediate dismissal for misconduct. |
| **2.4** Summarize the main personnel conduct issues addressed in the PPM. | All employees must<br>• Wear identification badges.<br>• Never engage in sexual harassment.<br>• Abstain from smoking and substance abuse.<br>• Keep personal telephone calls, visits, computer use, e-mailing, text messaging, and social networking to a minimum.<br>• Utilize Universal Precautions techniques while performing patient care functions.<br>• Maintain ethics as required in a healthcare setting. |
| **2.5** Provide examples of excused and unexcused absences according to PMG's attendance policy. | Excused absences include absences for<br>• Holidays or vacation.<br>• Jury duty.<br>• A death in the family.<br>• Weather-related emergencies.<br>• Other reasons preapproved by the practice manager. |

Unexcused absences include
- Unscheduled absences or lateness, such as taking an unscheduled personal day.
- Absences without proper notification, such as having a friend phone in your absence.
- Late arrivals or early departure, such as leaving a scheduled shift early.
- Other absences as defined by the practice manager.

| | |
|---|---|
| **2.6** Describe the steps used to screen routine and emergency telephone calls. | 1. Determine who the caller is.<br>2. Determine what the call is about.<br>3. Decide whether to transfer the call. The PSS handles all calls related to appointments, billing, and insurance. Other calls are transferred as described in the manual.<br>4. If the situation is a medical emergency, immediately transfer the call to a physician. Refer to PMG's list of symptoms and complaints that require emergency attention to determine whether a situation requires immediate action. |
| **2.7** Describe the PMG guidelines for the protection of patients' PHI in general, and when using information technology in particular. | General guidelines include safeguarding PHI during verbal communication, when photocopying or faxing, and when disposing of patient information.<br><br>Specific guidelines regarding information technology include protecting personal passwords, protecting the computer from viruses, safeguarding PHI that is printed or e-mailed, and securing PHI on laptop computers, tablets, smartphones, and PCs. |
| **2.8** List five tasks the PSS performs during each patient visit. | During each patient visit, the PSS<br>1. Greets the patient.<br>2. Gathers patient information.<br>3. Verifies insurance coverage.<br>4. Checks for preauthorization and referral requirements.<br>5. Concludes the visit by processing a payment or copayment if applicable and by scheduling a follow-up appointment as needed. |

| | |
|---|---|
| **2.9** Describe how the PSS uses Medisoft, the practice's billing program, in processing payments. | The PSS uses Medisoft in the payment process to perform the following tasks:<br>• Post charges, payments, and adjustments.<br>• Generate and submit insurance claims.<br>• Generate patient statements.<br>• Follow up on all outstanding insurance claims on a weekly basis.<br>• Follow up on all outstanding patient accounts on a monthly basis.<br>• Generate collection letters. |
| **2.10** List the required daily reports. | • Patient day sheet—provides a summary of patient activity on a given day.<br>• Procedure day sheet—lists all procedures performed on a particular day. |
| **2.11** Describe the different populations that Medicare, Medicaid, and workers' compensation plans serve. | Medicare is the federal government's insurance program for individuals age sixty-five and older and for some individuals with disabilities and end-stage renal disease (ESRD).<br><br>Medicaid is a state and federal assistance program that provides healthcare services for people who cannot afford them. Typically, recipients are individuals with low incomes who have children, are over age sixty-five, are blind, or have permanent disabilities.<br><br>Workers' compensation plans are government plans that pay for medical services when an individual is accidentally injured while performing his or her job or becomes ill due to the employment environment. |
| **2.12** Explain the purpose of the health plan information pages in the PPM. | The health plan information pages summarize the requirements of the major health plans with which PMG works. The information pages contain each plan's<br>• Contact information.<br>• Plan type.<br>• Coverage percentage.<br>• Precertification requirements.<br>• Deductible and copayment requirements. |

*For questions 1 through 15, write the letter that corresponds to the correct answer in the space provided.*

_____ 1. *[LO 2.8]* When a new patient telephones for an appointment, which of the following types of information is gathered during the phone call?
- **a.** referral number
- **b.** preauthorization number
- **c.** patient's date of birth
- **d.** patient's current medications

_____ 2. *[LO 2.9]* A transaction for a patient seen by a physician in a skilled nursing facility uses the POS (place of service) code:
- **a.** 11
- **b.** 21
- **c.** 31
- **d.** 33

_____ 3. *[LO 2.10]* Which daily log lists procedures performed, grouped by patient?
- **a.** practice day sheet
- **b.** procedure code day sheet
- **c.** patient day sheet
- **d.** patient statement

_____ 4. *[LO 2.12]* The Standard Health Care, Inc., PPO health plan covers what percentage of allowed services?
- **a.** 100 percent
- **b.** 90 percent
- **c.** 80 percent
- **d.** 70 percent

_____ 5. *[LO 2.12]* The policyholder's coinsurance amount for the Blue Cross and Blue Shield of Ohio Fee-for-Service Plan is:
- **a.** 20 percent
- **b.** 30 percent
- **c.** 25 percent
- **d.** 75 percent

_____ 6. *[LO 2.12]* The copayment amount for TRICARE is:
- **a.** $5.00
- **b.** $8.25
- **c.** $10.00
- **d.** $12.00

7. *[LO 2.1]* Which of the following type of outside entity does not have contact information stored in the PPM?
   a. laboratories
   b. accounting firms
   c. pharmacies
   d. nursing homes

8. *[LO 2.2]* When an employee of PMG has a grievance, the employee should talk to the practice manager within _____ days of the date of the problem.
   a. three
   b. five
   c. seven
   d. ten

9. *[LO 2.3]* Which of the following may be initiated by management for nondisciplinary reasons?
   a. discharge
   b. probation
   c. resignation
   d. termination

10. *[LO 2.4]* Employees who cannot make it to work because of inclement weather
    a. will be paid for the day
    b. will not be paid for the day
    c. will be paid at a 50 percent rate for the day
    d. will be given comp time for the day in lieu of pay

11. *[LO 2.5]* Which of the following is not an excused absence?
    a. an absence called in by a family member
    b. an absence for jury duty
    c. a death in the family
    d. a scheduled absence

12. *[LO 2.6]* According to the PMG telephone routing chart, when a patient calls for a prescription renewal, the employee should
    a. transfer the call to the physician
    b. transfer the call to the practice manager
    c. take a message for the physician
    d. take a message for the practice manager

_____ **13.** *[LO 2.7]* The PPM states that if someone asks for your password, you should
   **a.** say no
   **b.** say no and report the incident to the practice manager
   **c.** say no and immediately change your password
   **d.** say yes, but only in an emergency

_____ **14.** *[LO 2.8]* Before some procedures may be performed, a patient may need a _____ from his or her insurance carrier.
   **a.** referral
   **b.** premium
   **c.** preauthorization
   **d.** explanation of benefits

_____ **15.** *[LO 2.9]* If full payment is not received within _____ days, a patient's credit at PMG will be limited until arrangements are made to pay the full amount owed on the account.
   **a.** 30
   **b.** 60
   **c.** 90
   **d.** 120

## Critical Thinking Questions

*Answer the questions below in the space provided.*

16. *[LO 2.7]* Jennifer works as a patient services specialist at a medical office. Her best friend, Darleen, is a dental assistant in the same area. Jennifer and Darleen use several of the same social networking services. When one of Darleen's previous boyfriends comes in for an appointment at the medical office, Jennifer uses her private cell phone to copy the photo from his medical record to her social networking page and texts Darleen, saying, "Get ready. Guess who is here today...." Because Jennifer and Darleen are merely corresponding as usual, they do not feel they are violating patient privacy. Do you agree with their point of view? How can their offices ward off potential HIPAA violations?

_____

_____

_____

17. *[LO 2.4, LO 2.7]* Discuss ways to protect the use of passwords in an office setting. In what sense are passwords equivalent to legal signatures?

_____

_____

_____

18. *[LO 2.8]* When obtaining preregistration information from new patients, why is it important for a PSS to be knowledgeable about the medical practice's participation with different insurance carriers?

_____

_____

_____

19. *[LO 2.8]* What is the difference between a preauthorization and a referral?

_____

_____

_____

# On the Job

This section contains the jobs you will complete during your ten-day assignment at Polaris Medical Group (June 11 through June 22, 2018). Jobs are listed by day, and there are typically nine to fourteen jobs to complete for each day. Most days also contain Medisoft Training Topics. Each Training Topic describes a specific Medisoft feature that is needed to complete the jobs for that day.

While completing the jobs in Part 3, you will be using the source documents located in Part 4. In addition, you will be referring to sections of Part 2, Polaris Medical Group Policy and Procedure Manual, for specific information about insurance carriers, scheduling, billing, and other activities of the practice.

**IMPORTANT**!   As explained in the To the Student section of the Preface before you begin the jobs in Part 3, you must be sure that Medisoft® Version 19 is installed on your computer and that the Medisoft Student Data File is loaded. The Medisoft Student Data File, located at the book's website (www.mhhe.com/medisoft), contains all the base information needed to complete Part 3. Information about PMG's providers, established patients, and insurance affiliations is already set up in a working database contained in the Student Data File. Refer to the Preface for instructions on how to check whether the software and the Student Data File are installed on your computer and on how to install them if they are not.

Whenever you exit Medisoft, you will be reminded to back up your work. For easy reference, it is a good idea to create a separate backup file for each day of the simulation. In addition, if you are sharing a computer in an instructional environment, you will need to restore your backup file before you begin each new Medisoft session. Instructions on backing up and restoring data in Medisoft are provided in the To the Student section of the Preface and at the book's website.

## Using the Allowed Amounts Feature in Medisoft

Medisoft contains an option for storing allowed amounts for each procedure in its database. An allowed amount is the amount an insurance carrier agrees to pay for a given procedure. In some cases, the insurance carrier's allowed amount for a procedure may be the same amount as the provider's fee, as in an indemnity plan. In other instances, such as in a managed care plan or a Medicare plan, the insurance carrier's allowed amount will be less than the provider's fee, since the provider has agreed to a discounted fee schedule in return for other advantages offered by the plan.

In order to estimate how much the insurance carrier can be expected to pay on a claim and how much the patient will be responsible for, Medisoft needs to know the allowed amount for each procedure. Once the program knows the allowed amount, it is able to calculate the correct insurance adjustment (the difference between the provider's fee and the allowed amount). With both the allowed and adjustment amounts in place, the program estimates who can be expected to pay how much.

Allowed amounts can either be stored in the database at the time each procedure is set up, as in the case of the Polaris Medical Group database in this text/workbook, or they can be entered manually each time a payment is received from an insurance carrier. Allowed amounts are generally listed on the remittance advice (RA). In the PMG database, the allowed amounts for all procedures have already been entered in the Allowed Amounts tab of the Procedure/Payment/Adjustment dialog box for you. Figure 3-1 shows an example of the allowed amounts for a given procedure.

Once the allowed amounts table has been filled in, whenever a transaction is entered in the Transaction Entry dialog box, the corresponding allowed amount for that carrier is displayed automatically in the Allowed column (see Figure 3-2).

Similarly, when a payment is received from the insurance carrier and is applied to the transactions in the Apply Payment/Adjustments to Charges dialog box, Medisoft displays the allowed amount and corresponding adjustment in the Allowed and Adjustment columns (see Figure 3-3). The patient services specialist can compare the amounts displayed with the amounts on the RA to verify that the payment received is correct.

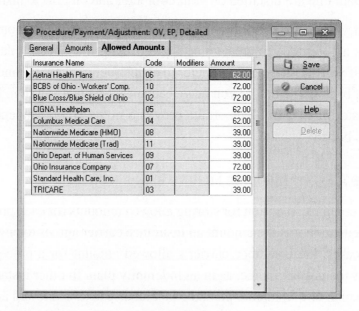

**FIGURE 3-1** Allowed Amounts Tab for Procedure 99213

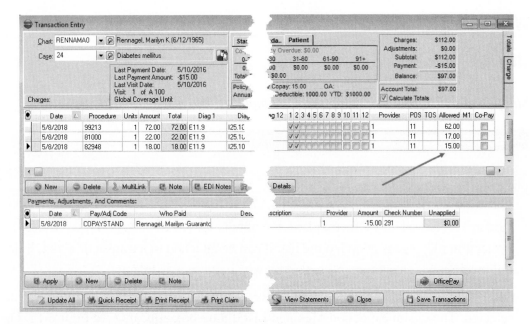

**FIGURE 3-2**   Transaction Entry Dialog Box with Allowed Amounts Displayed

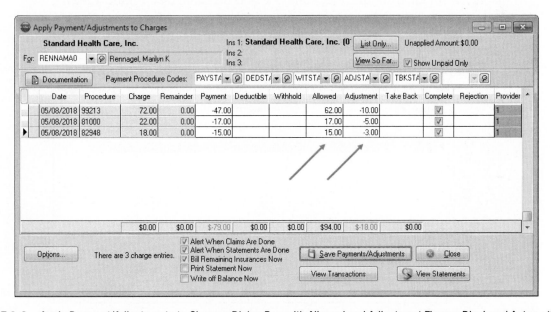

**FIGURE 3-3**   Apply Payment/Adjustments to Charges Dialog Box with Allowed and Adjustment Figures Displayed Automatically

In general, the Allowed Amounts feature makes the payment verification process easier and more accurate.

*Note:* In addition to filling in the Allowed Amounts table, in order for Medisoft to calculate the required adjustments automatically, the Calculate Disallowed Adjustment Amounts option must be checked off under the Payment Application tab in Program Options. In the PMG database, this option has already been selected as the default.

# WEEK 1

## Day 1

*Study the Medisoft Training Topic, and complete the jobs listed for today.*

---

### MEDISOFT TRAINING TOPIC 1:

### Claim Rejection Messages

The Claim Rejection Message List in Medisoft is used to store rejection codes and messages received on EOBs (explanation of benefits) or RAs (remittance advices). Once a rejection message is added to the list, it can be attached to a transaction and, if desired, printed on a patient statement to explain why a claim was rejected.

To add a message to the list, the Claim Rejection Messages option on the Lists menu is selected. The Claim Rejection Message List dialog box appears (see Figure T1-1).

To enter a message, the New button is selected. The Claim Rejection Message dialog box is displayed for entering the rejection code and message (see Figure T1-2).

---

**FIGURE T1-1** Claim Rejection Message List Dialog Box

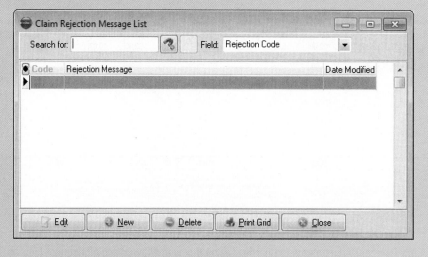

**FIGURE T1-2** Claim Rejection Message Dialog Box

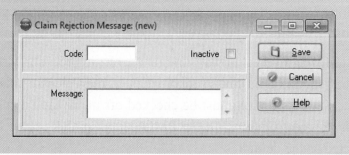

The code and message are taken from the EOB or RA. Examples of claim rejection messages are "These are noncovered services because this is not deemed a medical necessity by the payer" and "Claim denied as patient cannot be identified as our insured." The message can be up to 120 characters long. After the code and message are entered, the Save button is clicked to store the new entry.

Once a rejection message is added to the list, it can be attached to its corresponding transaction while applying the insurance payment through the Deposit List dialog box. After clicking the Apply button, the Apply Payment/Adjustments to Charges dialog box appears. To attach the message to the transaction, the rejection message code is entered in the Rejection field to the far right of the Apply Payment/Adjustments to Charges dialog box (see Figure T1-3).

It is also possible to print rejection messages on patient statements. To do so, a patient statement report must be reformatted so that it prints transaction statement notes. To reformat patient statements, the Medisoft Report Designer program (accessed by selecting the Design Custom Reports and Bills option on the Reports menu) must be used.

**FIGURE T1-3** Rejection Field in the Apply Payment/Adjustments to Charges Dialog Box

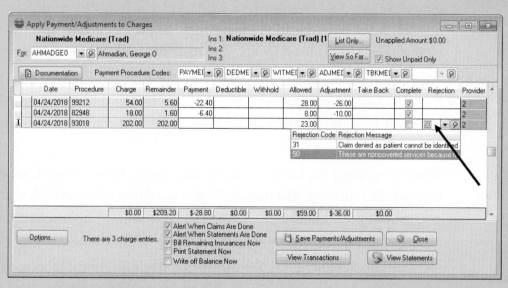

## ❑ Job 1

If you have not done so already, read the Polaris Medical Group Policy and Procedure Manual (Part 2).

## ❑ Job 2

Today is Monday, June 11, 2018. Before beginning, be sure to change the Medisoft Program Date to this date. Then open Office Hours and print today's schedules for Dr. Crebore and Dr. Mahabir. (You will also have to change the date in Office Hours.)

## ❑ Job 3

**Tip!**

**Job 3**

When you set up a new case, remember to edit the Insurance Coverage Percents by Service Classification boxes at the bottom of the Policy 1 tab in the Case dialog box, as different health plans pay different percentages for covered services. For instance, TRICARE pays for 100 percent of covered services, while Medicare generally pays for 80 percent. Insurance coverage percentages are given for each carrier in the health plan information pages (pages 77–87) in Part 2.

When you first view the Policy 1 tab, if the Insurance Coverage Percents boxes are not visible, use your mouse to extend the length of the dialog box so that the information comes into view.

Mary Anne Kopelman, the wife of Captain Arnold B. Kopelman, U.S. Army, arrives at the office for her appointment with Dr. Crebore. She is a new patient. Mary Anne has been experiencing shortness of breath and fatigue. Dr. Crebore examines Mary Anne and orders blood work.

Mary Anne is covered under her husband's TRICARE insurance policy. Her husband is not a patient at PMG. However, information about him needs to be entered in Medisoft because he is the guarantor for Mary Anne. Using the information on Source Document 1 (SD 1) located in Part 4, create a chart number and enter information about Arnold Kopelman in the Patient/Guarantor dialog box in Medisoft (Name, Address tab and Other Information tab).

Then complete the appropriate boxes in the Patient/Guarantor dialog box for Mary Anne Kopelman and establish a case for this office visit using SD 1. Note that basic information about Mary Anne was entered at the time she telephoned for an appointment.

When completing the Medicaid and Tricare tab in Mary Anne's Case dialog box, use the following information: Non-Availability Indicator: NA statement not needed; Branch of Service: Army; Sponsor Status: Active; Special Program: leave blank; Sponsor Grade: W2; Effective Dates: 6/1/2018 to 5/31/2019.

Once the case is created, use SD 2 to enter today's diagnosis, procedures, and payment (made with check 1011). Whenever you apply a copayment to the procedure charges, the standard practice at PMG is to apply the copayment to the patient's office visit procedure. In this case, the office visit procedure code is 99202. After applying the copayment, print a walkout receipt.

## ❑ Job 4

Angelo X. Daiute telephones to inquire whether PMG is accepting new patients. He has just moved to Fairview and would like to schedule an appointment for a routine comprehensive physical examination.

Establish Daiute as a patient in Medisoft using the information below. Then use Office Hours to schedule the appointment on June 14 with Dr. Crebore at 10:30 (forty-five minutes). You will create a case for him on the day of the appointment.

Angelo X. Daiute
22 Van Cortland Drive, Apt. 390
Fairview, OH 43773
Phone: 999-555-1758
Date of Birth: 1/5/1978
Sex: M
SS#: 756-99-2637
Employer: COSTINC
Status: Full-time
Work Phone: 999-555-4300
Race: White
Ethnicity: Hispanic
Language: English

Tip!

**Job 4**
The default date in Office Hours is the Windows System Date. You will need to change the date to enter the appointment.

## ❏ Job 5

A Medicare RA with a payment arrives (see SD 3) for Lydia P. Stephanos for her office visit on May 24, 2018. Notice that the RA contains a claim rejection message at the bottom. Before entering and applying the payment, add the rejection code and message to the Claim Rejection Messages list in Medisoft.

Then compare the procedure codes and amounts on the RA with those in the Transaction Entry dialog box in Medisoft. If the codes are correct, enter and apply the payment in Medisoft using the Enter Deposits/Payments option on the Activities menu. Lydia is covered by Nationwide Medicare (Traditional). When applying the payment ($0.00) for the rejected procedure in the Apply Payment/Adjustments to Charges dialog box, tab over to the Rejection field on the far right of the window to record the corresponding claim rejection code. Also, make sure the Print Statement Now check box at the bottom of the window is *not* checked. (Only the first three check boxes should be checked.)

*Note:* When applying a payment to charges in the Apply Payment/Adjustments to Charges dialog box, it is important to press Tab to move through each field of the grid. As you tab across each row, Medisoft calculates and fills in any automatic amounts for you, including allowed amounts and adjustments. Since the Remainder amount in column 4 changes depending on what is displayed in the other fields, you must tab past the end of the row for the Remainder amount to be accurate.

Copyright ©2016 McGraw-Hill Education

Case Studies for Use with Computers in the Medical Office **101**

**Tip !**

**Job 6**

To create a new case for Lydia Stephanos, use the Copy Case button to make a copy of her existing case. Then edit the Personal tab and the Diagnosis tab.

**Tip !**

**Job 7**

When adding Gregory Kavanaugh's new employer to the database, select Code in the Field drop-down box so that the entities in the Address List dialog box are listed alphabetically by code rather than by type (the default setting).

## ❑ Job 6

Lydia P. Stephanos has an office visit with Dr. Mahabir for treatment of a cyst. Create a new case for this visit and use SD 4 to enter the procedures and charges for the new case in Medisoft.

## ❑ Job 7

Gregory Kavanaugh has an office visit with Dr. Crebore for the routine monitoring of his CD4/CD8 ratio. While in the office, he tells you that his employer and insurance carrier have changed since his last visit. He completes a new patient information form (SD 5). Using this form, update his information in Medisoft. Note that his new employer is not in the database and will need to be added.

Also, since Gregory has changed insurance carriers, you must create a new case for today's visit, even though it is a routine office visit for an existing condition for which he has been previously treated. Use the Copy Case button to make a copy of the old case. Then update the employment and insurance information in the Personal and Policy 1 tabs respectively. The policy start and end dates for the new plan are 5/1/2018 – 12/31/2018. Refer to the health plan information page for the new insurance carrier for details on insurance coverage percentages. Note that Gregory has paid the deductible for the new insurance carrier.

After the new case has been created, enter today's procedures, charges, and payment using SD 6.

## ❑ Job 8

Victoria Ferrara, an attorney with a local firm, telephones for an appointment. She needs follow-up care for a wound. Schedule her for a fifteen-minute appointment on June 13 at 2:00.

## ❑ Job 9

An RA is transmitted from Standard Health Care for Martin Szinovacz's office visit on May 16, 2018 (SD 7). Record the deposit/payment in Medisoft and apply it to the appropriate transactions.

## ❑ Job 10

Cynthia Cashell phones the office. Her psoriasis has flared up and she would like an appointment with Dr. Crebore. Schedule her for a fifteen-minute office visit on June 20 at 10:30.

## ❑ Job 11

Dr. Mahabir examines Dan Connolly for his complaint of joint pain in the hips. Create a new case for today's visit. Using SD 8, record the procedure for the visit. Schedule a fifteen-minute follow-up office visit for June 22 at 10:00.

## ❑ Job 12

Cameron Trotta telephones to reschedule his appointment for his annual checkup. It is currently scheduled for June 12 at 3:00. Move the appointment to 2:00 on June 14.

## ❑ Job 13

Preview and then print a patient day sheet for June 11, 2018. For the Date Created range boxes, click to place a check mark in the Show all values of the Date Created field box so that the report prints correctly. (For the purposes of the jobs in this simulation, always click to place a check mark in the Show all values of the Date Created field box so that all Date Created values are included in the report.) Enter *06112018* in both the Date From range boxes. *Note:* These instructions must be followed each time a patient day sheet is printed (substituting a different date in the Date From range boxes).

## ❑ Job 14

Create insurance claims for June 11, 2018. In the Create Claims dialog box, enter *06112018* in both Range of Transaction Dates boxes. Change the status of the claims from Ready To Send to Sent. *Note:* These instructions must be followed each time claims are created (substituting a different date).

*A Note on Claim Status:* If claims were transmitted electronically, the claim status for each claim would automatically change from Ready To Send to Sent once the claims were sent. As it is not possible to actually send electronic claims while working on the jobs in this text/workbook, you will be asked to change the claim status manually from Ready To Send to Sent for the claims you create. To change the status of claims, use the Change Status button in the Claim Management dialog box.

The Sent status in the Claim Management dialog box is required when you create patient statements at the end of the simulation. The program generates remainder statements for patients whose claims have a Sent status. Therefore, if you do not change the status of the claims you create to Sent, you will not be able to generate any remainder statements toward the end.

**Tip!**

**Job 11**

Remember to select Dr. Mahabir as the provider in Office Hours before making the new appointment.

**Tip!**

**Job 14**

To change the status of a single claim in the Claim Management dialog box, click on the claim to select it and then click the Change Status button. To change the status of multiple claims, first select them in the Claim Management dialog box by holding down the CTRL key and clicking each claim to be included. Then click the Change Status button. Changes will apply to all claims that were selected.

# Daily Worksheet

## WEEK 1

## Day 1

*After completing all the jobs for Week 1 Day 1, answer the following questions in the spaces provided.*

1. What name is entered in the Policy Holder 1 box in the Policy 1 tab (in the Case folder) for Mary Anne Kopelman?

   _____

   _____

2. What are the total charges for Lydia Stephanos's June 11 office visit?

   _____

   _____

3. How many cases are there for Gregory Kavanaugh? Why?

   _____

   _____

4. What amount of the total charges on May 16 was Martin Szinovacz responsible for?

   _____

   _____

5. Who is Dr. Crebore's first appointment on June 14?

   _____

   _____

6. For Dan Connolly, for what amount of the total charges on June 11 is his secondary insurance carrier responsible?

   _____

   _____

7. What were the total check copayments made by patients for June 11?

   _____

   _____

# WEEK 1

## Day 2

*Study the Medisoft Training Topic, and complete the jobs listed for today.*

### Creating a Patient by Insurance Carrier Report and Exporting It to a PDF File

The Medisoft Reports menu contains a Standard Patient Lists option that can be used to create two convenient patient list reports: Patient by Diagnosis and Patient by Insurance Carrier. The Patient by Diagnosis report lists patients according to their primary diagnosis code, and the Patient by Insurance Carrier report lists patients according to their primary insurance carrier.

To generate a Patient by Insurance Carrier report, open the Reports menu, click Standard Patient Lists, and then click Patient by Insurance Carrier on the submenu that appears (see Figure T2-1).

**FIGURE T2-1**  Standard Patient Lists Option with Submenu

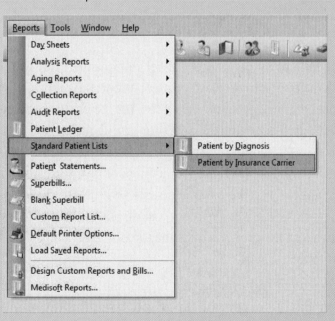

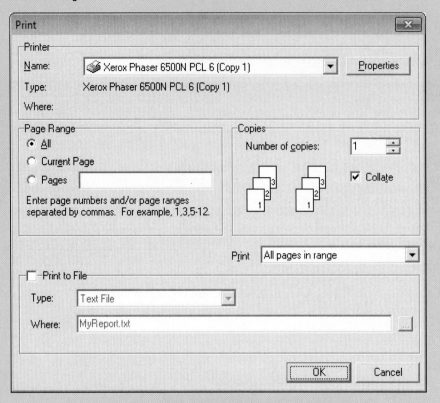

After clicking the Patient by Insurance Carrier option, the Print Report Where? dialog box displays, with the option to preview, print, or export the report. To preview the results of the report before printing it or exporting it to a file, select the preview option and click the Start button. A Search dialog box appears for setting the parameters of the report. The report can be generated without specifying a range of insurance carrier codes so that all carriers are included, or it can be created for a range of insurance carriers by selecting the appropriate code range. Once the parameters are set, the OK button is clicked, and the report (Patient Census by Carrier [Primary]) is displayed in the Print Preview window. After viewing the report, the printer icon at the top of the Print Preview window is clicked to send the report to the printer.

In addition to previewing and printing the report, the report can be exported to a PDF file (or other file type). To export the report, click the Print icon in the Print Preview toolbar. In the Print dialog box, click the Print to File box and select PDF File from the drop-down list in the Type field. Next, click the Lookup button located to the right of the Where field (see Figure T2-2). In the Save As dialog box, select a location for the file in the Save in field. Enter a name in the File name field (see Figure T2-3). Finally, click the Save button. You are returned to the Print dialog box. Click the OK button to save the report as a PDF file.

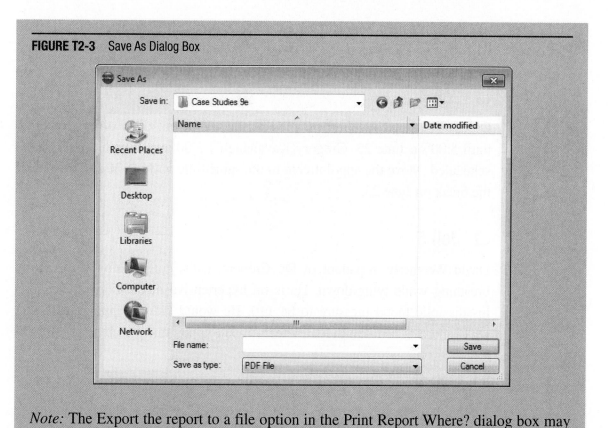

**FIGURE T2-3** Save As Dialog Box

*Note:* The Export the report to a file option in the Print Report Where? dialog box may also be used to save other types of reports as PDF files, such as the patient day sheet reports created at the end of each day in the simulation.

## ❏ Job 1

Change the Medisoft Program Date to June 12, 2018.

Print today's schedules for Dr. Crebore and Dr. Mahabir. Today is Tuesday, June 12, 2018.

## ❏ Job 2

Gloria Berkel-Rees telephones for an appointment with Dr. Mahabir. She is due for a three-month checkup on her chronic asthma. Schedule her for a fifteen-minute office visit on June 15 at 2:45.

## ❏ Job 3

A new patient, Wilma Estephan, arrives for her appointment with Dr. Mahabir. She has complained of pain during urination. Wilma is a Medicare HMO patient. Using SD 9, finish completing the patient information sections of Medisoft for Wilma and create a case for this visit. Then enter today's transactions using the encounter form found on SD 10. The copayment is paid with check 359. Print a walkout receipt.

## ❏ Job 4

Dr. Crebore stops by to inform you that she will be out of the office from 3:00 until 5:00 on June 25. Gregory Kavanaugh's 3:00 appointment must be rescheduled. Move the appointment to the same time on June 26 and then enter the break on June 25.

## ❏ Job 5

David Weatherly, a patient of Dr. Crebore, calls, complaining of difficulty breathing while lying down. He is on hypertensive medications and reports his diastolic blood pressure to be 110. He would like an appointment with Dr. Crebore. Schedule him for a fifteen-minute appointment on June 15 at 10:00.

## ❏ Job 6

Jimmy LeConey is seen by Dr. Crebore for flu-like symptoms. Jimmy's mother, Ann, reports that Jimmy is no longer covered by her insurance policy; he is now covered by his father's policy. Jimmy's father is not a patient at PMG. Using the information on SD 11, enter Jimmy's father as a guarantor.

Then create a new case for Jimmy and enter the new insurance information. Note that his father has met the deductible for the year ($500). His policy pays for 70 percent of covered services once the deductible is met. Finally, enter today's transactions using the information found on the encounter form (SD 12).

After the insurance carrier is billed and the RA is received, the guarantor (Jimmy's father) can be billed for the amount not paid by the carrier.

## ❏ Job 7

Dr. Mahabir has just finished examining Will Brown. Will complained of rectal bleeding. Dr. Mahabir performed an anoscopy and found external hemorrhoids. Since this is a new condition, you will need to create a new case. Then, using SD 13, enter today's transactions.

## ❏ Job 8

Roberta Yange-Sang telephones to make a follow-up appointment with Dr. Mahabir for an examination of her laceration. Schedule her for a fifteen-minute appointment on June 15 at 10:45.

## ❏ Job 9

An RA arrives with payment from Ohio Insurance Company (SD 14). Compare the procedure codes and amounts with those in Medisoft for each patient. If they are correct, use the Enter Deposits/Payments option to enter and apply the payment in Medisoft. While applying the payment in the Apply Payment/ Adjustments to Charges dialog box, apply Victoria Ferrara's payment first, and then Gregory Kavanaugh's. When applying Gregory's payment, click the Write off Balance Now check box at the bottom of the window to write off his remaining balance, which should be less than $10.00. As Gregory has switched insurance carriers, this is the last payment from this carrier for this case. (*Note:* A default code for small balance write-offs, ADJSMALBAL, has already been set up in the PMG procedure code database, and the maximum write-off amount to be used with the code is currently set at $10.00 in the Program Options dialog box.)

After applying Gregory Kavanaugh's payment, open the Transaction Entry window and locate the adjustment for the small balance write-off in the lower half of the window. Since the program has used the computer's system date for this transaction rather than the Medisoft Program Date of 6/12/2018, change the date in the Date field to 6/12/2018 and then save the change.

## ❏ Job 10

George Ahmadian calls to reschedule his appointment that is scheduled for tomorrow at 4:00. Move the appointment to 3:00 on June 14.

## ❏ Job 11

Dr. Mahabir has finished examining Alan Harcar, who is found to have an upper respiratory infection. Create a new case, enter today's transactions from SD 15, and print a walkout receipt. The copayment is paid with check 1201. Schedule Alan for a forty-five-minute appointment for a comprehensive physical examination (CPE) on June 15 at 4:00.

## ❏ Job 12

Generate a Patient by Insurance Carrier report that includes all insurance carriers. Select the option to preview the report, and then print it from the preview window. Next, generate the report again and export it to a PDF file. Save the file in the folder with your Medisoft backup files and name it patient_by_ins_list.pdf.

## ❏ Job 13

Preview and then print a patient day sheet for June 12, 2018. Under the Date Created range boxes, click to place a check mark in the Show all values of the Date Created field box so that all values are included. Enter *06122018* in both the Date From range boxes.

## ❏ Job 14

Create insurance claims for June 12, 2018. (Remember to enter *06122018* in both Range of Transaction Dates fields.) Notice how today's claims are added to the previous day's claims in the Claim Management dialog box, bringing the total to eight. Change the status of the new claims from Ready To Send to Sent.

# Daily Worksheet

## WEEK 1

## Day 2

*After completing all the jobs for Week 1 Day 2, answer the following questions in the spaces provided.*

1. What is the amount of the copayment for Wilma Estephan's primary insurance carrier?

   _____

   _____

2. Who is listed as the policyholder in Jimmy LeConey's influenza case?

   _____

   _____

3. What are the total charges for Jimmy LeConey's June 12 office visit?

   _____

   _____

4. What services were performed during Will Brown's office visit on June 12?

   _____

   _____

5. For what amount of the total charges on June 12 is Will Brown responsible?

   _____

   _____

6. Who is Dr. Mahabir's first appointment on June 15?

   _____

   _____

7. Which patients have Standard Health Care, Inc., for their insurance carrier?

   _____

   _____

8. What are the total insurance payments for June 12?

   _____

   _____

9. What is the amount of Alan Harcar's copayment for his June 12 office visit?

   _____

   _____

# WEEK 1

## Day 3

*Study the Medisoft Training Topic, and complete the jobs listed for today.*

### MEDISOFT TRAINING TOPIC 3:

### Adding a New Provider

When a new provider joins the medical practice, the provider's name and other data must be added to the provider list database in Medisoft. To add a new provider, select Provider on the Lists menu and then select Providers on the submenu. The Provider List dialog box is displayed (see Figure T3-1).

The Provider List dialog box lists the current providers in the database. To add a provider, the New button is clicked. The Provider dialog box is displayed. It contains three tabs for storing the new provider's information: Address, Reference, and Provider IDs (see Figure T3-2).

*Address Tab*  The Address tab, displayed in Figure T3-2, contains three panels. The top panel contains the Code field, used by the Medisoft program to identify the provider within the program. A provider code can be up to five characters long. If the Code field is left blank, Medisoft assigns a code automatically.

The second panel is used to enter the provider's name, address, and credentials. It also contains fields for the provider's e-mail address and phone numbers.

The third panel is used to record important details such as the provider's Medicare-participating status and license number. The Signature On File and Signature Date fields are used if the provider has signed an agreement with Medicare to accept Medicare charges.

---

**FIGURE T3-1**  Provider List Dialog Box

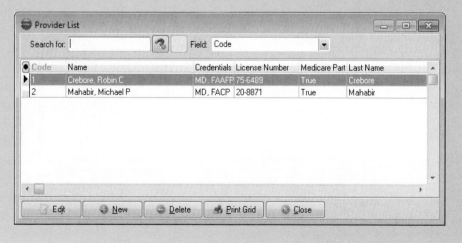

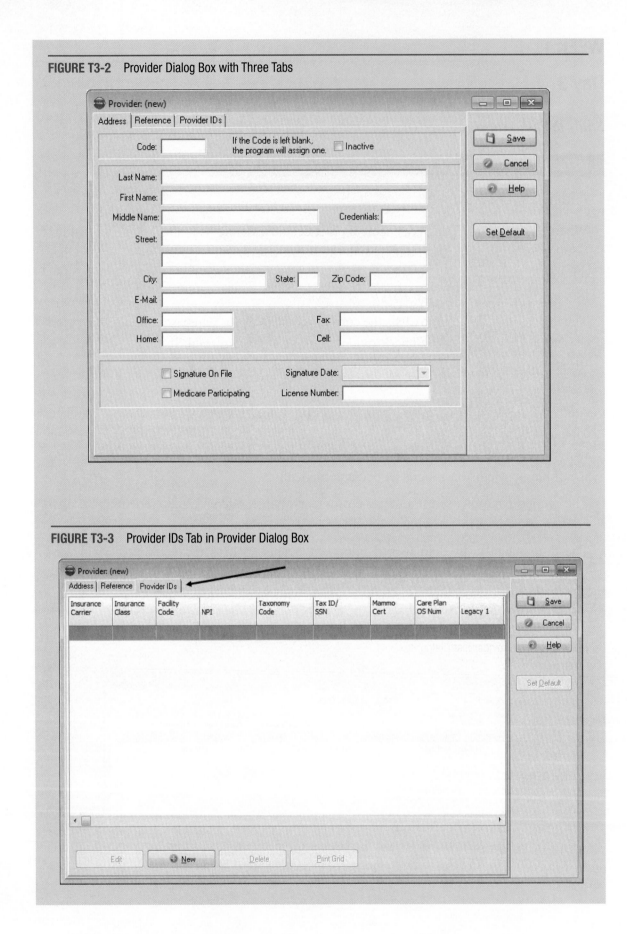

**FIGURE T3-2** Provider Dialog Box with Three Tabs

**FIGURE T3-3** Provider IDs Tab in Provider Dialog Box

***Reference*** The Reference tab is used to store data from the Default Pins and Default Group IDs tabs used in previous versions of Medisoft—data that were required prior to the use of the National Provider Identifier (NPI). In Version 16, these tabs were removed and replaced with the new Provider IDs tab. Therefore, the Reference tab is used for reference purposes only. For new providers, it is kept blank.

***Provider IDs*** The Provider IDs tab (see Figure T3-3) contains a grid with columns for reporting key details associated with a provider. The grid includes the following column headings: Insurance Carrier, Insurance Class, Facility Code, NPI, Taxonomy Code, Tax ID/SSN, Mammography Certificate, Care Plan Oversight Number, and Legacy 1, 2, and 3. To create an entry in the grid for a new provider, the New button is clicked.

***New Provider ID Dialog Box*** When the New button is clicked in the Provider IDs tab, the New Provider ID dialog box displays (see Figure T3-4). The New Provider ID dialog box contains four panels that are used to enter the provider's data. After the data are saved, the information is transferred to the various column headings in the Provider IDs tab.

The top panel in the New Provider ID dialog box is used to indicate whether the provider information in the database applies to all insurance carriers associated with the provider or to a specific insurance carrier or insurance class. If a specific carrier or class is required, the corresponding button is clicked and the specific carrier or class is selected from the drop-down list to the right of the button.

**FIGURE T3-4** New Provider ID Dialog Box

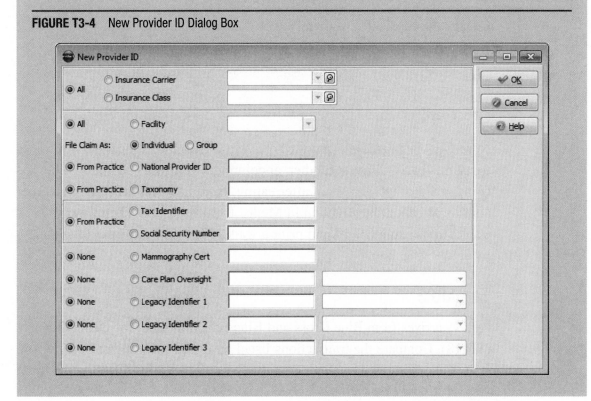

Similarly, the second and third panels contain buttons for indicating whether the provider information applies to all facilities associated with the provider or to a specific facility, whether the provider files claims as an individual or as part of a group, and whether to pull the provider's NPI, taxonomy code, and tax ID/Social Security number from the Practice IDs grid or from the specific numbers reported in the boxes within the panel.

The fourth panel contains fields for reporting a mammography certificate number, a care plan oversight number, and up to three legacy numbers, if the provider uses these numbers. If the provider does not use these numbers, the default setting None is selected for each item. After the data in the four panels of the New Provider ID dialog box are complete, the OK button is clicked and the data display as an entry line in the Provider IDs tab. A provider may have one entry line containing information that applies to all insurance carriers or individual entry lines containing information specific to particular insurance carriers. When the program creates claims, it pulls from the appropriate entry line for that provider.

After information in the three tabs of the Provider dialog box is complete, the Save button in the upper-right side of the dialog box is clicked to store the information in the database. The new provider now appears in the Provider List dialog box and can be selected for use elsewhere in the program as needed.

## ❑ Job 1

Change the Medisoft Program Date to June 13, 2018.

Print today's schedules for Dr. Crebore and Dr. Mahabir. Today is Wednesday, June 13, 2018.

## ❑ Job 2

Nora McAniff, a new patient who is employed by Argene Interiors on a part-time basis, arrives for her appointment with Dr. Mahabir. She has complained of stomach pain after eating. Nora is a Medicare patient. Enter additional patient information in Medisoft using SD 16. Then enter today's transactions using SD 17 and print a walkout receipt. Nora pays the copayment with check 984.

## ❑ Job 3

An RA arrives from Blue Cross and Blue Shield of Ohio for Diana O'Keefe (SD 18). Compare the transactions listed on the RA with those in Medisoft. If the RA is correct, enter and apply the payment in Medisoft using the Enter Deposits/Payments option.

## ❏ Job 4

Susan Jonas telephones to change the time of her daughter Felidia's June 20 appointment, which is currently scheduled for 11:00. Susan would like to bring Felidia in earlier so that she does not miss half of the school day. Move the appointment to the earliest available time on June 20.

## ❏ Job 5

Stewart Weintraub calls with an emergency. He has fallen off the ladder in his garage and is afraid he may have broken his arm. Dr. Mahabir meets him in the Emergency Department at St. Mary's Hospital. An X-ray reveals a closed oblique fracture of the left humerus. Dr. Carey, an orthopedic surgeon on staff at St. Mary's Hospital, performs the reduction, and a cast is applied.

Create a new case for the accident and enter the procedure and diagnosis in Medisoft using SD 19. Note that you will need to fill in the Condition tab since this case is for an accident. Note also that the insurance copayment is not collected, since this is a hospital emergency room visit.

## ❏ Job 6

Roger Deysenrothe telephones to say that he cannot remember the date and time of his son Floyd's appointment. Locate the appointment in Office Hours and tell Roger the date and time.

## ❏ Job 7

Sergeant Georgia Wu telephones to request a follow-up appointment with Dr. Crebore for her daughter Elizabeth. Elizabeth has a mild case of comedonal acne. Schedule a fifteen-minute appointment for June 18 at 4:15.

## ❏ Job 8

A Medicare RA arrives for George Ahmadian's May 23 office visit (SD 20). Part of the claim has been rejected. Compare the RA with the Medisoft transaction information for this visit. The encounter form for the office visit is SD 21. When you have discovered the problem, correct the transaction. Remember to enter the payment for procedure 82948 in the Enter Deposits/Payments area of Medisoft. When applying the insurance payment, leave the payment box for the corrected transaction blank for now.

## ❏ Job 9

Victoria Ferrara arrives for her follow-up visit with Dr. Crebore. She has an infected wound that needs to be checked. Using the information on SD 22, enter today's transaction.

**Tip!**

**Job 6**
To locate an appointment in Office Hours, use the Appointment List option on the Office Hours Lists menu.

## ❏ Job 10

The practice manager has given you a paper (SD 23) with information on a new provider who is to join the practice next month. You will need to add this initial information to the PMG database. Since Dr. Crebore and Dr. Mahabir are code numbers 1 and 2 in the database, assign code number 3 to the new provider.

## ❏ Job 11

Flora Torres-Gil telephones to schedule an appointment for her bursitis. Schedule a fifteen-minute office visit on June 19 at 9:45.

## ❏ Job 12

Print a patient day sheet for June 13, 2018.

## ❏ Job 13

Create insurance claims for June 13, 2018. Remember to change the status of the claims from Ready To Send to Sent.

Then create a new claim for George Ahmadian's corrected procedure for his visit on May 23, 2018. (In the Create Claims dialog box, enter *05232018* in both Range of Transaction Dates boxes and select George Ahmadian's chart number in both Chart Numbers boxes.) Change the status of the claim from Ready To Send to Sent.

# Daily Worksheet

## WEEK 1

### Day 3

*After completing all the jobs for Week 1 Day 3, answer the following questions in the spaces provided.*

1. What is the Medicare amount allowed for the June 13 procedure performed on Nora McAniff?
   _____
   _____

2. How much did Blue Cross and Blue Shield pay on Diana O'Keefe's account on June 13?
   _____
   _____

3. Who is Dr. Crebore's next patient after Felidia Jonas on June 20?
   _____
   _____

4. What POS code is used when entering Stewart Weintraub's June 13 transaction? What place of service does it indicate?
   _____
   _____

5. What is Victoria Ferrara's diagnosis for her office visit on June 13?
   _____
   _____

6. Who is Flora Torres-Gil's provider?
   _____
   _____

7. What were the total insurance and patient payments for June 13?
   _____
   _____

8. What is the balance owed by Diana O'Keefe for her rheumatoid arthritis case?
   _____
   _____

# WEEK 1

## Day 4

*Study the Medisoft Training Topic, and complete the jobs listed for today.*

---

**MEDISOFT TRAINING TOPIC 4:**

### Printing a Patient Face Sheet

Sometimes it is helpful to have a printout of a patient's case information. The Patient Face Sheet report in Medisoft pulls data from several tabs in the patient's Case dialog box into a single-page report. The patient's personal information, such as name, address, employer, date of birth, and so on, is listed at the top of the report. Below that is the case information, which includes fields for the case description, last visit date, referral, guarantor information, diagnoses, and details of the patient's insurance plan(s).

Although it is possible to produce a Patient Face Sheet using the Reports menu, it is more convenient to use the Face Sheet button located in the Case dialog box. After clicking the Face Sheet button, the Print Report Where? dialog box appears. (The usual Data Selection Questions dialog box does not display, since the patient and case have already been selected in the Case dialog box.) After an option is selected to preview, print, or export the report, the report is generated.

---

### ❑ Job 1

Change the Medisoft Program Date to June 14, 2018.

Print today's schedules for Dr. Crebore and Dr. Mahabir. Today is Thursday, June 14, 2018.

### ❑ Job 2

Diana O'Keefe calls to schedule an appointment. Schedule her for a fifteen-minute appointment on June 19 at 10:45.

### ❑ Job 3

An RA arrives with payment from Standard Health Care (SD 24). Compare the procedure codes and amounts with those in Medisoft. If they are correct, enter and apply the payment in Medisoft.

## ❏ Job 4

Angelo Daiute arrives for an annual exam with Dr. Crebore. Dr. Crebore would like to see Angelo in one week to recheck his blood pressure, which was elevated.

Enter Angelo's personal and insurance information in Medisoft, and then enter today's transactions using SDs 25 and 26. Angelo is a new patient, but his insurance deductible for this year has already been met. He pays the co-payment with check 3317.

Schedule Angelo for a fifteen-minute follow-up appointment on June 25 at 1:00.

## ❏ Job 5

Hector Valaquez telephones the office. He is not currently a patient. His sun-burned back is bothering him. He would like to know if the practice is accepting new patients and whether he can come in tomorrow. Establish Hector as a patient in Medisoft using the information below, and then schedule him for a fifteen-minute appointment with Dr. Crebore tomorrow at 9:00. A case will be created for him tomorrow after the appointment.

> Hector M. Valaquez
> 199 Transfer Street
> Highland, OH 45132
> Phone: 999-555-3364
> Date of Birth: 8/15/1990
> Sex: M
> SS#: 459-94-9934
> Race: White
> Ethnicity: Hispanic
> Language: English

## ❏ Job 6

The practice manager informs you that she would like case information on Daniel Connolly's chest pain case for billing purposes. Print out a Patient Face Sheet for her to refer to.

## ❏ Job 7

Dr. Crebore would like Gregory Kavanaugh to be examined by a neurologist to evaluate the seizures he has been experiencing. Check to see whether Gregory's insurance plan requires authorization before a referral to a specialist is made.

## ❏ Job 8

Rachel Atchely, a resident at Grandview Nursing Home, calls for a follow-up appointment for her cellulitis. Schedule her for a fifteen-minute appointment on June 20 at noon at Grandview. Enter *See at GNH* in the Note box as a reminder that Rachel is to be seen at Grandview Nursing Home.

## ❏ Job 9

Cameron Trotta arrives for his 2:00 appointment. Dr. Mahabir wants Cameron scheduled for a follow-up visit as he is due for a five-year flexible sigmoidoscopy (45330). Schedule a sixty-minute appointment for June 27 at 10:00. Using SD 27, enter the charges and copayment (check 869) and print a walkout receipt.

## ❏ Job 10

Seymour Colbs calls. He needs to change his appointment. He is currently scheduled for 4:00 tomorrow. He would like to come in earlier, if possible. Reschedule the appointment for 9:30 tomorrow with Dr. Crebore.

## ❏ Job 11

The practice has received a payment from the collection agency for Paul Ramos's account. Paul's account has an overdue amount of $205 that is more than 90 days past due. The statement included with the payment indicates that the agency has collected 50 percent of the amount owed, or $102.50, to date. After the agency subtracts its fee of 30 percent ($30.75), the amount paid to the provider is $71.75.

Post this amount to the patient's account using the payment code PAY-COLLECT (Patient Payment from Collections). In the Description box, key *Collections payment.* The payment is made with check number 10063. Remember to apply the payment to the patient's charges, and then save the transaction.

## ❏ Job 12

George Ahmadian has diabetes mellitus and hypertension. He has been experiencing increasing confusion, agitation, and short-term memory loss over the past two months. He has just been examined by Dr. Mahabir. Using SD 28, create a new case and enter today's transactions.

❑  ## Job 13

An RA arrives with payment from Standard Health Care (SD 29). Compare the procedure codes and amounts with those in Medisoft. If they are correct, enter and apply the payment in Medisoft.

❑  ## Job 14

Print a patient day sheet for June 14, 2018.

❑  ## Job 15

Create insurance claims for June 14, 2018. Change the status of the claims.

# Daily Worksheet

## WEEK 1

### Day 4

*After completing all the jobs for Week 1 Day 4, answer the following questions in the spaces provided.*

1. What is Angelo Daiute's account total after he pays his copayment on June 14?

   _____

   _____

2. What are the name and phone number for the secondary insurance company listed on Daniel Connolly's Patient Face Sheet for his chest pain case?

   _____

   _____

3. What procedure is Cameron Trotta scheduled for on June 27? How much time is scheduled for the appointment?

   _____

   _____

4. What time is Seymour Colbs's appointment on June 15?

   _____

   _____

5. What is George Ahmadian's diagnosis for his June 14 office visit?

   _____

   _____

6. What were the total procedure charges for June 14?

   _____

   _____

7. What were the total insurance payments for June 14?

   _____

   _____

## Day 5

*Study the Medisoft Training Topic, and complete the jobs listed for today.*

**MEDISOFT TRAINING TOPIC 5:**

### Using Quick Balance

Medisoft's Quick Balance feature simplifies the task of discovering the amount owed on a patient account. This feature can be accessed by pressing the Quick Balance speed button located on the toolbar (see Figure T5-1). If the Quick Balance feature is activated from within the Transaction Entry dialog box or the Patient/Guarantor dialog box, the information will be displayed for the patient who is currently selected. For example, if the Transaction Entry box lists Lydia Stephanos's data, pressing the Quick Balance button will display the balance on her account. A sample Quick Balance dialog box is shown in Figure T5-2.

The dialog box lists all the patients for whom this individual is guarantor. For example, the Quick Balance dialog box for Roger Deysenrothe lists Roger, his wife Mae, and his son Floyd, since Roger is the guarantor on all three accounts. The amount listed as the Guarantor Remainder Total is the amount owed by the guarantor *after* the insurance carrier has paid on the claim. If the insurance carrier has not yet paid, the balance for the account will be zero.

Note that the information can be printed from within the Quick Balance dialog box. In addition, the balance for another patient can be viewed by selecting a different chart number in the Chart field.

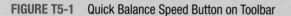

**FIGURE T5-1**   Quick Balance Speed Button on Toolbar

**FIGURE T5-2**   Quick Balance Dialog Box

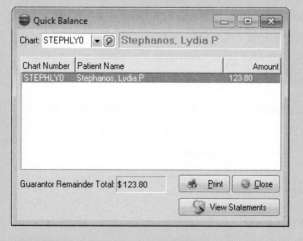

## ❏ Job 1

Change the Medisoft Program Date to June 15, 2018.

Print today's schedules for Dr. Crebore and Dr. Mahabir. Today is Friday, June 15, 2018.

## ❏ Job 2

Hector Valaquez, a new patient, is examined by Dr. Crebore. Enter patient information about Hector using SD 30, and record today's transactions using SD 31. Hector pays his copayment with check 3231 and needs a walkout receipt.

## ❏ Job 3

Seymour Colbs arrives for his office visit. Dr. Crebore removes the sutures in Seymour's hand. Enter today's transactions in Medisoft using SD 32. The copayment is paid with check 839. Print a walkout receipt.

## ❏ Job 4

David Weatherly, a patient of Dr. Crebore who is on hypertensive medication and who is experiencing difficulty breathing, arrives for his office visit. He is examined by Dr. Crebore. Using SD 33, create a new case and enter the transactions in Medisoft. The copayment is made with check 2312, and a walkout receipt is printed.

## ❏ Job 5

Victoria Ferrara telephones. She would like to know the balance due on her account. Use the Quick Balance shortcut key to determine the amount. Compare this amount with the information displayed in the Transaction Entry dialog box. Remember that the Quick Balance dialog box displays the amount owed *after* the insurance carrier has paid a claim. In Victoria's case, notice that only the first claim has been paid.

## ❏ Job 6

Myrna Beedon telephones. She reports that she has felt extremely tired for the past few days. She would like to see Dr. Mahabir. Schedule her for a fifteen-minute appointment on June 18 at 4:00.

## ❏ Job 7

Mae Deysenrothe calls to reschedule her appointment on June 18 at 10:00 with Dr. Mahabir. Reschedule her for June 20 at 2:15.

## ❏ Job 8

Review the audit/edit report received for Rachel Atchely's claim (SD 34). Rachel, who resides at the Grandview Nursing Home, is a patient of Dr. Mahabir. Dr. Mahabir's visit on May 23 was for a brief checkup. Identify the error in the procedure code and edit the transaction using the correct code (99307—Subseq. nursing facility care, pf.).

Then create a new claim for the visit. Remember to enter *05232018* in both Range of Transaction Dates boxes and to select Rachel Atchely's chart number in both Chart Number boxes. Change the status of the claim from Ready To Send to Sent.

## ❏ Job 9

Roberta Yange-Sang arrives for an examination of her laceration. Roberta is a Medicaid patient. During the visit, Dr. Mahabir notes that the wound is clear. Roberta is instructed to return in ten days for a recheck.

Enter today's transactions using SD 35 (the copayment is paid with check 240), print a walkout receipt, and schedule Roberta for a fifteen-minute follow-up appointment on June 25 at 10:00.

## ❏ Job 10

Gloria Berkel-Rees comes in for her three-month checkup with Dr. Mahabir. She has chronic asthma along with hay fever. She also needs drug therapy evaluation. Using SD 36, enter the charges. Note that the charge for procedure code 99070 (Supplies and materials) is set to 0.00 in the database as the amount varies depending on what supplies and materials are ordered. The amount charged for today's encounter is shown on the encounter form. Remember to record this amount in both the Amount and Allowed fields when you enter the transaction.

## ❏ Job 11

Chantalle Usdan calls the office to schedule a sigmoidoscopy. She has been referred to Dr. Mahabir by her primary care physician, Dr. Rachel Innanni.

Establish Chantalle as a patient in Medisoft using the information below. Schedule her for a sixty-minute appointment on June 20 at 10:00. A case can be created on the day of the visit.

> Chantalle E. Usdan
> 28 Fairview Blvd.
> Columbus, OH 43214

Phone: 999-555-4555
Date of Birth: 2/23/1962
Sex: F
SS#: 234-60-8721
Race: White
Ethnicity: Non-Hispanic
Language: English

## ❏ Job 12

Alan Harcar arrives for his comprehensive physical examination. Create a new case and record today's transactions using SD 37. (*Optional:* Use the Multi-Link feature to enter all the transactions except for the office visit code.) The copayment is made with check 1024. Print a walkout receipt.

## ❏ Job 13

Luther Jackson recently overpaid on his account. Not realizing that his deductible had been met, Luther sent a check for $72 for his May 30 office visit, which paid for services in full. Meanwhile, his insurance carrier, Ohio Insurance Company, sent a payment for 90 percent of the charges. (Ohio Insurance Company pays for 90 percent of covered services once the deductible has been met.) This means Luther paid 100 percent of the charges ($72.00) when he only owed 10 percent ($7.20).

Issue a refund to his account for the overpaid amount ($72.00 − $7.20 = $64.80). In the Pay/Adj Code box, use the adjustment code REFUNDPAT (Patient Refund). In the Description box, key *Overpaid-refund.* The refund is made with check 224. Remember to apply the adjustment to the corresponding charge, and then save the transaction.

## ❏ Job 14

Print a patient day sheet for June 15, 2018.

## ❏ Job 15

Create insurance claims for June 15, 2018. Change the status of the claims.

**Tip!**

**Job 13**

Adjustments are entered in the Transaction Entry dialog box the same way payments are. In the Payments, Adjustments, And Comments section, enter the date, an adjustment code, description, amount, and check number if applicable. Then click the Apply button to apply the adjustment to the corresponding charges, and save the transaction.

132    Part 3    On the Job

Copyright ©2016 McGraw-Hill Education

# Daily Worksheet

## WEEK 1

## Day 5

*After completing all the jobs for Week 1 Day 5, answer the following questions in the spaces provided.*

1. What is Hector Valaquez's primary insurance carrier? How much is his copayment?

   _____

   _____

2. For his June 15 office visit, for what amount of the charges was Seymour Colbs responsible?

   _____

   _____

3. What is the diagnosis for David Weatherly's June 15 office visit?

   _____

   _____

4. How much time is scheduled for Mae Deysenrothe's appointment on June 20?

   _____

   _____

5. What is the amount Medicaid owes for Roberta Yange-Sang's June 15 office visit?

   _____

   _____

6. What services were performed at Gloria Berkel-Rees's June 15 office visit?

   _____

   _____

7. What is the diagnosis for Alan Harcar's June 15 office visit?

   _____

   _____

8. What were the total number of procedures performed on June 15?

   _____

   _____

## End-of-Week-1 Job

### Printing a Copayment Report

The Medisoft Reports menu contains an option for printing a copayment report. The report creates an alphabetical listing of all patients who have made copayments and includes the date of each payment as well as the case number, payment code, and amount paid. The amount paid is further broken down into applied and unapplied amounts. A total line at the bottom lists the total copayment amount and total applied and unapplied amounts.

To generate a copayment report, open the Reports menu, click Analysis Reports, and then click Copayment Report on the submenu that appears. The Print Report Where? dialog box displays with the option to preview, print, or export the report. After selecting an option, the Start button is clicked. A Search dialog box appears for setting the parameters of the report. The report can be generated without parameters, or it can be created for a range of patients, dates, providers, and/or billing codes. After setting the parameters, click the OK button. Depending on which option was selected in the Print Report Where? dialog box, the report is displayed in the preview window, sent to the printer, or exported to a selected file type.

## ❏ Job 1

Print a copayment report for all patients for the period of June 11 through June 15, 2018.

# WEEK 2

## Day 1

*Study the Medisoft Training Topic, and complete the jobs listed for today.*

### MEDISOFT TRAINING TOPIC 7:

### Entering Prior Authorization Numbers

Sometimes insurance carriers require services to be authorized before they are performed. If preauthorization is not given, the claim will not be paid. Once preauthorization numbers are obtained from the insurance carrier, they are entered in Medisoft. This information is entered in the Prior Authorization Number box, which is found in the Miscellaneous tab of the Case folder (see Figure T7-1). From one to fifteen characters can be entered in the Prior Authorization Number box.

**FIGURE T7-1**   Miscellaneous Tab of Case Folder with Prior Authorization Number Box

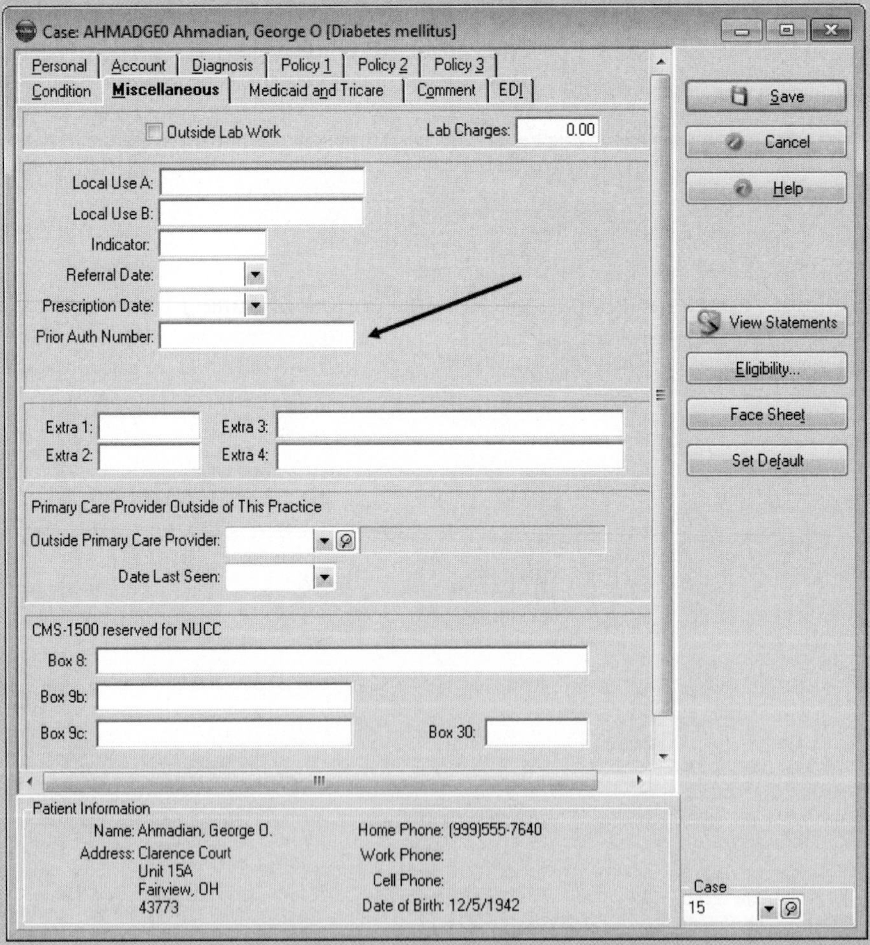

## ❏ Job 1

Change the Medisoft Program Date to June 18, 2018.

Print today's schedules for Dr. Crebore and Dr. Mahabir. Today is Monday, June 18, 2018.

## ❏ Job 2

There is a message from Myrna Beedon, a Medicare patient of Dr. Mahabir who has a history of congenital heart disease. She was scheduled for a 4:00 appointment today. After you relate the message to Dr. Mahabir, he orders her admitted to St. Mary's Hospital and visits her there. Enter the preauthorization number for Myrna's hospital admission, HA46230, in the appropriate box in the Case folder. Then enter the transactions using SD 38. Note that no copayment is collected since this is a hospital visit.

## ❏ Job 3

Dan Connolly calls to reschedule the appointment that is currently scheduled for June 22 at 10:00. Change the appointment to 2:45 on the same day.

## ❏ Job 4

Fran Ferrone is a new patient who has come in for her appointment with Dr. Crebore because of possible bronchitis. Fran is employed by Woodworkers Warehouse in Fairview. The company is not in the Medisoft database of employers, so you will need to add it, using the information on SD 39.

When you call Fran's insurance carrier to verify coverage, you learn that she has met the $500.00 deductible for the year. Complete the Other Information tab in the Patient/Guarantor dialog box for Fran and set up a case using SD 39. When completing the Policy 1 tab in the Case dialog box, remember to refer to the Health Plan Information Pages in Part 2 to obtain the correct insurance coverage percentages for her plan. Enter today's diagnosis and transactions using the encounter form found on SD 40.

## ❏ Job 5

Ann LeConey telephones. She needs an appointment with Dr. Mahabir for a recheck of an irritated patch of skin on her arm. Schedule her for a fifteen-minute appointment on June 20 at 4:30.

## ❏ Internet Activity

Go to the website for Aetna. Look up information on the different types of health plans offered. Explore the member and provider areas of the website.

## ❑ Job 6

Susan Jonas calls the office to say that her dermatitis has flared up and that she would like an appointment. Schedule her for a fifteen-minute appointment at 4:30 on June 21.

## ❑ Job 7

Jimmy Hellery is examined by Dr. Mahabir. He has complained of a severe sore throat and fever. Set up a new case. Enter the transactions in Medisoft using SD 41 and print a walkout receipt. The copayment is made with check 1019.

## ❑ Job 8

Roger Deysenrothe brings his son Floyd in for a tetanus vaccine. Create a new case. Using SD 42, record the transactions in Medisoft and print a walkout receipt. The copayment is made with check 1117.

## ❑ Job 9

A remittance advice has arrived from Will Brown's insurance carrier (SD 43). Review the RA, enter the payment, and apply it to Brown's account.

## ❑ Job 10

Georgia Wu brings her daughter Elizabeth in for an appointment with Dr. Crebore to check Elizabeth's mild case of comedonal acne of the cheeks. Enter the transactions in Medisoft, including the payment (made with check 1202), using SD 44. Print a walkout receipt.

## ❑ Job 11

Marilyn Rennagel, a patient of Dr. Crebore, calls for an appointment. She needs routine monitoring of her diabetes mellitus and stable coronary artery disease. Schedule her for a fifteen-minute appointment on June 22 at 3:00.

## ❑ Job 12

Print a patient day sheet for June 18, 2018.

## ❑ Job 13

Create insurance claims for June 18, 2018. Change the status of the claims.

# Daily Worksheet

## WEEK 2

### Day 1

*After completing all the jobs for Week 2 Day 1, answer the following questions in the spaces provided.*

1. What POS code is entered for Myrna Beedon's transactions on June 18?

   _____

   _____

2. Where is the preauthorization number for Myrna Beedon's hospital admission entered in Medisoft?

   _____

   _____

3. Who has the appointment with Dr. Mahabir before Ann LeConey on June 20?

   _____

   _____

4. What is the amount of the copayment Joan Hellery pays for her son Jimmy's visit on June 18?

   _____

   _____

5. What is Floyd Deysenrothe's diagnosis for his June 18 office visit?

   _____

   _____

6. What is the total amount of copayments made on June 18?

   _____

   _____

7. What are the total procedure charges for June 18?

   _____

   _____

8. What were the total insurance payments for June 18?

   _____

   _____

# WEEK 2

## Day 2

*Study the Medisoft Training Topics, and complete the jobs listed for today.*

**MEDISOFT TRAINING TOPIC 8:**

### Entering Additional Diagnosis Codes

Before a diagnosis code can be selected in the Diagnosis tab of the Case folder, it must be entered in the database. To add a diagnosis code to the database, select Diagnosis Codes from the Lists menu. The Diagnosis List dialog box is displayed. It lists all the diagnosis codes already entered. The codes are listed in numerical order by code number or alphabetically by description, depending on the setting in the Field box at the top of the dialog box.

To add a new diagnosis code, click the New button at the bottom of the dialog box. The Diagnosis: (new) dialog box is displayed (see Figure T8-1). Enter the diagnosis code in the Code box and a description of the diagnosis in the Description box (from one to 100 characters can be used). If the code is from ICD-9, click the Copy button to the right of the ICD-9 Code: field to copy the code and description to the ICD-9 fields. If the code is from ICD-10, click the copy button to the right of the ICD-10 Code: field to copy the information to the ICD-10 fields. Then click the Save button to add the code to the Medisoft database.

**FIGURE T8-1** Diagnosis Dialog Box

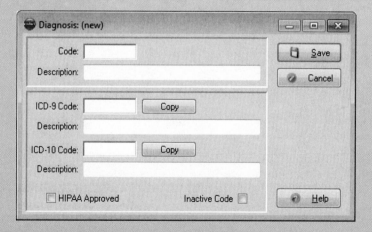

**MEDISOFT TRAINING TOPIC 9:**

### Adding a New Insurance Carrier

Whenever required, a new insurance carrier can be added to the database. To add a new carrier, select Insurance on the Lists menu, and then select Carriers on the submenu. The Insurance Carrier List dialog box is displayed (see Figure T9-1), listing the carriers currently in the database.

**FIGURE T9-1** Insurance Carrier List Dialog Box

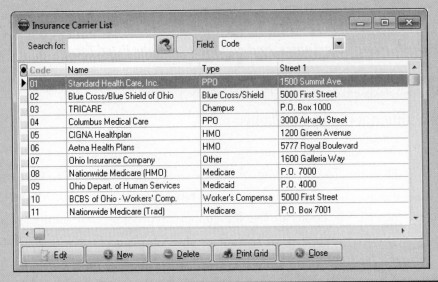

**FIGURE T9-2** Insurance Carrier Dialog Box with Four Tabs

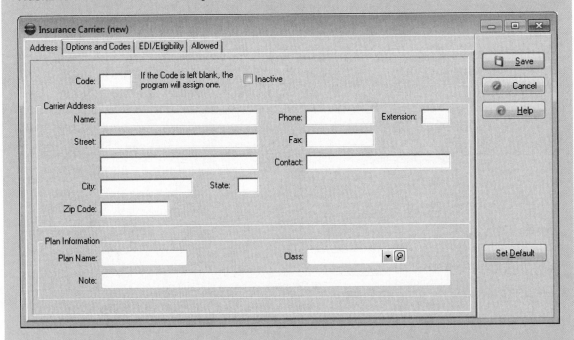

To add a new carrier, the New button is clicked. The Insurance Carrier: (new) dialog box is displayed. It contains four tabs for storing the new carrier's information: Address, Options and Codes, EDI/Eligibility, and Allowed (see Figure T9-2).

*Address*    The Address tab (shown in Figure T9-2) is divided into three panels. The top panel contains the Code field, used by the Medisoft program to identify the insurance carrier within the program. If no code is assigned, the program assigns one automatically. The second panel contains the insurance carrier's demographic information, including name, address, phone, fax, and a contact person. The third panel is used to enter plan information, including the plan name, the class (classes are categories of insurance carriers that a practice may create for organizational purposes), and any relevant notes about the plan.

***Options and Codes*** The Options and Codes tab (shown in Figure T9-3) contains two panels. The Options panel at the top contains various billing options. Several options apply to paper claims only:

**Procedure Code and Diagnosis Code Sets:** These fields specify which set of procedure and diagnosis codes the carrier requires. If the Diagnosis Code Set is ICD-10, the ICD-10 Effective Date should be completed.

**Patient, Insured, or Physician Signature on File:** These fields are used to control what is printed in specific boxes on the CMS-1500 form. Options include printing the words *Signature on File* if these fields have been activated in the patient and provider records; printing the party's name (patient, insured, or physician); or leaving the box blank, which is the default setting.

**Print PINS on Forms:** This field is used on paper claims to record an attending provider's PIN (when the attending provider is other than the usual assigned provider).

**Default Billing Method 1, 2, 3:** These fields identify whether claims for this carrier are to be printed on paper or transmitted electronically. Fields 1, 2, and 3 correspond to the billing methods for primary, secondary, and tertiary claims respectively.

The Default Payment Application Codes panel at the bottom of the Options and Codes tab is used to select the default codes to be used when entering payments, adjustments, withhold amounts, deductibles, and take backs for the new carrier. Codes are first created

---

**FIGURE T9-3** Options and Codes Tab

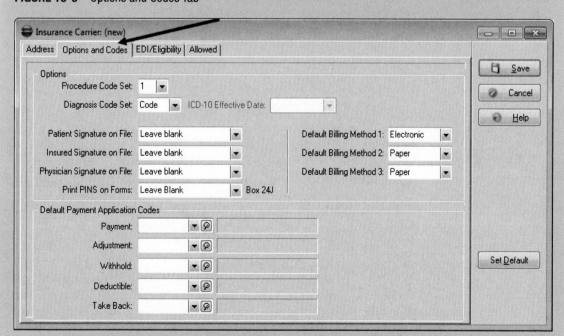

in the Procedure/Payment/Adjustment dialog box and then selected as defaults in the Options and Codes tab.

*EDI/Eligibility*   If the new carrier transmits claim information electronically and/or offers online eligibility verification for checking the status of a patient's insurance eligibility, this tab is used to select numbers or data connected with such transactions (see Figure T9-4). For example, the EDI Receiver field is for selecting the EDI receiver to which this insurance carrier's claims are sent. The first two panels are used to select primary receivers for primary claims and secondary receivers for secondary claims.

A third panel, Carrier EDI Settings, is used to record a variety of other details required for electronic claims. The Type field is used to report the type of plan, such as Other, Medicare, Medicaid, Tricare/Champus, HMO, PPO, and so on. The Delay Secondary Billing field is used to indicate whether a secondary claim form should be created at the same time as the primary claim is created (the default setting) or whether the billing should be delayed until an RA is received and a payment or adjustment has been made for the primary carrier. To delay billing, a check mark is displayed in the field. For most fields in this tab, the practice's electronic claims manual must be referred to in order to determine what data are required and the format to be used for the data.

*Allowed*   The fourth tab in the Insurance Carrier dialog box, the Allowed tab (see Figure T9-5), contains a table for storing the new insurance carrier's allowed amounts for each procedure code in the database. Amounts may be entered in the table manually, as in the case of the PMG database, or they may be stored by the program automatically, based on the amount the carrier last paid.

---

**FIGURE T9-4**   EDI/Eligibility Tab

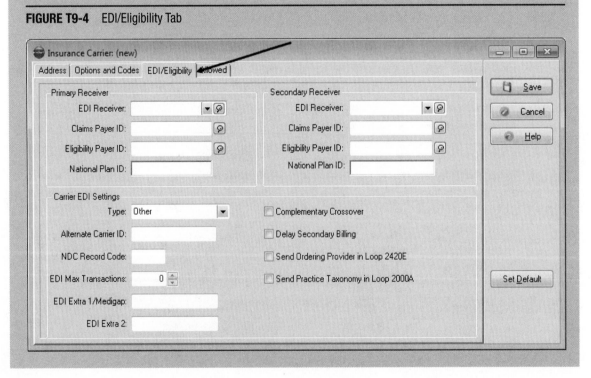

**FIGURE T9-5** Allowed Tab

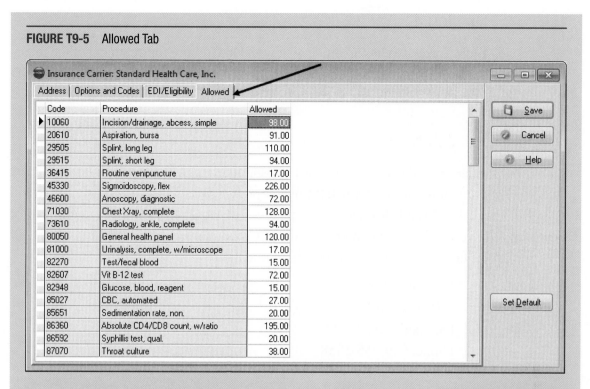

Information entered in this tab appears simultaneously in the Allowed Amounts tab of the Procedure/Payment/Adjustment dialog box (see Training Topic 13: Entering Additional Procedure Codes and Allowed Amounts). Allowed amounts can be entered through either dialog box.

After information on the new insurance carrier is entered in the four tabs of the Insurance Carrier dialog box, the Save button is clicked. The new carrier is now listed in the Insurance Carrier List dialog box and can be selected for use in the program as needed.

## ❏ Job 1

Change the Medisoft Program Date to June 19, 2018.

Print today's schedules for Dr. Crebore and Dr. Mahabir. Today is Tuesday, June 19, 2018.

## ❏ Job 2

Martin Szinovacz calls to schedule an appointment to have his blood pressure checked. Schedule him for a fifteen-minute appointment on June 22 at 9:15.

## ❏ Job 3

The practice manager has just handed you a list of additional diagnosis codes that need to be added to the database (SD 45). Enter the codes in Medisoft.

**Tip!**

**Job 3**

By default, diagnosis codes in the Diagnosis List dialog box are listed in alphabetical order by description. To list the codes in numerical order by code number, select Code 1 in the Field drop-down box.

## ❑ Job 4

Flora Torres-Gil has an office visit with Dr. Crebore for treatment of the recurrent bursitis in her left shoulder. Enter the transactions in Medisoft using SD 46. Flora pays with check 1309. Print a walkout receipt.

## ❑ Job 5

Eugene Kadar calls to request an appointment with one of the physicians. He is not currently a patient of the practice. Eugene has recurring sores on his lip. Establish Eugene as a patient in Medisoft. Then schedule him for a fifteen-minute appointment with Dr. Crebore on June 22 at 10:15. A case will be created on the day of the appointment.

> Eugene S. Kadar
> 8003 Oxford Lane
> Highland, OH 45132
> Phone: 999-555-5858
> Date of Birth: 6/1/85
> Sex: M
> SS#: 499-09-7453
> Race: White
> Ethnicity: Non-Hispanic
> Language: English

## ❑ Job 6

Jorge Martinez calls to ask whether he can change the time of his appointment with Dr. Mahabir on June 21. He has a meeting he must attend at work. Locate Jorge's current appointment in Medisoft and change it to 4:00 on the same day.

## ❑ Job 7

The new provider who is to join the practice next month has a contract with an insurance carrier not currently in the PMG database. Use the information contained in SDs 47 and 48 to add the new carrier. Fill in only those boxes for which information is provided. Otherwise, keep the default settings as they are. In the Address tab, use code number 12 for the new carrier, since that is the next number in sequence.

*Note:* For the purposes of this job, the codes to be selected in the Options and Codes tab have already been created and stored in the Procedure/Payment/ Adjustment dialog box for you. For information on creating codes, see Training Topic 13: Entering Additional Procedure Codes and Allowed Amounts.

## ❑ Job 8

Hanna Wong calls to complain of chest pain when lifting. Hanna is not currently a patient of the practice but would like an appointment as soon as possible. Enter the following information, obtained over the phone, into the patient information section of Medisoft, and then schedule Hanna for a sixty-minute appointment at 10:00 tomorrow with Dr. Mahabir.

> Hanna Z. Wong
> 22-B 22nd Avenue
> Highland, OH 45132
> Phone: 999-555-1122
> Date of Birth: 11/5/45
> Sex: F
> SS#: 015-98-2139
> Race: Asian
> Ethnicity: Non-Hispanic
> Language: English

## ❑ Job 9

Ann LeConey comes in for her appointment with Dr. Mahabir. He rechecks the irritated skin on her arm. Record the transactions using SD 56. The copayment is made with check 1834. Print a walkout receipt.

## ❑ Job 10

Print a patient day sheet for June 20, 2018.

## ❑ Job 11

Create insurance claims for June 20, 2018. Change the status of the claims.

# Daily Worksheet

## WEEK 2

### Day 3

*After completing all the jobs for Week 2 Day 3, answer the following questions in the spaces provided.*

1. Who is the guarantor for Felidia Jonas's impetigo case?

   _____

   _____

2. Of the total charges for her June 20 office visit, for what amount is Cynthia Cashell responsible?

   _____

   _____

3. What is entered in the Visit Series Authorization Number box in the Account tab of the Case folder for Chantalle Usdan?

   _____

   _____

4. What is the charge for Rachel Atchely's nursing home visit on June 20?

   _____

   _____

5. What is the amount of Ann LeConey's copayment on June 20?

   _____

   _____

6. What is the total of all patient payments for June 20 (including copayments)?

   _____

   _____

7. How many insurance claims were created on June 20?

   _____

   _____

# WEEK 2

## Day 4

*Study the Medisoft Training Topic, and complete the jobs listed for today.*

### Entering Additional Procedure Codes and Allowed Amounts

CPT codes are often updated and modified, and some are deleted. Before CPT codes can be selected in the Transaction Entry dialog box, they must be entered in the database. To add or modify CPT codes in Medisoft, select Procedure/Payment/Adjustment Codes from the Lists menu. The Procedure/Payment/Adjustment List dialog box is displayed. This box lists all the procedure, payment, and adjustment codes in the database. When the Field box at the top of the dialog box is set to Code 1, the codes are listed in numerical order. This setting can be changed to list the codes by description or type.

To add a new CPT code, click the New button at the bottom of the dialog box. The Procedure/Payment/Adjustment: (new) dialog box is displayed. The dialog box has three tabs: General, Amounts, and Allowed Amounts.

*General Tab*    The General tab is used to enter detailed information about the code (see Figure T13-1). It contains the following fields:

**Code 1:** The procedure code itself is entered in the Code 1 box. It can be from one to ten characters in length. After the code is entered and the Tab or Enter key is pressed, this code automatically appears in the Alternate Codes 2 and 3 boxes.

In some cases, these default entries in the Alternate Codes 2 and 3 boxes are deleted so that other alternate codes can be used. For example, some insurance carriers use different codes for the same procedure. The alternate code boxes allow these codes to be linked to the major code in Medisoft.

**Inactive:** Clicking the Inactive box designates a code as not in use. This option may be used when a code needs to be modified, but open transactions (transactions that have not been returned to a zero balance) use the unmodified code. Codes marked as inactive appear with a red inactive message next to them in the Transaction Entry dialog box. Codes marked as inactive cannot be used unless the Inactive box is unchecked, making the code active again.

**Description:** In the Description box, enter an appropriate description of from one to forty characters.

**Code Type:** The Code Type drop-down list offers a number of choices for type of code, such as Procedure charge, Check copayment, Adjustment, and Insurance payment.

**FIGURE T13-1** General Tab of the Procedure/Payment/Adjustment Dialog Box

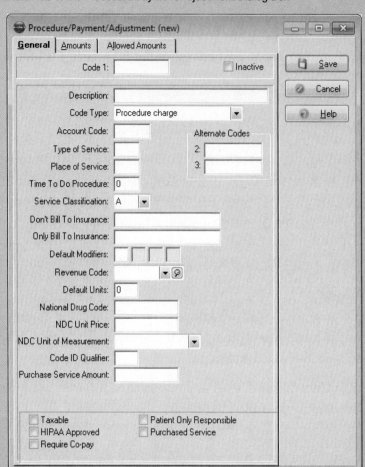

**Account Code:** Some practices group their procedure codes into account codes for reporting purposes. If an account code exists for the procedure code, it is entered in the Account Code box.

**Type of Service:** The appropriate type of service code is entered in the Type of Service box. Commonly used codes include:

1  Medical care

2  Surgery

3  Consultation

4  Diagnostic X-ray

5  Diagnostic lab

6  Radiation therapy

7  Anesthesia

8  Surgical assistance

9   Other medical

10  Blood charges

**Place of Service:** In the Place of Service box, enter the two-digit code that identifies the place the service was performed. Commonly used POS codes include:

11  Office

12  Home

13  Inpatient hospital

14  Outpatient hospital

15  Emergency room—hospital

16  Ambulatory surgical center

17  Birthing center

18  Skilled nursing facility

19  Nursing facility

20  Custodial care facility

**Time To Do Procedure:** Enter the approximate time, in minutes, required to perform the procedure. This information is used when determining the length of appointments scheduled in Office Hours. In the PMG database, only office visit procedure codes have been assigned time values.

**Service Classification:** This feature is available for assigning values (A–H) to procedures in order to classify them according to the category of service they represent. For example, A may be used for common procedures, B for surgery or lab charges, C for noncovered procedures, and so on. This feature is linked to the Insurance Coverage Percents by Service Classification field in the Policy tab of the Case dialog box, which determines the percentage of the charge amount that is billed to the insurance carrier as its share of the cost.

**Don't Bill To Insurance:** This feature allows you to restrict the printing of this particular code to certain insurance carriers. In the box, the code numbers of the insurance carriers that do not use this code are keyed. Enter the insurance carrier code numbers separated by commas.

**Only Bill To Insurance:** If a code is to be used only with certain insurance carriers, enter the codes of the insurance carriers, separated by commas.

**Default Modifiers:** If the procedure code always uses the same modifier(s), the modifiers can be entered in these boxes.

**Revenue Code:** If the practice is generating UB-04 claim forms, the revenue code for this procedure is entered.

**Default Units:** If applicable, the usual number of units for the procedure code can be entered.

The remaining fields are used in electronic claims:

**National Drug Code:** If the procedure has a national drug code assigned to it—for example, for reporting a prescription drug—the code is entered here.

**NDC Unit Price:** This box contains the unit price of the drug.

**NDC Unit of Measurement:** This box lists the appropriate unit of measurement.

**Code ID Qualifier:** If the National Drug Code has a qualifier indicating the type of code that is being transmitted, the qualifier is entered here.

**Purchase Service Amount:** The cost of the service purchased from a third party.

**Taxable:** This box is clicked if the code requires a tax charge.

**HIPAA Approved:** This box is linked to the Warn on Unapproved Codes option in the Program Options window. If the latter option is used, the HIPAA Approved box should be checked for each procedure code that is HIPAA compliant.

**Require Co-pay:** This box may be checked for a procedure that requires a copay (for example, an office visit code).

**Patient Only Responsible:** A check in the Patient Only Responsible box indicates that the patient alone, and not the insurance carrier, is responsible for the charges associated with the procedure.

**Purchased Service:** This box should be checked if the procedure is a service that is purchased from a third party—for example, lab work.

*Amounts Tab*   The Amounts tab contains information about the amount charged for the procedure (see Figure T13-2). It includes the following boxes:

**Charge Amounts A to Z:** The amount of the charge for the procedure is entered in the Charge Amounts A to Z boxes. Up to twenty-six different fees can be entered for each procedure. Box A is used to record the practice's normal charge for a procedure. Other boxes could be used to set up special pricing. For example, Box B could contain the fee for certain managed care plans that are paid a discounted amount.

The fees entered in the A to Z boxes are linked to the entry in the Price Code box in the Account tab within the Case folder. For example, if managed care fees are entered in the B box for each procedure code, managed care patients would also have B selected in the Price Code box. Then, when a charge is entered in the Transaction Entry dialog box, Medisoft automatically enters the fee listed in box B within the Amounts tab.

Polaris Medical Group uses a single fee schedule, so only box A is filled in. The actual amount the office receives for each procedure varies, however, depending on the type of insurance the patient has and the agreed-upon allowed amount for that procedure. The allowed amount paid by each carrier for a given procedure is entered in the Allowed Amounts tab of the Procedure/Payment/Adjustment dialog box, described below.

**FIGURE T13-2** Amounts Tab of the Procedure/Payment/Adjustment Dialog Box

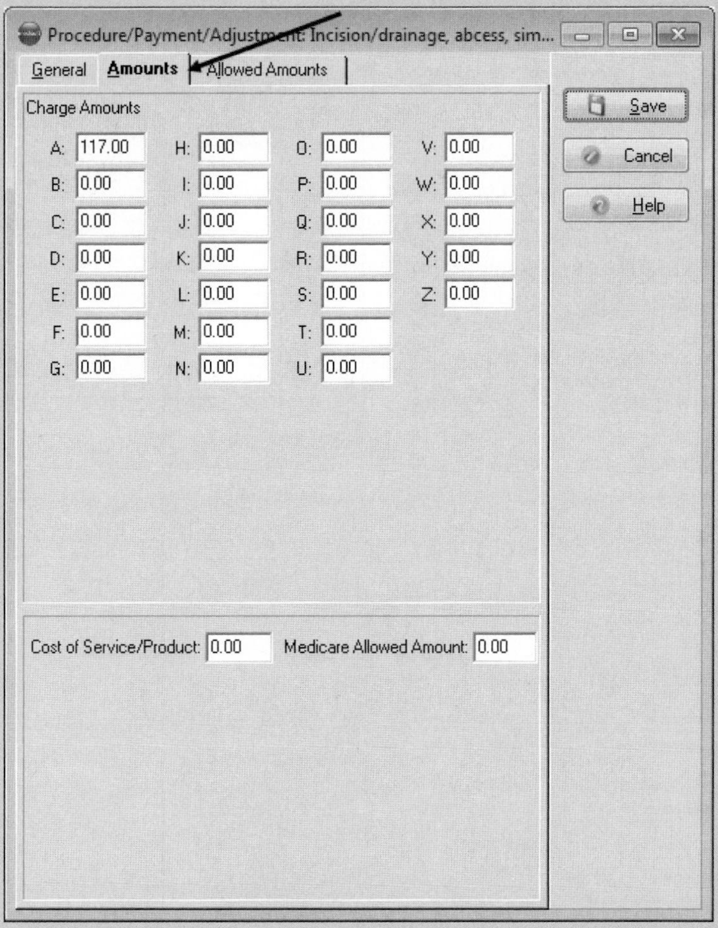

**Cost of Service/Product:** If there is an actual cost for the service or product, it is entered in the Cost of Service/Product box.

**Medicare Allowed Amount:** For Medicare-participating providers, the allowed amount for this procedure can be entered in the Medicare Allowed Amount box. For nonparticipating providers, the Medicare limiting charge is entered.

*Allowed Amounts Tab*    The Allowed Amounts tab (see Figure T13-3) keeps track of the amount allowed for the procedure charge, sorted by insurance carrier. This tab can be completed and kept up to date by the practice, or it can be automatically calculated by Medisoft based on the latest payments received from the insurance company.

The amount each insurance carrier agrees to pay for the procedure is recorded in the Amount column to the right of the carrier's name.

When the information entered in the three tabs is complete, pressing the Save button saves the information in the database. The new code is now listed in the Procedure/Payment/Adjustment List dialog box and can be selected for use in the Transaction Entry dialog box.

**FIGURE T13-3** Allowed Amounts Tab of the Procedure/Payment/Adjustment Dialog Box

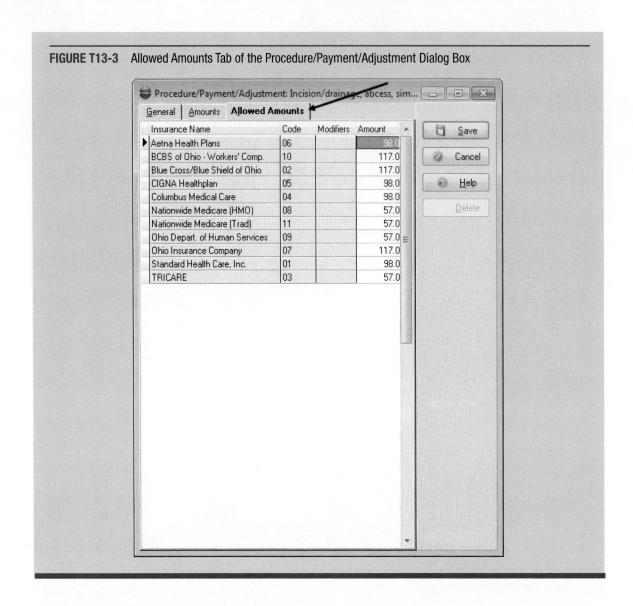

## ❑ Job 1

Change the Medisoft Program Date to June 21, 2018.

Print today's schedules for Dr. Crebore and Dr. Mahabir. Today is Thursday, June 21, 2018.

## ❑ Job 2

Hanna Wong, a new Medicare patient, sees Dr. Mahabir for the chest pain she has been experiencing when lifting. Dr. Mahabir examines Hanna and would like her to return on June 27 for a series of tests of heart function.

Use SD 57 to enter Hanna's information in Medisoft and to create a new case. Then enter today's transactions using SD 58. Hanna pays the copayment with check 840. Print a walkout receipt. Finally, schedule Hanna for a sixty-minute appointment on June 27 at 2:00.

## ❏ Job 3

Will Brown telephones to inquire about the balance due on his account. Research the information and inform him of the amount owed on his account, if any.

## ❏ Job 4

Review the audit/edit report found on SD 59. If there are any errors, correct them in Medisoft (for example, change an incorrect procedure code, an incorrect procedure charge, and so on).

## ❏ Job 5

Stewart Weintraub telephones. He is experiencing pain and stiffness in the arm that he fractured on June 13. Schedule him for a fifteen-minute appointment on June 26 at 3:15.

## ❏ Job 6

The practice manager has given you a list of new procedure codes (SD 60). Enter these codes in Medisoft. Fill in only those boxes for which information is provided on SD 60.

## ❏ Job 7

Jorge Martinez, a new patient, arrives for his appointment with Dr. Mahabir. He has been experiencing burning during urination. Using the information on SD 61, enter his information in Medisoft. Record the transactions and enter the payment (made with check 1819) using SD 62. Print a walkout receipt.

## ❏ Job 8

Susan Jonas is examined by Dr. Crebore for a patch of contact dermatitis. When you try to enter the transaction from the encounter form (SD 63), you notice that no ICD code has been marked. Look in Susan's chart for today (SD 64) to locate the reason for her visit and a description of her diagnosis (Problem 1). Create a new case for the visit, then locate the diagnosis code in Medisoft and enter it in the Diagnosis tab of the Case folder. Enter the transaction in Medisoft. Susan pays the copayment with check 349. Print a walkout receipt.

## ❏ Job 9

George Ahmadian telephones to request an appointment. He has a wart on his hand that he would like to have removed. Schedule him for a fifteen-minute appointment on June 25 at 9:45.

## ❏ Job 10

Print a patient day sheet for June 21, 2018.

## ❏ Job 11

Create insurance claims for June 21, 2018. Change the status of the claims.

# Daily Worksheet

## WEEK 2

### Day 4

*After completing all the jobs for Week 2 Day 4, answer the following questions in the spaces provided.*

1. What amount does Medicare owe for Hanna Wong's June 21 office visit after her copayment is deducted?

   _____

   _____

2. What is the amount William Brown owes on his account?

   _____

   _____

3. What is the description for procedure code 74290?

   _____

   _____

4. For what amount of Jorge Martinez's June 21 charges is his insurance carrier responsible after Martinez's copayment is deducted?

   _____

   _____

5. What is the amount of Susan Jonas's copayment on June 21?

   _____

   _____

6. What are the total procedure charges for June 21?

   _____

   _____

# WEEK 2

## Day 5

*Study the Medisoft Training Topics, and complete the jobs listed for today.*

---

**MEDISOFT TRAINING TOPIC 14:**

### Using Final Draft, Medisoft's Integrated Word Processor

Medisoft contains a fully integrated word processing program called Final Draft. Final Draft can be used to enter patient notes and narratives as well as letters and other documents used by the practice. Data from the Medisoft program can also be pulled into a Final Draft document using the Import File option on the File menu.

To use Final Draft, select the Final Draft option on the Activities menu. The main window of the program appears. To create a document, select New Document on the File menu (see Figure T14-1).

The menus on the menu bar at the top of the Final Draft window offer standard word processing features: text can be added, deleted, moved, copied, or replaced using the Edit menu; the default settings for font, line spacing, and page layout can be changed using the Format

---

**FIGURE T14-1**    Main Window of Final Draft Program with New Document Option Selected

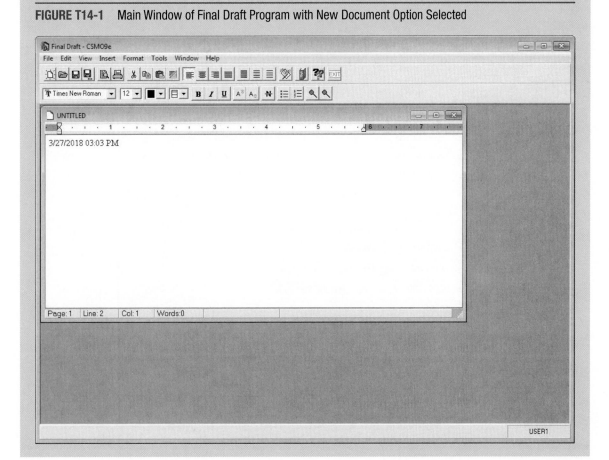

menu; and the spelling in a document can be checked using the Check Spelling option on the Tools menu. The File menu offers standard options for opening a new document, opening an existing document, saving a document (Save Document, Save As), and printing a document. To exit the program, select Exit on the File menu or click the X in the top-right corner of the Final Draft window. When you exit, you are returned to the Medisoft program.

## MEDISOFT TRAINING TOPIC 15:

## Changing an Insurance Carrier Code Set

While procedure and diagnosis codes used on insurance claims are specified by HIPAA, some insurance carriers use different code sets. For example, when ICD-10 became mandatory on October 1, 2015, some payers, such as automobile accident, disability, and workers' compensation, were not required to adopt the new code set, and continued to use ICD-9.

When it is necessary to change a payer's code set in Medisoft, the information is entered in the Insurance Carrier dialog box, which is accessed by clicking Insurance and then Carriers on the Lists menu. This displays the Insurance Carrier dialog box. Within the Insurance Carrier dialog box, code sets are listed on the Options and Codes tab (see Figure T15-1).

**FIGURE T15-1** Options and Codes Tab of the Insurance Carrier List Dialog Box

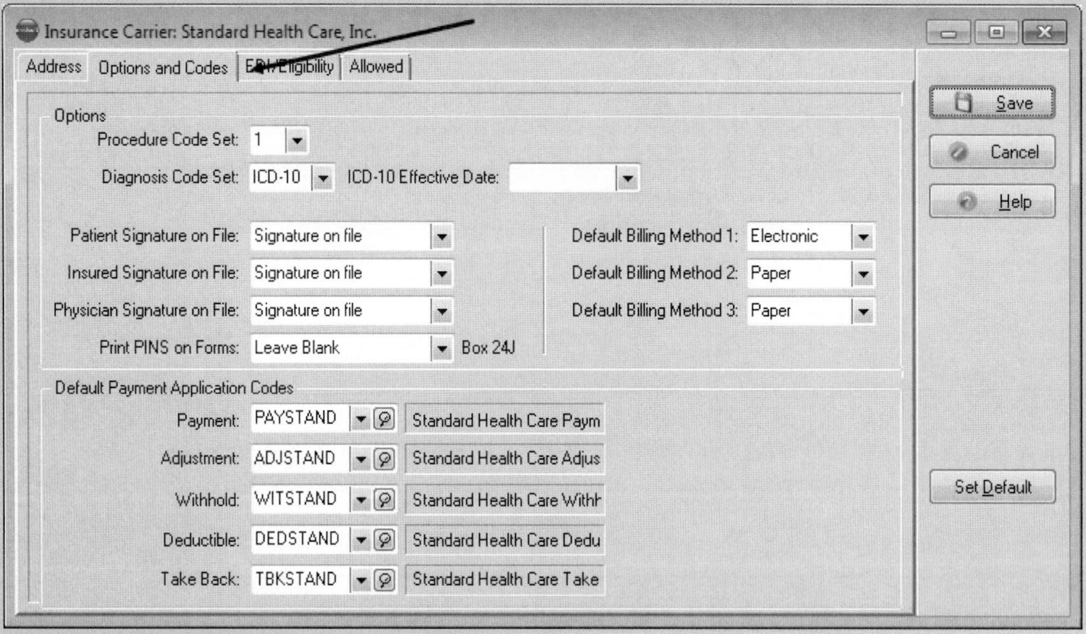

The Procedure Code Set field lists procedure code sets used by the practice. The sets are listed by a numeric code, such as 1, 2, or 3. The Diagnosis Code Set field lists code sets by name, such as ICD-9, ICD-10, etc. If ICD-10 was effective on a date other than October 1, 2015, a date should be entered in the ICD-10 Effective Date field.

## ❏ Job 1

Change the Medisoft Program Date to June 22, 2018.

Print today's schedules for Dr. Crebore and Dr. Mahabir. Today is Friday, June 22, 2018.

## ❏ Job 2

Martin Szinovacz has his blood pressure checked by Dr. Crebore. Enter the transaction in Medisoft using SD 65.

## ❏ Job 3

Fran Ferrone calls for an appointment. She is still complaining of a cough that keeps her awake at night. Schedule her for a fifteen-minute appointment on June 27 at 3:45.

She also requests a copy of the office's Notice of Privacy Practices. Use the Final Draft word processor to write a cover letter for mailing the Notice of Privacy Practices brochure. Start the letter with Polaris Medical Group's name and address, followed by Fran Ferrone's name and address (see SD 39) and the date. After a salutation, the note should say, "Enclosed please find a copy of the Polaris Medical Group's Notice of Privacy Practices brochure, as requested. We look forward to seeing you at your next appointment on June 27." End the letter with the standard closing, "Sincerely," and add your name and title (Patient Services Specialist). Run a spell check, and then print the letter. Use the Save Document option on the File menu to save it under the file name "Ferrone_cover." Select Letter as the File Type. When the Document Information for Untitled dialog box appears, click OK to accept the default settings.

## ❏ Job 4

Eugene Kadar, a new patient, is examined by Dr. Crebore. Eugene is complaining of painful recurring sores on his lip. Using the information on SD 66, enter the information in Medisoft. Enter today's transactions using SD 67. Eugene pays with check 2039. Print a walkout receipt.

## ❏ Job 5

William Nisinson arrives at the office with workers' compensation paperwork. He is not a patient of PMG and does not have an appointment. He works for Dan's Hardware as a driver and has been injured on the job. While unloading a delivery, he fell off the back of the truck. A radiological examination by Dr. Mahabir reveals a fractured ankle, and a splint is applied.

Using SD 68, establish William as a patient in Medisoft. Additional information to be entered in the Case folder is as follows:

*Policy tab:* Dr. Mahabir accepts assignment. The insurance carrier pays 100 percent of charges (boxes A–H).

*Condition tab:* The date of the injury is June 22, 2018. It is employment-related. The accident is categorized as a Work injury/Non-collision. In the Dates Unable to Work section, enter **06222018** in the From box.

*Miscellaneous tab:* Because this is a workers' compensation case, William must have an authorization number from his employer. Enter **Emp. Auth. #213-D** in the Local Use A box. (The remaining boxes in the Miscellaneous tab may be left blank.)

The insurance carrier for this case, Blue Cross Blue Shield Workers' Compensation, is no longer using ICD-9 for diagnosis coding. Change the Diagnosis Code Set entry in the Options and Codes tab of the Insurance Carrier dialog box to ICD-10, with an effective date of 1/1/2018.

Then enter today's transactions using SD 69.

Also, schedule William for a fifteen-minute follow-up appointment four weeks from today at 10:00.

### ❏ Internet Activity

Go to the website for the Ohio Bureau of Workers' Compensation. Look up information on the claim filing process.

### ❏ Job 6

Dan Connolly arrives for a follow-up visit for his hip pain with Dr. Mahabir. Enter the transactions using SD 70.

### ❏ Job 7

Yomo Hirosha, a patient of Dr. Mahabir, has been admitted to the Emergency Department of St. Mary's Hospital with complaints of chest pains. He has a history of myocardial infarction in April. Dr. Mahabir examines Yomo in the emergency room. Record the transaction in Medisoft using SD 71. Since this is a hospital visit, no copayment is collected.

**Tip!**

**Job 8**

Create a new case for Marilyn Rennagel's diabetes mellitus so that the new insurance carrier can be billed separately.

### ❏ Job 8

Marilyn Rennagel arrives for her appointment with Dr. Crebore. Marilyn has changed jobs and insurance carriers since her last office visit. Using the information on SD 72, update her information in Medisoft. She has met her deductible with the new carrier. Then enter today's transactions using SD 73.

## ❏ Job 9

Will Brown arrives in the office without an appointment. He is experiencing rectal bleeding again and would like to see Dr. Mahabir. Dr. Mahabir is currently at St. Mary's Hospital, but Dr. Crebore can fit Will in after she is finished with her current patient. Record today's transactions from the encounter form (SD 74).

## ❏ Job 10

Wilma Estephan calls to report that she is still experiencing pain during urination. Schedule her for the first available fifteen-minute appointment with Dr. Mahabir on June 25.

## ❏ Job 11

An RA arrives with payment from Standard Health Care for Angelo Daiute's office visit on June 14, 2018 (SD 75). Compare the procedure codes and amounts with those in Medisoft. If they are correct, enter the payment in Medisoft.

## ❏ Job 12

The bank has returned Cynthia Cashell's $125 check due to nonsufficient funds. The check was written to cover services received on June 18. In the Charges section of the Transaction Entry dialog box, post a returned check fee to Cynthia Cashell's account using the NSFFEE billing code that is set up in the database.

Then make an adjustment for the amount of the returned check in the Payments, Adjustments, And Comments section using the NSF adjustment code. In the Description box, key ***Returned check.*** Remember to apply the adjustment to the corresponding charges, and then save the transaction.

## ❏ Job 13

Print a patient day sheet for June 22, 2018.

## ❏ Job 14

Create insurance claims for June 22, 2018. Change the status of the claims.

**Tip!**

**Job 9**

When entering the procedure charge for Will Brown in the Transaction Entry dialog box, remember to select the correct provider in the Provider field for today's visit.

# Daily Worksheet

## WEEK 2

### Day 5

*After completing all the jobs for Week 2 Day 5, answer the following questions in the spaces provided.*

1.  What is the description for the ICD-10-CM code for Eugene Kadar's diagnosis?

    _____

    _____

2.  What amount does Eugene Kadar's insurance carrier now owe for his June 22 office visit?

    _____

    _____

3.  What is entered in the Local Use A box in the Miscellaneous tab of the Case folder for William Nisinson?

    _____

    _____

4.  For what amount of Dan Connolly's June 22 charges is Medicare responsible?

    _____

    _____

5.  What POS code is entered for Yomo Hirosha's transactions for June 22?

    _____

    _____

6.  What code is entered in the Provider box in the Transaction Entry dialog box for William Brown's June 22 office visit?

    _____

    _____

7.  What is the amount of the returned check fee in Cynthia Cashell's account?

    _____

    _____

8.  What are the total insurance payments for June 22?

    _____

    _____

## End-of-Month and Follow-Up Jobs

*Complete the jobs listed below.*

### ❏ Job 1

Change the Medisoft Program Date to June 30, 2018, and use SDs 76 through 86 to enter the insurance payments in Medisoft.

*Note:* When applying payments in the Apply Payment/Adjustments to Charges dialog box, remember to tab to the end of each row so that the Remainder amount in column 4 is updated.

### ❏ Job 2

Find all the patients who are insured under a CIGNA or Aetna capitated plan who were treated by Polaris Medical Group in May and June 2018. Since capitation payments arrived from CIGNA (see capitation payments in SDs 85 and 86, entered in Job 1 above), the charges in individual patient accounts must be written off so that patient accounts have zero balances.

*Hint:* In the Claim Management dialog box, the List Only button can be used to display only claims that match a specific insurance carrier. Use this button to display the list of patients insured under CIGNA and then Aetna who currently have claims. (Although capitated plans do not pay insurance claims, they request that claims be sent to them as they require the data for their records.) Make a note of each capitated patient's chart number for the two insurance carriers.

Then use the Enter Deposits/Payments option to enter a zero payment amount deposit for CIGNA. Select Insurance in the Payor Type field, Electronic in the Payment Method field, and 0.00 in the Payment Amount field. Apply the zero amount deposit in the Apply Payment/Adjustments to Charges dialog box to adjust the account of each CIGNA patient to a zero balance by entering an amount in the *Adjustment* column equal to the amount already displayed in the *Remainder* column.

Create a zero payment amount deposit for Aetna and follow the same steps to adjust the accounts for each Aetna patient.

After finishing your work in the Apply Payment/Adjustments to Charges dialog box for both groups of patients, change the status of the claims for these patients from Sent to Done.

**Tip!**

**Job 2**
Although Alan Harcar has two separate claims with CIGNA (claim numbers 46 and 58) for visits on 6/12/2018 and 6/15/2018, the transactions for both days appear together in the Apply Payment/Adjustments to Charges dialog box as you apply the zero amount deposit.

**Tip!**

**Job 2**
To display the list of Done claims in the Claim Management dialog box, click the List Only Claims That Match button and uncheck the Exclude Done check box in the Claim Status section.

## ❏ Job 3

Create remainder statements for all patients with outstanding balances greater than $5.00. Change the status of the statements from Ready To Send to Sent.

## ❏ Job 4

Using the patient day sheets for June 11 through 22, add up the total charges, receipts, and adjustments for the ten-day period. Make a note of these totals.

Now print a practice analysis report for June 11 through 22, 2018. Add the total charges, payments, and adjustments.

Compare the totals on the practice analysis with the totals for the day sheets you have for the same time period. The amounts on the practice analysis should agree with the amounts from the totaled day sheets.

## ❏ Job 5

Print a patient aging report through June 30, 2018, using the Medisoft Reports feature on the Reports menu. Within the Medisoft Reports window, select the report entitled "Date Accurate Patient Aging by Date of Service" in the Aging Power Pack folder to create the report. (*Hint:* Double-click on the Aging Power Pack folder to display its contents, and then double-click on the report title. It may take several minutes before the Search window for entering the parameters of the report displays.)

## ❏ JOB 6

It is still June 30. Looking at the aging report created in Job 5, determine which patient account(s) are more than 90 days past due. Create a collection tickler for each patient. Then create and print collection letters.

## ❏ JOB 7

It is now July 3. Paul Ramos calls and asks to speak to a billing specialist. He would like to know if PMG offers any payment plans, since he cannot pay his balance in full. Set up a payment plan for $25 a month, to be paid on the 15th of every month, starting July 15. Assign the code $25 to the plan, and enter "$25 a month" in the Description field. The payment is due every 30 days. Once you have created the plan, assign Paul Ramos to the payment plan (located in the Payment Plan tab of the Patient/Guarantor dialog box).

# Source Documents

T his section contains the source documents referred to in Part 3, On the Job. These documents represent typical paperwork found in medical practices and include patient information forms, encounter forms, physician's notes, chart notes, remittance advices, and audit/edit reports. Following is a numerical list of the source documents in Part 4:

| Doc. No. | Page No. | Form Type | Subject |
|---|---|---|---|
| 1 | 182 | Patient Information | Mary Anne Kopelman |
| 2 | 183 | Encounter | Mary Anne Kopelman |
| 3 | 184 | RA | Medicare |
| 4 | 185 | Encounter | Lydia Stephanos |
| 5 | 186 | Patient Information | Gregory Kavanaugh |
| 6 | 187 | Encounter | Gregory Kavanaugh |
| 7 | 188 | RA | Standard Health Care |
| 8 | 189 | Encounter | Daniel Connolly |
| 9 | 190 | Patient Information | Wilma Estephan |
| 10 | 191 | Encounter | Wilma Estephan |
| 11 | 192 | Patient Information | James LeConey |
| 12 | 193 | Encounter | James LeConey |
| 13 | 194 | Encounter | William Brown |
| 14 | 195 | RA | Ohio Insurance Company |
| 15 | 196 | Encounter | Alan Harcar |
| 16 | 197 | Patient Information | Nora McAniff |
| 17 | 198 | Encounter | Nora McAniff |
| 18 | 199 | RA | Blue Cross Blue Shield |
| 19 | 200 | Hospital Visit Codes | Stewart Weintraub |
| 20 | 201 | RA | Medicare |
| 21 | 202 | Encounter | George Ahmadian |
| 22 | 203 | Encounter | Victoria Ferrara |
| 23 | 204 | New Provider Notes | Dr. Sylvia T. Serto |
| 24 | 205 | RA | Standard Health Care |
| 25 | 206 | Patient Information | Angelo Daiute |
| 26 | 207 | Encounter | Angelo Daiute |
| 27 | 208 | Encounter | Cameron Trotta |
| 28 | 209 | Encounter | George Ahmadian |

| 29 | 210 | RA | Standard Health Care |
|----|-----|----|----|
| 30 | 211 | Patient Information | Hector Valaquez |
| 31 | 212 | Encounter | Hector Valaquez |
| 32 | 213 | Encounter | Seymour Colbs |
| 33 | 214 | Encounter | David Weatherly |
| 34 | 215 | Audit/Edit Report | Medicare |
| 35 | 216 | Encounter | Roberta Yange-Sang |
| 36 | 217 | Encounter | Gloria Berkel-Rees |
| 37 | 218 | Encounter | Alan Harcar |
| 38 | 219 | Hospital Visit Codes | Myrna Beedon |
| 39 | 220 | Patient Information | Fran Ferrone |
| 40 | 221 | Encounter | Fran Ferrone |
| 41 | 222 | Encounter | Jimmy Hellery |
| 42 | 223 | Encounter | Floyd Deysenrothe |
| 43 | 224 | RA | Blue Cross Blue Shield |
| 44 | 225 | Encounter | Elizabeth Wu |
| 45 | 226 | ICD Codes | Additions |
| 46 | 227 | Encounter | Flora Torres-Gil |
| 47 | 228 | New Carrier Notes | Ohio Maxcare PPO |
| 48 | 229 | New Carrier Fee Schedule | Ohio Maxcare PPO |
| 49 | 230 | Encounter | Diana O'Keefe |
| 50 | 231 | Encounter | Felidia Jonas |
| 51 | 232 | Encounter | Cynthia Cashell |
| 52 | 233 | Patient Information | Chantalle Usdan |
| 53 | 234 | Encounter | Chantalle Usdan |
| 54 | 235 | Encounter | Rachel Atchely |
| 55 | 236 | Encounter | Mae Deysenrothe |
| 56 | 237 | Encounter | Ann LeConey |
| 57 | 238 | Patient Information | Hanna Wong |
| 58 | 239 | Encounter | Hanna Wong |
| 59 | 240 | Audit/Edit Report | Medicare |
| 60 | 241 | CPT Codes | Additions |
| 61 | 242 | Patient Information | Jorge Martinez |
| 62 | 243 | Encounter | Jorge Martinez |
| 63 | 244 | Encounter | Susan Jonas |
| 64 | 245 | Chart Notes | Susan Jonas |
| 65 | 246 | Encounter | Martin Szinovacz |
| 66 | 247 | Patient Information | Eugene Kadar |
| 67 | 248 | Encounter | Eugene Kadar |
| 68 | 249 | Patient Information | William Nisinson |
| 69 | 250 | Encounter | William Nisinson |
| 70 | 251 | Encounter | Daniel Connolly |
| 71 | 252 | Hospital Visit Codes | Yomo Hirosha |

| 72 | 253 | Patient Information | Marilyn Rennagel |
| 73 | 254 | Encounter | Marilyn Rennagel |
| 74 | 255 | Encounter | William Brown |
| 75 | 256 | RA | Standard Health Care |
| 76 | 257 | RA | Ohio Insurance Company |
| 77 | 258 | RA | Standard Health Care |
| 78 | 259 | RA | Blue Cross Blue Shield |
| 79 | 260 | RA | Workers' Compensation |
| 80 | 261 | RA | Medicare HMO |
| 81 | 262 | RA | TRICARE |
| 82 | 263 | RA | Medicare |
| 83 | 264 | RA | Medicaid |
| 84 | 265 | RA | Columbus Medical Care |
| 85 | 266 | RA | Aetna |
| 86 | 267 | RA | CIGNA |

# PATIENT INFORMATION FORM

### THIS SECTION REFERS TO PATIENT ONLY

| Name: Mary Anne C. Kopelman | Sex: F | Marital Status: ☐ S ☒ M ☐ D ☐ W | Birth Date: 9/7/87 |
|---|---|---|---|

| Address: 45 Mason Street | SS#: 465-99-0022 | | |
|---|---|---|---|

| City: Hopewell | State: OH | Zip: 43746 | Employer: | Phone: |
|---|---|---|---|---|

| Home Phone: 999-555-6877 | Employer's Address: | |
|---|---|---|

| Work Phone: | City: | State: | Zip: |
|---|---|---|---|

| Race: | | Ethnicity: | Language: English |
|---|---|---|---|
| __American Indian or Alaska Native | __Other | __Hispanic or Latino | |
| __Asian | __Native Hawaiian or Other Pacific Islander | X Non-Hispanic or Latino | |
| __Black or African American | | __Declined | |
| X White | __Declined | | |

| Spouse's Name: Arnold B. Kopelman | Spouse's Employer: U.S. Army, Fort Tyrone (full-time) | |
|---|---|---|

| Emergency Contact: Arnold B. Kopelman | Relationship: Husband | Phone #: 999-555-6877 |
|---|---|---|

### FILL IN IF PATIENT IS A MINOR

| Parent/Guardian's Name: | Sex: | Marital Status: ☐ S ☐ M ☐ D ☐ W | Birth Date: |
|---|---|---|---|

| Phone: | SS#: | | |
|---|---|---|---|

| Address: | Employer: | Phone: |
|---|---|---|

| City: | State: | Zip: | Employer's Address: | | |
|---|---|---|---|---|---|

| Student Status: | City: | State: | Zip: |
|---|---|---|---|

### INSURANCE INFORMATION

| Primary Insurance Company: TRICARE | Secondary Insurance Company: |
|---|---|

| Subscriber's Name: Arnold B. Kopelman | Birth Date: 4/10/87 | Subscriber's Name: | Birth Date: |
|---|---|---|---|

| Plan: TRICARE | SS#: 230-56-9874 | Plan: |
|---|---|---|

| Policy #: 230-56-9874 | Group #: USA9947 | Policy #: | Group #: |
|---|---|---|---|

| Copayment/Deductible: $10 copay | Price Code: A | |
|---|---|---|

### OTHER INFORMATION

| Reason for visit: shortness of breath, fatigue | Allergy to Medication (list): |
|---|---|

| Name of referring physician: | If auto accident, list date and state in which it occurred: |
|---|---|

I authorize treatment and agree to pay all fees and charges for the person named above. I agree to pay all charges shown by statements, promptly upon their presentation, unless credit arrangements are agreed upon in writing.

I authorize payment directly to POLARIS MEDICAL GROUP of insurance benefits otherwise payable to me. I hereby authorize the release of any medical information necessary in order to process a claim for payment in my behalf.

| Mary Anne Kopelman | 6/11/18 |
|---|---|
| (Patient's Signature/Parent or Guardian's Signature) | (Date) |

I plan to make payment of my medical expenses as follows (check one or more):

X Insurance (as above)     X Cash/Check/Credit/Debit Card     ____Medicare     ____Medicaid     ____Workers' Comp.

# ENCOUNTER FORM

**6/11/2018**       **10:00am**
DATE              TIME

**Dr. Robin Crebore**
PROVIDER

**Mary Anne C. Kopelman**
PATIENT NAME

**KOPELMA0**
CHART #

| OFFICE VISITS - SYMPTOMATIC - NEW | | |
|---|---|---|
| 99201 | OF--New Patient Minimal | |
| 99202 | OF--New Patient Low | X |
| 99203 | OF--New Patient Detailed | |
| 99204 | OF--New Patient Moderate | |
| 99205 | OF--New Patient High | |
| **OFFICE VISITS - SYMPTOMATIC - ESTABLISHED** | | |
| 99211 | OF--Established Patient Minimal | |
| 99212 | OF--Established Patient Low | |
| 99213 | OF--Established Patient Detailed | |
| 99214 | OF--Established Patient Moderate | |
| 99215 | OF--Established Patient High | |
| **PREVENTIVE VISITS - NEW** | | |
| 99381 | Under 1 Year | |
| 99382 | 1 - 4 Years | |
| 99383 | 5 - 11 Years | |
| 99384 | 12 - 17 Years | |
| 99385 | 18 - 39 Years | |
| 99386 | 40 - 64 Years | |
| 99387 | 65 Years & Up | |
| **PREVENTIVE VISITS - ESTABLISHED** | | |
| 99391 | Under 1 Year | |
| 99392 | 1 - 4 Years | |
| 99393 | 5 - 11 Years | |
| 99394 | 12 - 17 Years | |
| 99395 | 18 - 39 Years | |
| 99396 | 40 - 64 Years | |
| 99397 | 65 Years & Up | |
| **HOSPITAL/NURSING HOME VISITS** | | |
| 99221 | Initial hospital care, det. | |
| 99222 | Initial hospital care, comp. | |
| 99223 | Initial hospital care, high | |
| 99281 | ER Visit, min. | |
| 99282 | ER Visit, low | |
| 99283 | ER Visit, det. | |
| 99284 | ER Visit, moderate | |
| 99285 | ER Visit, high | |
| 99307 | Subseq. nursing facility care, pf. | |
| | | |

| PROCEDURES | | |
|---|---|---|
| 10060 | Incision/drainage, abscess | |
| 20610 | Aspiration, bursa | |
| 29505 | Splint, long leg | |
| 29515 | Splint, short leg | |
| 36415 | Routine venipuncture | X |
| 45330 | Sigmoidoscopy, flex | |
| 46600 | Anoscopy, diagnostic | |
| 71030 | Chest x-ray, complete | |
| 73610 | Radiology, ankle, complete | |
| 93000 | Routine ECG | |
| 93018 | Cardiovascular stress test | |
| 99070 | Supplies and materials | |
| **LABORATORY** | | |
| 80050 | General health panel | X |
| 81000 | Urinalysis, complete | |
| 82270 | Blood, occult, feces screening | |
| 82607 | Vitamin B-12 test | |
| 82948 | Glucose, blood reagent | |
| 85027 | CBC, automated | |
| 85651 | Sedimentation rate test, manual | |
| 86360 | Absolute CD4/CD8 ratio | |
| 86592 | Syphilis test | |
| 87070 | Throat culture | |
| 87088 | Urine culture | |
| 88150 | Cytopathology, cervical or vaginal | |
| **INJECTIONS** | | |
| 90471 | Immunization administration | |
| 90472 | Immunization administration, 2nd | |
| 90658 | Influenza injection, ages >3 | |
| 90702 | DT immunization, ages <7 | |
| 90703 | Tetanus immunization | |
| 90707 | MMR immunization | |
| 96372 | Therapeutic injection | |
| 90723 | DTaP - HepB - IPV | |
| 90732 | Pneumococcal immunization | |
| | | |
| | | |

## POLARIS MEDICAL GROUP

| REFERRING PHYSICIAN | NPI |
|---|---|
| | |

AUTHORIZATION #

DIAGNOSIS
**D50.9**

PAYMENT AMOUNT
**$10 copay, check #1011**

NOTES

Nationwide Medicare
P.O. Box 7000
Columbus, OH 43214

Polaris Medical Group
2100 Grace Avenue
Columbus, OH 43214

**Practice ID:** 10-123456

**Date Prepared:** 6/7/18                             **EFT Number:** 3642987

| Patient's Name | Dates of Service From - Thru | POS | Proc | Qty | Charge Amount | Allowed Amount | Patient Resp. | Amt. Paid Provider |
|---|---|---|---|---|---|---|---|---|
| Stephanos, Lydia | 05/24/18 – 05/24/18 | 11 | 99397 | 1 | $155.00 | $118.00 | $118.00 | $00.00** |
| Stephanos, Lydia | 05/24/18 – 05/24/18 | 11 | 93000 | 1 | $84.00 | $29.00 | $5.80 | $23.20 |

**96: This procedure is not covered by Nationwide Medicare.

* * * * * * *     *EFT transmitted in the amount of $23.20*    * * * * * * *

# ENCOUNTER FORM

| | |
|---|---|
| **6/11/2018**  DATE | **10:00am**  TIME |
| **Lydia Stephanos**  PATIENT NAME | |

| | |
|---|---|
| **Dr. Michael Mahabir**  PROVIDER | |
| **STEPHLY0**  CHART # | |

### OFFICE VISITS - SYMPTOMATIC - NEW
| | | |
|---|---|---|
| 99201 | OF--New Patient Minimal | |
| 99202 | OF--New Patient Low | |
| 99203 | OF--New Patient Detailed | |
| 99204 | OF--New Patient Moderate | |
| 99205 | OF--New Patient High | |

### OFFICE VISITS - SYMPTOMATIC - ESTABLISHED
| | | |
|---|---|---|
| 99211 | OF--Established Patient Minimal | |
| 99212 | OF--Established Patient Low | |
| 99213 | OF--Established Patient Detailed | X |
| 99214 | OF--Established Patient Moderate | |
| 99215 | OF--Established Patient High | |

### PREVENTIVE VISITS - NEW
| | | |
|---|---|---|
| 99381 | Under 1 Year | |
| 99382 | 1 - 4 Years | |
| 99383 | 5 - 11 Years | |
| 99384 | 12 - 17 Years | |
| 99385 | 18 - 39 Years | |
| 99386 | 40 - 64 Years | |
| 99387 | 65 Years & Up | |

### PREVENTIVE VISITS - ESTABLISHED
| | | |
|---|---|---|
| 99391 | Under 1 Year | |
| 99392 | 1 - 4 Years | |
| 99393 | 5 - 11 Years | |
| 99394 | 12 - 17 Years | |
| 99395 | 18 - 39 Years | |
| 99396 | 40 - 64 Years | |
| 99397 | 65 Years & Up | |

### HOSPITAL/NURSING HOME VISITS
| | | |
|---|---|---|
| 99221 | Initial hospital care, det. | |
| 99222 | Initial hospital care, comp. | |
| 99223 | Initial hospital care, high | |
| 99281 | ER Visit, min. | |
| 99282 | ER Visit, low | |
| 99283 | ER Visit, det. | |
| 99284 | ER Visit, moderate | |
| 99285 | ER Visit, high | |
| 99307 | Subseq. nursing facility care, pf. | |
| | | |

### PROCEDURES
| | | |
|---|---|---|
| 10060 | Incision/drainage, abscess | X |
| 20610 | Aspiration, bursa | |
| 29505 | Splint, long leg | |
| 29515 | Splint, short leg | |
| 36415 | Routine venipuncture | |
| 45330 | Sigmoidoscopy, flex | |
| 46600 | Anoscopy, diagnostic | |
| 71030 | Chest x-ray, complete | |
| 73610 | Radiology, ankle, complete | |
| 93000 | Routine ECG | |
| 93018 | Cardiovascular stress test | |
| 99070 | Supplies and materials | |

### LABORATORY
| | | |
|---|---|---|
| 80050 | General health panel | |
| 81000 | Urinalysis, complete | |
| 82270 | Blood, occult, feces screening | |
| 82607 | Vitamin B-12 test | |
| 82948 | Glucose, blood reagent | |
| 85027 | CBC, automated | |
| 85651 | Sedimentation rate test, manual | |
| 86360 | Absolute CD4/CD8 ratio | |
| 86592 | Syphilis test | |
| 87070 | Throat culture | |
| 87088 | Urine culture | |
| 88150 | Cytopathology, cervical or vaginal | |

### INJECTIONS
| | | |
|---|---|---|
| 90471 | Immunization administration | |
| 90472 | Immunization administration, 2nd | |
| 90658 | Influenza injection, ages >3 | |
| 90702 | DT immunization, ages <7 | |
| 90703 | Tetanus immunization | |
| 90707 | MMR immunization | |
| 96372 | Therapeutic injection | |
| 90723 | DTaP - HepB - IPV | |
| 90732 | Pneumococcal immunization | |
| | | |
| | | |

## POLARIS MEDICAL GROUP

| | | NOTES |
|---|---|---|
| REFERRING PHYSICIAN | NPI | |
| AUTHORIZATION # | | |
| DIAGNOSIS  **L72.3** | | |
| PAYMENT AMOUNT | | |

## PATIENT INFORMATION FORM

### THIS SECTION REFERS TO PATIENT ONLY

| Name: Gregory W. Kavanaugh | Sex: M | Marital Status: ☒ S ☐ M ☐ D ☐ W | Birth Date: 12/15/92 |
|---|---|---|---|

| Address: 54 Grove St., Apt. 20 | SS#: 677-98-0078 |
|---|---|

| City: Germantown | State: OH | Zip: 45327 | Employer: Computer Consultants (full-time) | Phone: 999-555-3333 |
|---|---|---|---|---|

| Home Phone: 999-555-2626 | Employer's Address: 130 Parkway South |
|---|---|

| Work Phone: | City: Columbus | State: OH | Zip: 43214 |
|---|---|---|---|

| Race: | Ethnicity: | Language: English |
|---|---|---|
| __American Indian or Alaska Native  __Other | __Hispanic or Latino | |
| __Asian  __Native Hawaiian or Other Pacific Islander | X Non-Hispanic or Latino | |
| __Black or African American | __Declined | |
| X White  __Declined | | |

| Spouse's Name: | Spouse's Employer: |
|---|---|

| Emergency Contact: Ron Kavanaugh | Relationship: brother | Phone #: 999-555-0036 |
|---|---|---|

### FILL IN IF PATIENT IS A MINOR

| Parent/Guardian's Name: | Sex: | Marital Status: ☐ S ☐ M ☐ D ☐ W | Birth Date: |
|---|---|---|---|

| Phone: | SS#: |
|---|---|

| Address: | Employer: | Phone: |
|---|---|---|

| City: | State: | Zip: | Employer's Address: |
|---|---|---|---|

| Student Status: | City: | State: | Zip: |
|---|---|---|---|

### INSURANCE INFORMATION

| Primary Insurance Company: Standard Health Care, Inc. | Secondary Insurance Company: |
|---|---|

| Subscriber's Name: Gregory W. Kavanaugh | Birth Date: 12/15/92 | Subscriber's Name: | Birth Date: |
|---|---|---|---|

| Plan: PPO | SS#: 677-98-0078 | Plan: |
|---|---|---|

| Policy #: 000-GK9878 | Group #: CCTAA | Policy #: | Group #: |
|---|---|---|---|

| Copayment/Deductible: $15 / $1,000 | Price Code: A | |
|---|---|---|

### OTHER INFORMATION

| Reason for visit: routine monitoring | Allergy to Medication (list): |
|---|---|

| Name of referring physician: | If auto accident, list date and state in which it occurred: |
|---|---|

I authorize treatment and agree to pay all fees and charges for the person named above. I agree to pay all charges shown by statements, promptly upon their presentation, unless credit arrangements are agreed upon in writing.

I authorize payment directly to POLARIS MEDICAL GROUP of insurance benefits otherwise payable to me. I hereby authorize the release of any medical information necessary in order to process a claim for payment in my behalf.

| Gregory W. Kavanaugh | 6/11/18 |
|---|---|
| (Patient's Signature/Parent or Guardian's Signature) | (Date) |

I plan to make payment of my medical expenses as follows (check one or more):

X Insurance (as above)　　X Cash/Check/Credit/Debit Card　　____ Medicare　　____ Medicaid　　____ Workers' Comp.

# ENCOUNTER FORM

**6/11/2018**          **10:30am**
DATE                   TIME

**Gregory W. Kavanaugh**
PATIENT NAME

**Dr. Robin Crebore**
PROVIDER

**KAVANGRO**
CHART #

| OFFICE VISITS - SYMPTOMATIC - NEW | | |
|---|---|---|
| 99201 | OF--New Patient Minimal | |
| 99202 | OF--New Patient Low | |
| 99203 | OF--New Patient Detailed | |
| 99204 | OF--New Patient Moderate | |
| 99205 | OF--New Patient High | |
| **OFFICE VISITS - SYMPTOMATIC - ESTABLISHED** | | |
| 99211 | OF--Established Patient Minimal | |
| 99212 | OF--Established Patient Low | X |
| 99213 | OF--Established Patient Detailed | |
| 99214 | OF--Established Patient Moderate | |
| 99215 | OF--Established Patient High | |
| **PREVENTIVE VISITS - NEW** | | |
| 99381 | Under 1 Year | |
| 99382 | 1 - 4 Years | |
| 99383 | 5 - 11 Years | |
| 99384 | 12 - 17 Years | |
| 99385 | 18 - 39 Years | |
| 99386 | 40 - 64 Years | |
| 99387 | 65 Years & Up | |
| **PREVENTIVE VISITS - ESTABLISHED** | | |
| 99391 | Under 1 Year | |
| 99392 | 1 - 4 Years | |
| 99393 | 5 - 11 Years | |
| 99394 | 12 - 17 Years | |
| 99395 | 18 - 39 Years | |
| 99396 | 40 - 64 Years | |
| 99397 | 65 Years & Up | |
| **HOSPITAL/NURSING HOME VISITS** | | |
| 99221 | Initial hospital care, det. | |
| 99222 | Initial hospital care, comp. | |
| 99223 | Initial hospital care, high | |
| 99281 | ER Visit, min. | |
| 99282 | ER Visit, low | |
| 99283 | ER Visit, det. | |
| 99284 | ER Visit, moderate | |
| 99285 | ER Visit, high | |
| 99307 | Subseq. nursing facility care, pf. | |
| | | |
| | | |

| PROCEDURES | | |
|---|---|---|
| 10060 | Incision/drainage, abscess | |
| 20610 | Aspiration, bursa | |
| 29505 | Splint, long leg | |
| 29515 | Splint, short leg | |
| 36415 | Routine venipuncture | X |
| 45330 | Sigmoidoscopy, flex | |
| 46600 | Anoscopy, diagnostic | |
| 71030 | Chest x-ray, complete | |
| 73610 | Radiology, ankle, complete | |
| 93000 | Routine ECG | |
| 93018 | Cardiovascular stress test | |
| 99070 | Supplies and materials | |
| **LABORATORY** | | |
| 80050 | General health panel | |
| 81000 | Urinalysis, complete | |
| 82270 | Blood, occult, feces screening | |
| 82607 | Vitamin B-12 test | |
| 82948 | Glucose, blood reagent | |
| 85027 | CBC, automated | |
| 85651 | Sedimentation rate test, manual | |
| 86360 | Absolute CD4/CD8 ratio | X |
| 86592 | Syphilis test | |
| 87070 | Throat culture | |
| 87088 | Urine culture | |
| 88150 | Cytopathology, cervical or vaginal | |
| **INJECTIONS** | | |
| 90471 | Immunization administration | |
| 90472 | Immunization administration, 2nd | |
| 90658 | Influenza injection, ages >3 | |
| 90702 | DT immunization, ages <7 | |
| 90703 | Tetanus immunization | |
| 90707 | MMR immunization | |
| 96372 | Therapeutic injection | |
| 90723 | DTaP - HepB - IPV | |
| 90732 | Pneumococcal immunization | |
| | | |
| | | |
| | | |

## POLARIS MEDICAL GROUP

NOTES

| REFERRING PHYSICIAN | NPI |
|---|---|

AUTHORIZATION #

DIAGNOSIS
**B20**

PAYMENT AMOUNT
**$15 copay, check #200**

Standard Health Care
1500 Summit Avenue, Suite 500
Cincinnati, OH 45000

Polaris Medical Group
2100 Grace Avenue
Columbus, OH 43214

Practice ID: 01-234567

Date Prepared: 6/11/18                                    EFT Number: 267498

| Patient's Name | Dates of Service From - Thru | POS | Proc | Qty | Charge Amount | Allowed Amount | Patient Resp. | Amt. Paid Provider |
|---|---|---|---|---|---|---|---|---|
| Szinovacz, Martin | 5/16/18 – 5/16/18 | 11 | 99213 | 1 | $72.00 | $62.00 | $15.00 | $47.00 |

\* \* \* \* \* \* \* \*    *EFT transmitted in the amount of $47.00*    \* \* \* \* \* \* \* \*

# ENCOUNTER FORM

| | |
|---|---|
| **6/11/2018**     **2:00pm** | **Dr. Michael Mahabir** |
| DATE        TIME | PROVIDER |
| **Daniel Connolly** | **CONNODA0** |
| PATIENT NAME | CHART # |

| OFFICE VISITS - SYMPTOMATIC - NEW | | |
|---|---|---|
| 99201 | OF--New Patient Minimal | |
| 99202 | OF--New Patient Low | |
| 99203 | OF--New Patient Detailed | |
| 99204 | OF--New Patient Moderate | |
| 99205 | OF--New Patient High | |

| OFFICE VISITS - SYMPTOMATIC - ESTABLISHED | | |
|---|---|---|
| 99211 | OF--Established Patient Minimal | |
| 99212 | OF--Established Patient Low | |
| 99213 | OF--Established Patient Detailed | |
| 99214 | OF--Established Patient Moderate | X |
| 99215 | OF--Established Patient High | |

| PREVENTIVE VISITS - NEW | | |
|---|---|---|
| 99381 | Under 1 Year | |
| 99382 | 1 - 4 Years | |
| 99383 | 5 - 11 Years | |
| 99384 | 12 - 17 Years | |
| 99385 | 18 - 39 Years | |
| 99386 | 40 - 64 Years | |
| 99387 | 65 Years & Up | |

| PREVENTIVE VISITS - ESTABLISHED | | |
|---|---|---|
| 99391 | Under 1 Year | |
| 99392 | 1 - 4 Years | |
| 99393 | 5 - 11 Years | |
| 99394 | 12 - 17 Years | |
| 99395 | 18 - 39 Years | |
| 99396 | 40 - 64 Years | |
| 99397 | 65 Years & Up | |

| HOSPITAL/NURSING HOME VISITS | | |
|---|---|---|
| 99221 | Initial hospital care, det. | |
| 99222 | Initial hospital care, comp. | |
| 99223 | Initial hospital care, high | |
| 99281 | ER Visit, min. | |
| 99282 | ER Visit, low | |
| 99283 | ER Visit, det. | |
| 99284 | ER Visit, moderate | |
| 99285 | ER Visit, high | |
| 99307 | Subseq. nursing facility care, pf. | |
| | | |
| | | |

| PROCEDURES | | |
|---|---|---|
| 10060 | Incision/drainage, abscess | |
| 20610 | Aspiration, bursa | |
| 29505 | Splint, long leg | |
| 29515 | Splint, short leg | |
| 36415 | Routine venipuncture | |
| 45330 | Sigmoidoscopy, flex | |
| 46600 | Anoscopy, diagnostic | |
| 71030 | Chest x-ray, complete | |
| 73610 | Radiology, ankle, complete | |
| 93000 | Routine ECG | |
| 93018 | Cardiovascular stress test | |
| 99070 | Supplies and materials | |

| LABORATORY | | |
|---|---|---|
| 80050 | General health panel | |
| 81000 | Urinalysis, complete | |
| 82270 | Blood, occult, feces screening | |
| 82607 | Vitamin B-12 test | |
| 82948 | Glucose, blood reagent | |
| 85027 | CBC, automated | |
| 85651 | Sedimentation rate test, manual | |
| 86360 | Absolute CD4/CD8 ratio | |
| 86592 | Syphilis test | |
| 87070 | Throat culture | |
| 87088 | Urine culture | |
| 88150 | Cytopathology, cervical or vaginal | |

| INJECTIONS | | |
|---|---|---|
| 90471 | Immunization administration | |
| 90472 | Immunization administration, 2nd | |
| 90658 | Influenza injection, ages >3 | |
| 90702 | DT immunization, ages <7 | |
| 90703 | Tetanus immunization | |
| 90707 | MMR immunization | |
| 96372 | Therapeutic injection | |
| 90723 | DTaP - HepB - IPV | |
| 90732 | Pneumococcal immunization | |
| | | |
| | | |
| | | |

| POLARIS MEDICAL GROUP | | NOTES |
|---|---|---|
| REFERRING PHYSICIAN | NPI | |
| AUTHORIZATION # | | |
| DIAGNOSIS **M25.559** | | |
| PAYMENT AMOUNT | | |

# PATIENT INFORMATION FORM

| THIS SECTION REFERS TO PATIENT ONLY | | | |
|---|---|---|---|
| Name:<br>Wilma T. Estephan | Sex:<br>F | Marital Status:<br>☐ S ☐ M ☐ D ☒ W | Birth Date:<br>1/9/33 |

| | | |
|---|---|---|
| Address:<br>22 Horace Mann Road | SS#:<br>009-10-9988 | |

| City:<br>Highland | State:<br>OH | Zip:<br>45132 | Employer: | Phone: |
|---|---|---|---|---|

| Home Phone:<br>999-555-2387 | Employer's Address: | | |
|---|---|---|---|

| Work Phone: | City: | State: | Zip: |
|---|---|---|---|

| Race:<br>__American Indian or Alaska Native   __Other<br>__Asian   __Native Hawaiian or<br>__Black or African American   Other Pacific Islander<br>X White   __Declined | Ethnicity:<br>__Hispanic or Latino<br>X Non-Hispanic or Latino<br>__Declined | Language:<br>English |
|---|---|---|

| Spouse's Name: | Spouse's Employer: |
|---|---|

| Emergency Contact:<br>Joan Hause | Relationship:<br>daughter | Phone #:<br>999-302-4609 |
|---|---|---|

| FILL IN IF PATIENT IS A MINOR | | | |
|---|---|---|---|
| Parent/Guardian's Name: | Sex: | Marital Status:<br>☐ S ☐ M ☐ D ☐ W | Birth Date: |
| Phone: | SS#: | | |
| Address: | Employer: | | Phone: |
| City:     State:     Zip: | Employer's Address: | | |
| Student Status: | City:     State:     Zip: | | |

| INSURANCE INFORMATION | |
|---|---|
| Primary Insurance Company:<br>Nationwide Medicare HMO | Secondary Insurance Company: |
| Subscriber's Name:     Birth Date:<br>Wilma T. Estephan     1-9-33 | Subscriber's Name:     Birth Date: |
| Plan:     SS#:<br>HMO     009-10-9988 | Plan: |
| Policy #:     Group #:<br>009-10-9988A | Policy #:     Group #: |
| Copayment/Deductible:     Price Code:<br>$5 copay     A | |

| OTHER INFORMATION | |
|---|---|
| Reason for visit:<br>pain upon urination | Allergy to Medication (list): |
| Name of referring physician: | If auto accident, list date and state in which<br>it occurred: |

I authorize treatment and agree to pay all fees and charges for the person named above. I agree to pay all charges shown by statements, promptly upon their presentation, unless credit arrangements are agreed upon in writing.

I authorize payment directly to POLARIS MEDICAL GROUP of insurance benefits otherwise payable to me. I hereby authorize the release of any medical information necessary in order to process a claim for payment in my behalf.

| Wilma T. Estephan | 6/12/18 |
|---|---|
| (Patient's Signature/Parent or Guardian's Signature) | (Date) |

I plan to make payment of my medical expenses as follows (check one or more):

_____Insurance (as above)     X Cash/Check/Credit/Debit Card     X Medicare     _____Medicaid     _____Workers' Comp.

# ENCOUNTER FORM

| | |
|---|---|
| 6/12/2018    9:30am | Dr. Michael Mahabir |
| DATE          TIME | PROVIDER |
| Wilma T. Estephan | ESTEPWIO |
| PATIENT NAME | CHART # |

| OFFICE VISITS - SYMPTOMATIC - NEW | | |
|---|---|---|
| 99201 | OF--New Patient Minimal | |
| 99202 | OF--New Patient Low | X |
| 99203 | OF--New Patient Detailed | |
| 99204 | OF--New Patient Moderate | |
| 99205 | OF--New Patient High | |
| **OFFICE VISITS - SYMPTOMATIC - ESTABLISHED** | | |
| 99211 | OF--Established Patient Minimal | |
| 99212 | OF--Established Patient Low | |
| 99213 | OF--Established Patient Detailed | |
| 99214 | OF--Established Patient Moderate | |
| 99215 | OF--Established Patient High | |
| **PREVENTIVE VISITS - NEW** | | |
| 99381 | Under 1 Year | |
| 99382 | 1 - 4 Years | |
| 99383 | 5 - 11 Years | |
| 99384 | 12 - 17 Years | |
| 99385 | 18 - 39 Years | |
| 99386 | 40 - 64 Years | |
| 99387 | 65 Years & Up | |
| **PREVENTIVE VISITS - ESTABLISHED** | | |
| 99391 | Under 1 Year | |
| 99392 | 1 - 4 Years | |
| 99393 | 5 - 11 Years | |
| 99394 | 12 - 17 Years | |
| 99395 | 18 - 39 Years | |
| 99396 | 40 - 64 Years | |
| 99397 | 65 Years & Up | |
| **HOSPITAL/NURSING HOME VISITS** | | |
| 99221 | Initial hospital care, det. | |
| 99222 | Initial hospital care, comp. | |
| 99223 | Initial hospital care, high | |
| 99281 | ER Visit, min. | |
| 99282 | ER Visit, low | |
| 99283 | ER Visit, det. | |
| 99284 | ER Visit, moderate | |
| 99285 | ER Visit, high | |
| 99307 | Subseq. nursing facility care, pf. | |
| | | |

| PROCEDURES | | |
|---|---|---|
| 10060 | Incision/drainage, abscess | |
| 20610 | Aspiration, bursa | |
| 29505 | Splint, long leg | |
| 29515 | Splint, short leg | |
| 36415 | Routine venipuncture | |
| 45330 | Sigmoidoscopy, flex | |
| 46600 | Anoscopy, diagnostic | |
| 71030 | Chest x-ray, complete | |
| 73610 | Radiology, ankle, complete | |
| 93000 | Routine ECG | |
| 93018 | Cardiovascular stress test | |
| 99070 | Supplies and materials | |
| **LABORATORY** | | |
| 80050 | General health panel | |
| 81000 | Urinalysis, complete | X |
| 82270 | Blood, occult, feces screening | |
| 82607 | Vitamin B-12 test | |
| 82948 | Glucose, blood reagent | |
| 85027 | CBC, automated | |
| 85651 | Sedimentation rate test, manual | |
| 86360 | Absolute CD4/CD8 ratio | |
| 86592 | Syphilis test | |
| 87070 | Throat culture | |
| 87088 | Urine culture | X |
| 88150 | Cytopathology, cervical or vaginal | |
| **INJECTIONS** | | |
| 90471 | Immunization administration | |
| 90472 | Immunization administration, 2nd | |
| 90658 | Influenza injection, ages >3 | |
| 90702 | DT immunization, ages <7 | |
| 90703 | Tetanus immunization | |
| 90707 | MMR immunization | |
| 96372 | Therapeutic injection | |
| 90723 | DTaP - HepB - IPV | |
| 90732 | Pneumococcal immunization | |
| | | |
| | | |

## POLARIS MEDICAL GROUP

| | | NOTES |
|---|---|---|
| REFERRING PHYSICIAN | NPI | |
| AUTHORIZATION # | | |
| DIAGNOSIS **N30.20** | | |
| PAYMENT AMOUNT **$5 copay, check #359** | | |

# PATIENT INFORMATION FORM

## THIS SECTION REFERS TO PATIENT ONLY

| Name: James I. LeConey | | | Sex: M | Marital Status: ☒ S ☐ M ☐ D ☐ W | Birth Date: 6/30/02 |
|---|---|---|---|---|---|

| Address: 27 Ballard Drive | | | SS#: 887-68-4256 | | |
|---|---|---|---|---|---|

| City: Fairview | State: OH | Zip: 43773 | Employer: | | Phone: |
|---|---|---|---|---|---|

| Home Phone: 999-555-2398 | Employer's Address: |
|---|---|

| Work Phone: | City: | State: | Zip: |
|---|---|---|---|

**Race:**
__American Indian or Alaska Native   __Other
__Asian   __Native Hawaiian or Other Pacific Islander
__Black or African American
X White   __Declined

**Ethnicity:**
__Hispanic or Latino
X Non-Hispanic or Latino
__Declined

**Language:** English

| Spouse's Name: | Spouse's Employer: |
|---|---|

| Emergency Contact: Ann LeConey | Relationship: mother | Phone #: 999-555-2398 |
|---|---|---|

## FILL IN IF PATIENT IS A MINOR

| Parent/Guardian's Name: Brian Howard (father) | | | Sex: M | Marital Status: ☐ S ☐ M ☒ D ☐ W | Birth Date: 1/8/73 |
|---|---|---|---|---|---|

| Phone: 999-555-3124 | SS#: 350-26-0419 | |
|---|---|---|

| Address: 2349 Sheffield Way | Employer: The Columbus World Press (full-time) | Phone: |
|---|---|---|

| City: Columbus | State: OH | Zip: 43214 | Employer's Address: 2399 Overland Way | | |
|---|---|---|---|---|---|

| Student Status: | City: Columbus | State: OH | Zip: 43214 |
|---|---|---|---|

## INSURANCE INFORMATION

| Primary Insurance Company: Blue Cross & Blue Shield of Ohio | Secondary Insurance Company: |
|---|---|

| Subscriber's Name: Brian Howard | Birth Date: 1/8/73 | Subscriber's Name: | Birth Date: |
|---|---|---|---|

| Plan: Traditional | SS#: 350-26-0419 | Plan: |
|---|---|---|

| Policy #: XGS7612979 | Group #: 67544 | Policy #: | Group #: |
|---|---|---|---|

| Copayment/Deductible: $500 deductible | Price Code: A | |
|---|---|---|

## OTHER INFORMATION

| Reason for visit: flu | Allergy to Medication (list): |
|---|---|

| Name of referring physician: | If auto accident, list date and state in which it occurred: |
|---|---|

I authorize treatment and agree to pay all fees and charges for the person named above. I agree to pay all charges shown by statements, promptly upon their presentation, unless credit arrangements are agreed upon in writing.

I authorize payment directly to POLARIS MEDICAL GROUP of insurance benefits otherwise payable to me. I hereby authorize the release of any medical information necessary in order to process a claim for payment in my behalf.

| Ann LeConey | 6/12/18 |
|---|---|
| (Patient's Signature/Parent or Guardian's Signature) | (Date) |

I plan to make payment of my medical expenses as follows (check one or more):

X Insurance (as above)     X Cash/Check/Credit/Debit Card     ____ Medicare     ____ Medicaid     ____ Workers' Comp.

# ENCOUNTER FORM

| | |
|---|---|
| **6/12/2018**     **9:30am** | **Dr. Michael Mahabir** |
| DATE       TIME | PROVIDER |
| **James I. LeConey** | **LECONJIO** |
| PATIENT NAME | CHART # |

| OFFICE VISITS - SYMPTOMATIC - NEW | | |
|---|---|---|
| 99201 | OF--New Patient Minimal | |
| 99202 | OF--New Patient Low | |
| 99203 | OF--New Patient Detailed | |
| 99204 | OF--New Patient Moderate | |
| 99205 | OF--New Patient High | |

| OFFICE VISITS - SYMPTOMATIC - ESTABLISHED | | |
|---|---|---|
| 99211 | OF--Established Patient Minimal | |
| 99212 | OF--Established Patient Low | |
| 99213 | OF--Established Patient Detailed | |
| 99214 | OF--Established Patient Moderate | X |
| 99215 | OF--Established Patient High | |

| PREVENTIVE VISITS - NEW | | |
|---|---|---|
| 99381 | Under 1 Year | |
| 99382 | 1 - 4 Years | |
| 99383 | 5 - 11 Years | |
| 99384 | 12 - 17 Years | |
| 99385 | 18 - 39 Years | |
| 99386 | 40 - 64 Years | |
| 99387 | 65 Years & Up | |

| PREVENTIVE VISITS - ESTABLISHED | | |
|---|---|---|
| 99391 | Under 1 Year | |
| 99392 | 1 - 4 Years | |
| 99393 | 5 - 11 Years | |
| 99394 | 12 - 17 Years | |
| 99395 | 18 - 39 Years | |
| 99396 | 40 - 64 Years | |
| 99397 | 65 Years & Up | |

| HOSPITAL/NURSING HOME VISITS | | |
|---|---|---|
| 99221 | Initial hospital care, det. | |
| 99222 | Initial hospital care, comp. | |
| 99223 | Initial hospital care, high | |
| 99281 | ER Visit, min. | |
| 99282 | ER Visit, low | |
| 99283 | ER Visit, det. | |
| 99284 | ER Visit, moderate | |
| 99285 | ER Visit, high | |
| 99307 | Subseq. nursing facility care, pf. | |

| PROCEDURES | | |
|---|---|---|
| 10060 | Incision/drainage, abscess | |
| 20610 | Aspiration, bursa | |
| 29505 | Splint, long leg | |
| 29515 | Splint, short leg | |
| 36415 | Routine venipuncture | |
| 45330 | Sigmoidoscopy, flex | |
| 46600 | Anoscopy, diagnostic | |
| 71030 | Chest x-ray, complete | |
| 73610 | Radiology, ankle, complete | |
| 93000 | Routine ECG | |
| 93018 | Cardiovascular stress test | |
| 99070 | Supplies and materials | |

| LABORATORY | | |
|---|---|---|
| 80050 | General health panel | |
| 81000 | Urinalysis, complete | |
| 82270 | Blood, occult, feces screening | |
| 82607 | Vitamin B-12 test | |
| 82948 | Glucose, blood reagent | |
| 85027 | CBC, automated | |
| 85651 | Sedimentation rate test, manual | |
| 86360 | Absolute CD4/CD8 ratio | |
| 86592 | Syphilis test | |
| 87070 | Throat culture | |
| 87088 | Urine culture | |
| 88150 | Cytopathology, cervical or vaginal | |

| INJECTIONS | | |
|---|---|---|
| 90471 | Immunization administration | |
| 90472 | Immunization administration, 2nd | |
| 90658 | Influenza injection, ages >3 | |
| 90702 | DT immunization, ages <7 | |
| 90703 | Tetanus immunization | |
| 90707 | MMR immunization | |
| 96372 | Therapeutic injection | |
| 90723 | DTaP - HepB - IPV | |
| 90732 | Pneumococcal immunization | |
| | | |
| | | |
| | | |

## POLARIS MEDICAL GROUP

| | | NOTES |
|---|---|---|
| REFERRING PHYSICIAN | NPI | |
| AUTHORIZATION # | | |
| DIAGNOSIS | | |
| **J11.1** | | |
| PAYMENT AMOUNT | | |

# ENCOUNTER FORM

**6/12/2018**          **9:30am**
DATE                    TIME

**Dr. Michael Mahabir**
PROVIDER

**William A. Brown**
PATIENT NAME

**BROWNWI0**
CHART #

| OFFICE VISITS - SYMPTOMATIC - NEW | | |
|---|---|---|
| 99201 | OF--New Patient Minimal | |
| 99202 | OF--New Patient Low | |
| 99203 | OF--New Patient Detailed | |
| 99204 | OF--New Patient Moderate | |
| 99205 | OF--New Patient High | |
| **OFFICE VISITS - SYMPTOMATIC - ESTABLISHED** | | |
| 99211 | OF--Established Patient Minimal | |
| 99212 | OF--Established Patient Low | |
| 99213 | OF--Established Patient Detailed | |
| 99214 | OF--Established Patient Moderate | X |
| 99215 | OF--Established Patient High | |
| **PREVENTIVE VISITS - NEW** | | |
| 99381 | Under 1 Year | |
| 99382 | 1 - 4 Years | |
| 99383 | 5 - 11 Years | |
| 99384 | 12 - 17 Years | |
| 99385 | 18 - 39 Years | |
| 99386 | 40 - 64 Years | |
| 99387 | 65 Years & Up | |
| **PREVENTIVE VISITS - ESTABLISHED** | | |
| 99391 | Under 1 Year | |
| 99392 | 1 - 4 Years | |
| 99393 | 5 - 11 Years | |
| 99394 | 12 - 17 Years | |
| 99395 | 18 - 39 Years | |
| 99396 | 40 - 64 Years | |
| 99397 | 65 Years & Up | |
| **HOSPITAL/NURSING HOME VISITS** | | |
| 99221 | Initial hospital care, det. | |
| 99222 | Initial hospital care, comp. | |
| 99223 | Initial hospital care, high | |
| 99281 | ER Visit, min. | |
| 99282 | ER Visit, low | |
| 99283 | ER Visit, det. | |
| 99284 | ER Visit, moderate | |
| 99285 | ER Visit, high | |
| 99307 | Subseq. nursing facility care, pf. | |
| | | |
| | | |

| PROCEDURES | | |
|---|---|---|
| 10060 | Incision/drainage, abscess | |
| 20610 | Aspiration, bursa | |
| 29505 | Splint, long leg | |
| 29515 | Splint, short leg | |
| 36415 | Routine venipuncture | |
| 45330 | Sigmoidoscopy, flex | |
| 46600 | Anoscopy, diagnostic | X |
| 71030 | Chest x-ray, complete | |
| 73610 | Radiology, ankle, complete | |
| 93000 | Routine ECG | |
| 93018 | Cardiovascular stress test | |
| 99070 | Supplies and materials | |
| **LABORATORY** | | |
| 80050 | General health panel | |
| 81000 | Urinalysis, complete | |
| 82270 | Blood, occult, feces screening | X |
| 82607 | Vitamin B-12 test | |
| 82948 | Glucose, blood reagent | |
| 85027 | CBC, automated | |
| 85651 | Sedimentation rate test, manual | |
| 86360 | Absolute CD4/CD8 ratio | |
| 86592 | Syphilis test | |
| 87070 | Throat culture | |
| 87088 | Urine culture | |
| 88150 | Cytopathology, cervical or vaginal | |
| **INJECTIONS** | | |
| 90471 | Immunization administration | |
| 90472 | Immunization administration, 2nd | |
| 90658 | Influenza injection, ages >3 | |
| 90702 | DT immunization, ages <7 | |
| 90703 | Tetanus immunization | |
| 90707 | MMR immunization | |
| 96372 | Therapeutic injection | |
| 90723 | DTaP - HepB - IPV | |
| 90732 | Pneumococcal immunization | |
| | | |
| | | |

## POLARIS MEDICAL GROUP

NOTES

REFERRING PHYSICIAN

NPI

AUTHORIZATION #

DIAGNOSIS
**K64.4**

PAYMENT AMOUNT

Ohio Insurance Company
1600 Galleria Way
Cleveland, OH 44000

Polaris Medical Group
2100 Grace Avenue
Columbus, OH 43214

Practice ID: 09-012345

Date Prepared: 6/11/18                                    EFT Number: 0164297

| Patient's Name | Dates of Service From - Thru | POS | Proc | Qty | Charge Amount | Allowed Amount | Patient Resp. | Amt. Paid Provider |
|---|---|---|---|---|---|---|---|---|
| Ferrara, Victoria | 5/8/18 – 5/8/18 | 11 | 99212 | 1 | $54.00 | $54.00 | $5.40 | $48.60 |
| Kavanaugh, Gregory | 4/12/18 – 4/12/18 | 11 | 99213 | 1 | $72.00 | $72.00 | $7.20 | $64.80 |
| Totals | | | | | $126.00 | $126.00 | $12.60 | $113.40 |

\* \* \* \* \* \* \*    *EFT transmitted in the amount of $113.40*    \* \* \* \* \* \* \*

# ENCOUNTER FORM

| | |
|---|---|
| **6/12/2018**　　　**11:30am** | **Dr. Michael Mahabir** |
| DATE　　　　　　　TIME | PROVIDER |
| **Alan J. Harcar** | **HARCAALO** |
| PATIENT NAME | CHART # |

| OFFICE VISITS - SYMPTOMATIC - NEW | | |
|---|---|---|
| 99201 | OF--New Patient Minimal | |
| 99202 | OF--New Patient Low | |
| 99203 | OF--New Patient Detailed | |
| 99204 | OF--New Patient Moderate | |
| 99205 | OF--New Patient High | |
| **OFFICE VISITS - SYMPTOMATIC - ESTABLISHED** | | |
| 99211 | OF--Established Patient Minimal | |
| 99212 | OF--Established Patient Low | X |
| 99213 | OF--Established Patient Detailed | |
| 99214 | OF--Established Patient Moderate | |
| 99215 | OF--Established Patient High | |
| **PREVENTIVE VISITS - NEW** | | |
| 99381 | Under 1 Year | |
| 99382 | 1 - 4 Years | |
| 99383 | 5 - 11 Years | |
| 99384 | 12 - 17 Years | |
| 99385 | 18 - 39 Years | |
| 99386 | 40 - 64 Years | |
| 99387 | 65 Years & Up | |
| **PREVENTIVE VISITS - ESTABLISHED** | | |
| 99391 | Under 1 Year | |
| 99392 | 1 - 4 Years | |
| 99393 | 5 - 11 Years | |
| 99394 | 12 - 17 Years | |
| 99395 | 18 - 39 Years | |
| 99396 | 40 - 64 Years | |
| 99397 | 65 Years & Up | |
| **HOSPITAL/NURSING HOME VISITS** | | |
| 99221 | Initial hospital care, det. | |
| 99222 | Initial hospital care, comp. | |
| 99223 | Initial hospital care, high | |
| 99281 | ER Visit, min. | |
| 99282 | ER Visit, low | |
| 99283 | ER Visit, det. | |
| 99284 | ER Visit, moderate | |
| 99285 | ER Visit, high | |
| 99307 | Subseq. nursing facility care, pf. | |
| | | |
| | | |

| PROCEDURES | | |
|---|---|---|
| 10060 | Incision/drainage, abscess | |
| 20610 | Aspiration, bursa | |
| 29505 | Splint, long leg | |
| 29515 | Splint, short leg | |
| 36415 | Routine venipuncture | |
| 45330 | Sigmoidoscopy, flex | |
| 46600 | Anoscopy, diagnostic | |
| 71030 | Chest x-ray, complete | |
| 73610 | Radiology, ankle, complete | |
| 93000 | Routine ECG | |
| 93018 | Cardiovascular stress test | |
| 99070 | Supplies and materials | |
| **LABORATORY** | | |
| 80050 | General health panel | |
| 81000 | Urinalysis, complete | |
| 82270 | Blood, occult, feces screening | |
| 82607 | Vitamin B-12 test | |
| 82948 | Glucose, blood reagent | |
| 85027 | CBC, automated | |
| 85651 | Sedimentation rate test, manual | |
| 86360 | Absolute CD4/CD8 ratio | |
| 86592 | Syphilis test | |
| 87070 | Throat culture | |
| 87088 | Urine culture | |
| 88150 | Cytopathology, cervical or vaginal | |
| **INJECTIONS** | | |
| 90471 | Immunization administration | |
| 90472 | Immunization administration, 2nd | |
| 90658 | Influenza injection, ages >3 | |
| 90702 | DT immunization, ages <7 | |
| 90703 | Tetanus immunization | |
| 90707 | MMR immunization | |
| 96372 | Therapeutic injection | |
| 90723 | DTaP - HepB - IPV | |
| 90732 | Pneumococcal immunization | |
| | | |
| | | |

| POLARIS MEDICAL GROUP | | NOTES |
|---|---|---|
| REFERRING PHYSICIAN | NPI | |
| AUTHORIZATION # | | |
| DIAGNOSIS<br>J11.1 | | |
| PAYMENT AMOUNT<br>**$18.00 copay, check #1201** | | |

# PATIENT INFORMATION FORM

### THIS SECTION REFERS TO PATIENT ONLY

| | | | |
|---|---|---|---|
| **Name:** Nora B. McAniff | **Sex:** F | **Marital Status:** ☐ S ☒ M ☐ D ☐ W | **Birth Date:** 5/1/53 |

| | |
|---|---|
| **Address:** 2300 First Avenue, Apt. D-40 | **SS#:** 504-00-6758 |

| | | | | |
|---|---|---|---|---|
| **City:** Jackson | **State:** OH | **Zip:** 45640 | **Employer:** Argene Interiors (part-time) | **Phone:** |

| | |
|---|---|
| **Home Phone:** 999-555-2309 | **Employer's Address:** 1700 Watertown Avenue |

| | | | |
|---|---|---|---|
| **Work Phone:** 999-555-6978 | **City:** Jackson | **State:** OH | **Zip:** 45640 |

**Race:**

___American Indian or Alaska Native     ___Other

___Asian                                               ___Native Hawaiian or

___Black or African American                  Other Pacific Islander

_X_ White                                             ___Declined

**Ethnicity:**

___Hispanic or Latino

_X_Non-Hispanic or Latino

___Declined

**Language:** English

| | |
|---|---|
| **Spouse's Name:** John McAniff | **Spouse's Employer:** Town of Jackson |

| | | |
|---|---|---|
| **Emergency Contact:** John McAniff | **Relationship:** Husband | **Phone #:** 999-555-1022 |

### FILL IN IF PATIENT IS A MINOR

| | | | |
|---|---|---|---|
| **Parent/Guardian's Name:** | **Sex:** | **Marital Status:** ☐ S ☐ M ☐ D ☐ W | **Birth Date:** |

| | |
|---|---|
| **Phone:** | **SS#:** |

| | | |
|---|---|---|
| **Address:** | **Employer:** | **Phone:** |

| | | | |
|---|---|---|---|
| **City:** | **State:** | **Zip:** | **Employer's Address:** |

| | | | |
|---|---|---|---|
| **Student Status:** | **City:** | **State:** | **Zip:** |

### INSURANCE INFORMATION

| | |
|---|---|
| **Primary Insurance Company:** Nationwide Medicare HMO | **Secondary Insurance Company:** |

| | | |
|---|---|---|
| **Subscriber's Name:** Nora B. McAniff | **Birth Date:** 5/1/53 | **Subscriber's Name:**            **Birth Date:** |

| | | |
|---|---|---|
| **Plan:** HMO | **SS#:** 504-00-6758 | **Plan:** |

| | | |
|---|---|---|
| **Policy #:** 504-00-6758BSA | **Group #:** | **Policy #:**            **Group #:** |

| | |
|---|---|
| **Copayment/Deductible:** $5 copay | **Price Code:** A |

### OTHER INFORMATION

| | |
|---|---|
| **Reason for visit:** stomach pain | **Allergy to Medication (list):** |

| | |
|---|---|
| **Name of referring physician:** | **If auto accident, list date and state in which it occurred:** |

I authorize treatment and agree to pay all fees and charges for the person named above. I agree to pay all charges shown by statements, promptly upon their presentation, unless credit arrangements are agreed upon in writing.

I authorize payment directly to POLARIS MEDICAL GROUP of insurance benefits otherwise payable to me. I hereby authorize the release of any medical information necessary in order to process a claim for payment in my behalf.

| | |
|---|---|
| _Nora B. McAniff_ | 6/13/18 |
| (Patient's Signature/Parent or Guardian's Signature) | (Date) |

I plan to make payment of my medical expenses as follows (check one or more):

_____Insurance (as above)     _X_ Cash/Check/Credit/Debit Card     _X_ Medicare     _____Medicaid     _____Workers' Comp.

# ENCOUNTER FORM

| 6/13/2018 | 9:00am | Dr. Michael Mahabir |
|-----------|--------|---------------------|
| DATE | TIME | PROVIDER |

| Nora B. McAniff | MCANIN00 |
|-----------------|----------|
| PATIENT NAME | CHART # |

| OFFICE VISITS - SYMPTOMATIC - NEW | | |
|---|---|---|
| 99201 | OF--New Patient Minimal | |
| 99202 | OF--New Patient Low | X |
| 99203 | OF--New Patient Detailed | |
| 99204 | OF--New Patient Moderate | |
| 99205 | OF--New Patient High | |
| **OFFICE VISITS - SYMPTOMATIC - ESTABLISHED** | | |
| 99211 | OF--Established Patient Minimal | |
| 99212 | OF--Established Patient Low | |
| 99213 | OF--Established Patient Detailed | |
| 99214 | OF--Established Patient Moderate | |
| 99215 | OF--Established Patient High | |
| **PREVENTIVE VISITS - NEW** | | |
| 99381 | Under 1 Year | |
| 99382 | 1 - 4 Years | |
| 99383 | 5 - 11 Years | |
| 99384 | 12 - 17 Years | |
| 99385 | 18 - 39 Years | |
| 99386 | 40 - 64 Years | |
| 99387 | 65 Years & Up | |
| **PREVENTIVE VISITS - ESTABLISHED** | | |
| 99391 | Under 1 Year | |
| 99392 | 1 - 4 Years | |
| 99393 | 5 - 11 Years | |
| 99394 | 12 - 17 Years | |
| 99395 | 18 - 39 Years | |
| 99396 | 40 - 64 Years | |
| 99397 | 65 Years & Up | |
| **HOSPITAL/NURSING HOME VISITS** | | |
| 99221 | Initial hospital care, det. | |
| 99222 | Initial hospital care, comp. | |
| 99223 | Initial hospital care, high | |
| 99281 | ER Visit, min. | |
| 99282 | ER Visit, low | |
| 99283 | ER Visit, det. | |
| 99284 | ER Visit, moderate | |
| 99285 | ER Visit, high | |
| 99307 | Subseq. nursing facility care, pf. | |
| | | |

| PROCEDURES | | |
|---|---|---|
| 10060 | Incision/drainage, abscess | |
| 20610 | Aspiration, bursa | |
| 29505 | Splint, long leg | |
| 29515 | Splint, short leg | |
| 36415 | Routine venipuncture | |
| 45330 | Sigmoidoscopy, flex | |
| 46600 | Anoscopy, diagnostic | |
| 71030 | Chest x-ray, complete | |
| 73610 | Radiology, ankle, complete | |
| 93000 | Routine ECG | |
| 93018 | Cardiovascular stress test | |
| 99070 | Supplies and materials | |
| **LABORATORY** | | |
| 80050 | General health panel | |
| 81000 | Urinalysis, complete | |
| 82270 | Blood, occult, feces screening | |
| 82607 | Vitamin B-12 test | |
| 82948 | Glucose, blood reagent | |
| 85027 | CBC, automated | |
| 85651 | Sedimentation rate test, manual | |
| 86360 | Absolute CD4/CD8 ratio | |
| 86592 | Syphilis test | |
| 87070 | Throat culture | |
| 87088 | Urine culture | |
| 88150 | Cytopathology, cervical or vaginal | |
| **INJECTIONS** | | |
| 90471 | Immunization administration | |
| 90472 | Immunization administration, 2nd | |
| 90658 | Influenza injection, ages >3 | |
| 90702 | DT immunization, ages <7 | |
| 90703 | Tetanus immunization | |
| 90707 | MMR immunization | |
| 96372 | Therapeutic injection | |
| 90723 | DTaP - HepB - IPV | |
| 90732 | Pneumococcal immunization | |
| | | |
| | | |
| | | |

## POLARIS MEDICAL GROUP

| REFERRING PHYSICIAN | NPI | NOTES |
|---|---|---|
| AUTHORIZATION # | | |
| DIAGNOSIS<br>K21.0 | | |
| PAYMENT AMOUNT<br>$5.00 copay, check #984 | | |

Blue Cross Blue Shield of Ohio
5000 First Street
Worthington, OH 43085

Polaris Medical Group
2100 Grace Avenue
Columbus, OH 43214

Practice ID: 04-5678901

Date Prepared: 6/11/18                                      EFT Number: 123896362

| Patient's Name | Dates of Service From - Thru | POS | Proc | Qty | Charge Amount | Allowed Amount | Patient Resp. | Amt. Paid Provider |
|---|---|---|---|---|---|---|---|---|
| O'Keefe, Diana | 5/16/18 – 5/16/18 | 11 | 99211 | 1 | $36.00 | $36.00 | $10.80 | $25.20 |
| O'Keefe, Diana | 5/16/18 – 5/16/18 | 11 | 85651 | 1 | $24.00 | $24.00 | $7.20 | $16.80 |
| Totals | | | | | $60.00 | $60.00 | $18.00 | $42.00 |

* * * * * * *    *EFT transmitted in the amount of $42.00*    * * * * * * *

## Diagnosis and Procedure Codes: Hospital Visit

Patient:  Stewart Weintraub

Subject:  Hospital Visit, 6/13/18

ICD:  S42.309A

CPT:  99283

Nationwide Medicare
P.O. Box 7001
Columbus, OH 43214


Polaris Medical Group
2100 Grace Avenue
Columbus, OH 43214

Practice ID: 10-123456

Date Prepared: 6/7/18                                      EFT Number: 3642987


| Patient's Name | Dates of Service From - Thru | POS | Proc | Qty | Charge Amount | Allowed Amount | Patient Resp. | Amt. Paid Provider |
|---|---|---|---|---|---|---|---|---|
| Ahmadian, George | 4/24/18 – 4/24/18 | 11 | 99385 | 1 | $215.00 | **A | $106.00 | **A |
| Ahmadian, George | 4/24/18 – 4/24/18 | 11 | 82948 | 1 | $18.00 | $8.00 | $1.60 | $6.40 |

| | | | | | | | | |
|---|---|---|---|---|---|---|---|---|
| Totals | | | | | $233.00 | $8.00 | $107.60 | $6.40 |

**A  This procedure is denied for this patient.


* * * * * * *  *EFT transmitted in the amount of $6.40*  * * * * * * *

# ENCOUNTER FORM

| | | |
|---|---|---|
| **5/23/2018** | **9:00am** | **Dr. Michael Mahabir** |
| DATE | TIME | PROVIDER |
| **George O. Ahmadian** | | **AHMADGEO** |
| PATIENT NAME | | CHART # |

| OFFICE VISITS - SYMPTOMATIC - NEW | | |
|---|---|---|
| 99201 | OF--New Patient Minimal | |
| 99202 | OF--New Patient Low | |
| 99203 | OF--New Patient Detailed | |
| 99204 | OF--New Patient Moderate | |
| 99205 | OF--New Patient High | |
| **OFFICE VISITS - SYMPTOMATIC - ESTABLISHED** | | |
| 99211 | OF--Established Patient Minimal | |
| 99212 | OF--Established Patient Low | |
| 99213 | OF--Established Patient Detailed | X |
| 99214 | OF--Established Patient Moderate | |
| 99215 | OF--Established Patient High | |
| **PREVENTIVE VISITS - NEW** | | |
| 99381 | Under 1 Year | |
| 99382 | 1 - 4 Years | |
| 99383 | 5 - 11 Years | |
| 99384 | 12 - 17 Years | |
| 99385 | 18 - 39 Years | |
| 99386 | 40 - 64 Years | |
| 99387 | 65 Years & Up | |
| **PREVENTIVE VISITS - ESTABLISHED** | | |
| 99391 | Under 1 Year | |
| 99392 | 1 - 4 Years | |
| 99393 | 5 - 11 Years | |
| 99394 | 12 - 17 Years | |
| 99395 | 18 - 39 Years | |
| 99396 | 40 - 64 Years | |
| 99397 | 65 Years & Up | |
| **HOSPITAL/NURSING HOME VISITS** | | |
| 99221 | Initial hospital care, det. | |
| 99222 | Initial hospital care, comp. | |
| 99223 | Initial hospital care, high | |
| 99281 | ER Visit, min. | |
| 99282 | ER Visit, low | |
| 99283 | ER Visit, det. | |
| 99284 | ER Visit, moderate | |
| 99285 | ER Visit, high | |
| 99307 | Subseq. nursing facility care, pf. | |
| | | |
| | | |

| PROCEDURES | | |
|---|---|---|
| 10060 | Incision/drainage, abscess | |
| 20610 | Aspiration, bursa | |
| 29505 | Splint, long leg | |
| 29515 | Splint, short leg | |
| 36415 | Routine venipuncture | |
| 45330 | Sigmoidoscopy, flex | |
| 46600 | Anoscopy, diagnostic | |
| 71030 | Chest x-ray, complete | |
| 73610 | Radiology, ankle, complete | |
| 93000 | Routine ECG | |
| 93018 | Cardiovascular stress test | |
| 99070 | Supplies and materials | |
| **LABORATORY** | | |
| 80050 | General health panel | |
| 81000 | Urinalysis, complete | |
| 82270 | Blood, occult, feces screening | |
| 82607 | Vitamin B-12 test | |
| 82948 | Glucose, blood reagent | X |
| 85027 | CBC, automated | |
| 85651 | Sedimentation rate test, manual | |
| 86360 | Absolute CD4/CD8 ratio | |
| 86592 | Syphilis test | |
| 87070 | Throat culture | |
| 87088 | Urine culture | |
| 88150 | Cytopathology, cervical or vaginal | |
| **INJECTIONS** | | |
| 90471 | Immunization administration | |
| 90472 | Immunization administration, 2nd | |
| 90658 | Influenza injection, ages >3 | |
| 90702 | DT immunization, ages <7 | |
| 90703 | Tetanus immunization | |
| 90707 | MMR immunization | |
| 96372 | Therapeutic injection | |
| 90723 | DTaP - HepB - IPV | |
| 90732 | Pneumococcal immunization | |
| | | |
| | | |

| **POLARIS MEDICAL GROUP** | | NOTES |
|---|---|---|
| REFERRING PHYSICIAN | NPI | |
| AUTHORIZATION # | | |
| DIAGNOSIS **E11.9, I10** | | |
| PAYMENT AMOUNT | | |

# ENCOUNTER FORM

| | |
|---|---|
| **6/13/2018** DATE | **2:00pm** TIME |
| **Dr. Robin Crebore** PROVIDER | |

| | |
|---|---|
| **Victoria A. Ferrara** PATIENT NAME | **FERRAVIO** CHART # |

| OFFICE VISITS - SYMPTOMATIC - NEW | | |
|---|---|---|
| 99201 | OF--New Patient Minimal | |
| 99202 | OF--New Patient Low | |
| 99203 | OF--New Patient Detailed | |
| 99204 | OF--New Patient Moderate | |
| 99205 | OF--New Patient High | |

| OFFICE VISITS - SYMPTOMATIC - ESTABLISHED | | |
|---|---|---|
| 99211 | OF--Established Patient Minimal | |
| 99212 | OF--Established Patient Low | X |
| 99213 | OF--Established Patient Detailed | |
| 99214 | OF--Established Patient Moderate | |
| 99215 | OF--Established Patient High | |

| PREVENTIVE VISITS - NEW | | |
|---|---|---|
| 99381 | Under 1 Year | |
| 99382 | 1 - 4 Years | |
| 99383 | 5 - 11 Years | |
| 99384 | 12 - 17 Years | |
| 99385 | 18 - 39 Years | |
| 99386 | 40 - 64 Years | |
| 99387 | 65 Years & Up | |

| PREVENTIVE VISITS - ESTABLISHED | | |
|---|---|---|
| 99391 | Under 1 Year | |
| 99392 | 1 - 4 Years | |
| 99393 | 5 - 11 Years | |
| 99394 | 12 - 17 Years | |
| 99395 | 18 - 39 Years | |
| 99396 | 40 - 64 Years | |
| 99397 | 65 Years & Up | |

| HOSPITAL/NURSING HOME VISITS | | |
|---|---|---|
| 99221 | Initial hospital care, det. | |
| 99222 | Initial hospital care, comp. | |
| 99223 | Initial hospital care, high | |
| 99281 | ER Visit, min. | |
| 99282 | ER Visit, low | |
| 99283 | ER Visit, det. | |
| 99284 | ER Visit, moderate | |
| 99285 | ER Visit, high | |
| 99307 | Subseq. nursing facility care, pf. | |
| | | |
| | | |

| PROCEDURES | | |
|---|---|---|
| 10060 | Incision/drainage, abscess | |
| 20610 | Aspiration, bursa | |
| 29505 | Splint, long leg | |
| 29515 | Splint, short leg | |
| 36415 | Routine venipuncture | |
| 45330 | Sigmoidoscopy, flex | |
| 46600 | Anoscopy, diagnostic | |
| 71030 | Chest x-ray, complete | |
| 73610 | Radiology, ankle, complete | |
| 93000 | Routine ECG | |
| 93018 | Cardiovascular stress test | |
| 99070 | Supplies and materials | |

| LABORATORY | | |
|---|---|---|
| 80050 | General health panel | |
| 81000 | Urinalysis, complete | |
| 82270 | Blood, occult, feces screening | |
| 82607 | Vitamin B-12 test | |
| 82948 | Glucose, blood reagent | |
| 85027 | CBC, automated | |
| 85651 | Sedimentation rate test, manual | |
| 86360 | Absolute CD4/CD8 ratio | |
| 86592 | Syphilis test | |
| 87070 | Throat culture | |
| 87088 | Urine culture | |
| 88150 | Cytopathology, cervical or vaginal | |

| INJECTIONS | | |
|---|---|---|
| 90471 | Immunization administration | |
| 90472 | Immunization administration, 2nd | |
| 90658 | Influenza injection, ages >3 | |
| 90702 | DT immunization, ages <7 | |
| 90703 | Tetanus immunization | |
| 90707 | MMR immunization | |
| 96372 | Therapeutic injection | |
| 90723 | DTaP - HepB - IPV | |
| 90732 | Pneumococcal immunization | |
| | | |
| | | |

## POLARIS MEDICAL GROUP

| | | NOTES |
|---|---|---|
| REFERRING PHYSICIAN | NPI | |
| AUTHORIZATION # | | |
| DIAGNOSIS **S31.000A** | | |
| PAYMENT AMOUNT | | |

**Preliminary information on Dr. Sylvia Serto, 6/13/2018**

**Address Tab**

Sylvia T. Serto, MD, FACP

2100 Grace Avenue

Columbus, OH 43214

Office Phone: 999 555-9800

Fax: 999 555-9801

Dr. Serto is a Medicare-participating provider, and she accepts assignment for Medicare and Medicaid (signature date: 1/1/2018).

License Number: 86-5991

**Reference Tab**

*Leave blank*

**Provider IDs Tab (New Provider ID Data)**

*Panel 1:* Her provider ID data apply to all insurance carriers and classes in the database.

*Panel 2:* Her data apply to all facilities with which she works.

Dr. Serto files claims as an individual, using NPI 1287654321 and Taxonomy Code 207R00000X.

*Panel 3:* Her Tax Identifier is EIN 22-7294401.

*Panel 4:* No additional IDs are required.

Standard Health Care
1500 Summit Avenue, Suite 500
Cincinnati, OH 45000

Polaris Medical Group
2100 Grace Avenue
Columbus, OH 43214

Practice ID: 01-234567

Date Prepared: 6/12/18                                    EFT Number: 0347869

| Patient's Name | Dates of Service From - Thru | POS | Proc | Qty | Charge Amount | Allowed Amount | Patient Resp. | Amt. Paid Provider |
|---|---|---|---|---|---|---|---|---|
| Rennagel, Marilyn | 5/8/18 – 5/8/18 | 11 | 99213 | 1 | $72.00 | $62.00 | $15.00 | $47.00 |
| Rennagel, Marilyn | 5/8/18 – 5/8/18 | 11 | 81000 | 1 | $22.00 | $17.00 | $0.00 | $17.00 |
| Rennagel, Marilyn | 5/8/18 – 5/8/18 | 11 | 82948 | 1 | $18.00 | $15.00 | $0.00 | $15.00 |
| Totals | | | | | $112.00 | $94.00 | $15.00 | $79.00 |

* * * * * * *     *EFT transmitted in the amount of $79.00*     * * * * * * *

# PATIENT INFORMATION FORM

## THIS SECTION REFERS TO PATIENT ONLY

| Name: Angelo X. Daiute | Sex: M | Marital Status: ☐ S ☒ M ☐ D ☐ W | Birth Date: 1/5/78 |
|---|---|---|---|

| Address: 22 Van Cortland Drive, Apt. 390 | SS#: 756-99-2637 | | |
|---|---|---|---|

| City: Fairview | State: OH | Zip: 43773 | Employer: COSTINC (full-time) | Phone: |
|---|---|---|---|---|

| Home Phone: 999-555-1758 | Employer's Address: 3504 Overland Avenue | | |
|---|---|---|---|

| Work Phone: 999-555-4300 | City: Columbus | State: OH | Zip: 43214 |
|---|---|---|---|

**Race:**

__American Indian or Alaska Native    __Other
__Asian    __Native Hawaiian or Other Pacific Islander
__Black or African American
X White    __Declined

**Ethnicity:**

X Hispanic or Latino
__Non-Hispanic or Latino
__Declined

**Language:** English

| Spouse's Name: Mary Daiute | Spouse's Employer: not employed |
|---|---|

| Emergency Contact: Mary Daiute | Relationship: wife | Phone #: 999-555-1758 |
|---|---|---|

## FILL IN IF PATIENT IS A MINOR

| Parent/Guardian's Name: | Sex: | Marital Status: ☐ S ☐ M ☐ D ☐ W | Birth Date: |
|---|---|---|---|

| Phone: | SS#: | | |
|---|---|---|---|

| Address: | Employer: | Phone: |
|---|---|---|

| City: | State: | Zip: | Employer's Address: |
|---|---|---|---|

| Student Status: | City: | State: | Zip: |
|---|---|---|---|

## INSURANCE INFORMATION

| Primary Insurance Company: Standard Health Care | Secondary Insurance Company: |
|---|---|

| Subscriber's Name: Angelo X. Daiute | Birth Date: 1/5/78 | Subscriber's Name: | Birth Date: |
|---|---|---|---|

| Plan: PPO | SS#: 756-99-2637 | Plan: |
|---|---|---|

| Policy #: 000-AD9876 | Group #: CSTAA | Policy #: | Group #: |
|---|---|---|---|

| Copayment/Deductible: $15 / $1,000 | Price Code: A | |
|---|---|---|

## OTHER INFORMATION

| Reason for visit: comprehensive physical examination | Allergy to Medication (list): |
|---|---|

| Name of referring physician: | If auto accident, list date and state in which it occurred: |
|---|---|

I authorize treatment and agree to pay all fees and charges for the person named above. I agree to pay all charges shown by statements, promptly upon their presentation, unless credit arrangements are agreed upon in writing.

I authorize payment directly to **POLARIS MEDICAL GROUP** of insurance benefits otherwise payable to me. I hereby authorize the release of any medical information necessary in order to process a claim for payment in my behalf.

| Angelo X. Daiute | 6/14/18 |
|---|---|
| (Patient's Signature/Parent or Guardian's Signature) | (Date) |

I plan to make payment of my medical expenses as follows (check one or more):

X Insurance (as above)    X Cash/Check/Credit/Debit Card    ____ Medicare    ____ Medicaid    ____ Workers' Comp.

# ENCOUNTER FORM

| | |
|---|---|
| **6/14/2018**  **10:30am** | **Dr. Robin Crebore** |
| DATE  TIME | PROVIDER |
| **Angelo X. Daiute** | **DAIUTANO** |
| PATIENT NAME | CHART # |

| OFFICE VISITS - SYMPTOMATIC - NEW | | |
|---|---|---|
| 99201 | OF--New Patient Minimal | |
| 99202 | OF--New Patient Low | |
| 99203 | OF--New Patient Detailed | |
| 99204 | OF--New Patient Moderate | |
| 99205 | OF--New Patient High | |

| OFFICE VISITS - SYMPTOMATIC - ESTABLISHED | | |
|---|---|---|
| 99211 | OF--Established Patient Minimal | |
| 99212 | OF--Established Patient Low | |
| 99213 | OF--Established Patient Detailed | |
| 99214 | OF--Established Patient Moderate | |
| 99215 | OF--Established Patient High | |

| PREVENTIVE VISITS - NEW | | |
|---|---|---|
| 99381 | Under 1 Year | |
| 99382 | 1 - 4 Years | |
| 99383 | 5 - 11 Years | |
| 99384 | 12 - 17 Years | |
| 99385 | 18 - 39 Years | |
| 99386 | 40 - 64 Years | X |
| 99387 | 65 Years & Up | |

| PREVENTIVE VISITS - ESTABLISHED | | |
|---|---|---|
| 99391 | Under 1 Year | |
| 99392 | 1 - 4 Years | |
| 99393 | 5 - 11 Years | |
| 99394 | 12 - 17 Years | |
| 99395 | 18 - 39 Years | |
| 99396 | 40 - 64 Years | |
| 99397 | 65 Years & Up | |

| HOSPITAL/NURSING HOME VISITS | | |
|---|---|---|
| 99221 | Initial hospital care, det. | |
| 99222 | Initial hospital care, comp. | |
| 99223 | Initial hospital care, high | |
| 99281 | ER Visit, min. | |
| 99282 | ER Visit, low | |
| 99283 | ER Visit, det. | |
| 99284 | ER Visit, moderate | |
| 99285 | ER Visit, high | |
| 99307 | Subseq. nursing facility care, pf. | |

| PROCEDURES | | |
|---|---|---|
| 10060 | Incision/drainage, abscess | |
| 20610 | Aspiration, bursa | |
| 29505 | Splint, long leg | |
| 29515 | Splint, short leg | |
| 36415 | Routine venipuncture | X |
| 45330 | Sigmoidoscopy, flex | |
| 46600 | Anoscopy, diagnostic | |
| 71030 | Chest x-ray, complete | |
| 73610 | Radiology, ankle, complete | |
| 93000 | Routine ECG | X |
| 93018 | Cardiovascular stress test | |
| 99070 | Supplies and materials | |

| LABORATORY | | |
|---|---|---|
| 80050 | General health panel | X |
| 81000 | Urinalysis, complete | X |
| 82270 | Blood, occult, feces screening | |
| 82607 | Vitamin B-12 test | |
| 82948 | Glucose, blood reagent | |
| 85027 | CBC, automated | |
| 85651 | Sedimentation rate test, manual | |
| 86360 | Absolute CD4/CD8 ratio | |
| 86592 | Syphilis test | |
| 87070 | Throat culture | |
| 87088 | Urine culture | |
| 88150 | Cytopathology, cervical or vaginal | |

| INJECTIONS | | |
|---|---|---|
| 90471 | Immunization administration | |
| 90472 | Immunization administration, 2nd | |
| 90658 | Influenza injection, ages >3 | |
| 90702 | DT immunization, ages <7 | |
| 90703 | Tetanus immunization | |
| 90707 | MMR immunization | |
| 96372 | Therapeutic injection | |
| 90723 | DTaP - HepB - IPV | |
| 90732 | Pneumococcal immunization | |

| POLARIS MEDICAL GROUP | | NOTES |
|---|---|---|
| REFERRING PHYSICIAN | NPI | |
| AUTHORIZATION # | | |
| DIAGNOSIS  **Z00.00** | | |
| PAYMENT AMOUNT  **$15.00 copay, check #3317** | | |

# ENCOUNTER FORM

| 6/14/2018 | 2:00pm | Dr. Michael Mahabir |
|---|---|---|
| DATE | TIME | PROVIDER |

| Cameron T. Trotta | | TROTTCA0 |
|---|---|---|
| PATIENT NAME | | CHART # |

| OFFICE VISITS - SYMPTOMATIC - NEW | | |
|---|---|---|
| 99201 | OF--New Patient Minimal | |
| 99202 | OF--New Patient Low | |
| 99203 | OF--New Patient Detailed | |
| 99204 | OF--New Patient Moderate | |
| 99205 | OF--New Patient High | |
| **OFFICE VISITS - SYMPTOMATIC - ESTABLISHED** | | |
| 99211 | OF--Established Patient Minimal | |
| 99212 | OF--Established Patient Low | |
| 99213 | OF--Established Patient Detailed | |
| 99214 | OF--Established Patient Moderate | |
| 99215 | OF--Established Patient High | |
| **PREVENTIVE VISITS - NEW** | | |
| 99381 | Under 1 Year | |
| 99382 | 1 - 4 Years | |
| 99383 | 5 - 11 Years | |
| 99384 | 12 - 17 Years | |
| 99385 | 18 - 39 Years | |
| 99386 | 40 - 64 Years | |
| 99387 | 65 Years & Up | |
| **PREVENTIVE VISITS - ESTABLISHED** | | |
| 99391 | Under 1 Year | |
| 99392 | 1 - 4 Years | |
| 99393 | 5 - 11 Years | |
| 99394 | 12 - 17 Years | |
| 99395 | 18 - 39 Years | |
| 99396 | 40 - 64 Years | X |
| 99397 | 65 Years & Up | |
| **HOSPITAL/NURSING HOME VISITS** | | |
| 99221 | Initial hospital care, det. | |
| 99222 | Initial hospital care, comp. | |
| 99223 | Initial hospital care, high | |
| 99281 | ER Visit, min. | |
| 99282 | ER Visit, low | |
| 99283 | ER Visit, det. | |
| 99284 | ER Visit, moderate | |
| 99285 | ER Visit, high | |
| 99307 | Subseq. nursing facility care, pf. | |

| PROCEDURES | | |
|---|---|---|
| 10060 | Incision/drainage, abscess | |
| 20610 | Aspiration, bursa | |
| 29505 | Splint, long leg | |
| 29515 | Splint, short leg | |
| 36415 | Routine venipuncture | X |
| 45330 | Sigmoidoscopy, flex | |
| 46600 | Anoscopy, diagnostic | |
| 71030 | Chest x-ray, complete | |
| 73610 | Radiology, ankle, complete | |
| 93000 | Routine ECG | X |
| 93018 | Cardiovascular stress test | |
| 99070 | Supplies and materials | |
| **LABORATORY** | | |
| 80050 | General health panel | X |
| 81000 | Urinalysis, complete | X |
| 82270 | Blood, occult, feces screening | X |
| 82607 | Vitamin B-12 test | |
| 82948 | Glucose, blood reagent | |
| 85027 | CBC, automated | |
| 85651 | Sedimentation rate test, manual | |
| 86360 | Absolute CD4/CD8 ratio | |
| 86592 | Syphilis test | |
| 87070 | Throat culture | |
| 87088 | Urine culture | |
| 88150 | Cytopathology, cervical or vaginal | |
| **INJECTIONS** | | |
| 90471 | Immunization administration | |
| 90472 | Immunization administration, 2nd | |
| 90658 | Influenza injection, ages >3 | |
| 90702 | DT immunization, ages <7 | |
| 90703 | Tetanus immunization | |
| 90707 | MMR immunization | |
| 96372 | Therapeutic injection | |
| 90723 | DTaP - HepB - IPV | |
| 90732 | Pneumococcal immunization | |
| | | |
| | | |
| | | |

## POLARIS MEDICAL GROUP

| REFERRING PHYSICIAN | NPI | NOTES |
|---|---|---|
| AUTHORIZATION # | | |
| DIAGNOSIS | | |
| Z00.00 | | |
| PAYMENT AMOUNT | | |
| $18.00 copay, check #869 | | |

# ENCOUNTER FORM

| | |
|---|---|
| **6/14/2018**  **3:00pm** | **Dr. Michael Mahabir** |
| DATE  TIME | PROVIDER |
| **George O. Ahmadian** | **AHMADGE0** |
| PATIENT NAME | CHART # |

| OFFICE VISITS - SYMPTOMATIC - NEW | | |
|---|---|---|
| 99201 | OF--New Patient Minimal | |
| 99202 | OF--New Patient Low | |
| 99203 | OF--New Patient Detailed | |
| 99204 | OF--New Patient Moderate | |
| 99205 | OF--New Patient High | |

| OFFICE VISITS - SYMPTOMATIC - ESTABLISHED | | |
|---|---|---|
| 99211 | OF--Established Patient Minimal | |
| 99212 | OF--Established Patient Low | |
| 99213 | OF--Established Patient Detailed | |
| 99214 | OF--Established Patient Moderate | |
| 99215 | OF--Established Patient High | X |

| PREVENTIVE VISITS - NEW | | |
|---|---|---|
| 99381 | Under 1 Year | |
| 99382 | 1 - 4 Years | |
| 99383 | 5 - 11 Years | |
| 99384 | 12 - 17 Years | |
| 99385 | 18 - 39 Years | |
| 99386 | 40 - 64 Years | |
| 99387 | 65 Years & Up | |

| PREVENTIVE VISITS - ESTABLISHED | | |
|---|---|---|
| 99391 | Under 1 Year | |
| 99392 | 1 - 4 Years | |
| 99393 | 5 - 11 Years | |
| 99394 | 12 - 17 Years | |
| 99395 | 18 - 39 Years | |
| 99396 | 40 - 64 Years | |
| 99397 | 65 Years & Up | |

| HOSPITAL/NURSING HOME VISITS | | |
|---|---|---|
| 99221 | Initial hospital care, det. | |
| 99222 | Initial hospital care, comp. | |
| 99223 | Initial hospital care, high | |
| 99281 | ER Visit, min. | |
| 99282 | ER Visit, low | |
| 99283 | ER Visit, det. | |
| 99284 | ER Visit, moderate | |
| 99285 | ER Visit, high | |
| 99307 | Subseq. nursing facility care, pf. | |
| | | |
| | | |

| PROCEDURES | | |
|---|---|---|
| 10060 | Incision/drainage, abscess | |
| 20610 | Aspiration, bursa | |
| 29505 | Splint, long leg | |
| 29515 | Splint, short leg | |
| 36415 | Routine venipuncture | |
| 45330 | Sigmoidoscopy, flex | |
| 46600 | Anoscopy, diagnostic | |
| 71030 | Chest x-ray, complete | |
| 73610 | Radiology, ankle, complete | |
| 93000 | Routine ECG | |
| 93018 | Cardiovascular stress test | |
| 99070 | Supplies and materials | |

| LABORATORY | | |
|---|---|---|
| 80050 | General health panel | |
| 81000 | Urinalysis, complete | |
| 82270 | Blood, occult, feces screening | |
| 82607 | Vitamin B-12 test | |
| 82948 | Glucose, blood reagent | |
| 85027 | CBC, automated | |
| 85651 | Sedimentation rate test, manual | |
| 86360 | Absolute CD4/CD8 ratio | |
| 86592 | Syphilis test | |
| 87070 | Throat culture | |
| 87088 | Urine culture | |
| 88150 | Cytopathology, cervical or vaginal | |

| INJECTIONS | | |
|---|---|---|
| 90471 | Immunization administration | |
| 90472 | Immunization administration, 2nd | |
| 90658 | Influenza injection, ages >3 | |
| 90702 | DT immunization, ages <7 | |
| 90703 | Tetanus immunization | |
| 90707 | MMR immunization | |
| 96372 | Therapeutic injection | |
| 90723 | DTaP - HepB - IPV | |
| 90732 | Pneumococcal immunization | |

## POLARIS MEDICAL GROUP

| | | NOTES |
|---|---|---|
| REFERRING PHYSICIAN | NPI | |
| AUTHORIZATION # | | |
| DIAGNOSIS  **G30.9** | | |
| PAYMENT AMOUNT | | |

Standard Health Care
1500 Summit Avenue, Suite 500
Cincinnati, OH 45000

Polaris Medical Group
2100 Grace Avenue
Columbus, OH 43214

Practice ID: 01-234567

Date Prepared: 6/13/18                                     EFT Number: 035102

| Patient's Name | Dates of Service From - Thru | POS | Proc | Qty | Charge Amount | Allowed Amount | Patient Resp. | Amt. Paid Provider |
|---|---|---|---|---|---|---|---|---|
| Szinovacz, Martin G | 5/24/18 – 5/24/18 | 11 | 99395 | 1 | $178.00 | $137.00 | $15.00 | $122.00 |
| Szinovacz, Martin G | 5/24/18 – 5/24/18 | 11 | 36415 | 1 | $22.00 | $17.00 | $0.00 | $17.00 |
| Szinovacz, Martin G | 5/24/18 – 5/24/18 | 11 | 80050 | 1 | $143.00 | $120.00 | $0.00 | $120.00 |
| Szinovacz, Martin G | 5/24/18 – 5/24/18 | 11 | 81000 | 1 | $22.00 | $17.00 | $0.00 | $17.00 |
| Szinovacz, Martin G | 5/24/18 – 5/24/18 | 11 | 93000 | 1 | $84.00 | $70.00 | $0.00 | $70.00 |

| Totals | | | | | $449.00 | $361.00 | $15.00 | $346.00 |

\* \* \* \* \* \* \*     *EFT transmitted in the amount of $346.00*     \* \* \* \* \* \* \*

# PATIENT INFORMATION FORM

## THIS SECTION REFERS TO PATIENT ONLY

| Name: Hector M. Valaquez | Sex: M | Marital Status: ☐ S ☒ M ☐ D ☐ W | Birth Date: 8/15/90 |
|---|---|---|---|

| Address: 199 Transfer Street | SS#: 459-94-9934 | |
|---|---|---|

| City: Highland | State: OH | Zip: 45132 | Employer: COSTINC (full-time) | Phone: |
|---|---|---|---|---|

| Home Phone: 999-555-3364 | Employer's Address: 3504 Overland Avenue | |
|---|---|---|

| Work Phone: 999-555-4300 | City: Columbus | State: OH | Zip: 43214 |
|---|---|---|---|

Race:

__American Indian or Alaska Native   __Other

__Asian   __Native Hawaiian or

__Black or African American   Other Pacific Islander

X White   __Declined

Ethnicity:

X Hispanic or Latino

__Non-Hispanic or Latino

__Declined

Language: English

| Spouse's Name: Juanita T. Valaquez | Spouse's Employer: Hapgood School District |
|---|---|

| Emergency Contact: Juanita T. Valaquez | Relationship: wife | Phone #: 999-555-3364 |
|---|---|---|

## FILL IN IF PATIENT IS A MINOR

| Parent/Guardian's Name: | Sex: | Marital Status: ☐ S ☐ M ☐ D ☐ W | Birth Date: |
|---|---|---|---|

| Phone: | SS#: | |
|---|---|---|

| Address: | Employer: | Phone: |
|---|---|---|

| City: | State: | Zip: | Employer's Address: |
|---|---|---|---|

| Student Status: | City: | State: | Zip: |
|---|---|---|---|

## INSURANCE INFORMATION

| Primary Insurance Company: Aetna Health Plans | Secondary Insurance Company: |
|---|---|

| Subscriber's Name: Hector M. Valaquez | Birth Date: 8/15/90 | Subscriber's Name: | Birth Date: |
|---|---|---|---|

| Plan: Ohio HMO, capitated | SS#: 459-94-9934 | Plan: |
|---|---|---|

| Policy #: 134GG | Group #: COS 41 | Policy #: | Group #: |
|---|---|---|---|

| Copayment/Deductible: $15 copay | Price Code: A | |
|---|---|---|

## OTHER INFORMATION

| Reason for visit: sunburn | Allergy to Medication (list): |
|---|---|

| Name of referring physician: | If auto accident, list date and state in which it occurred: |
|---|---|

I authorize treatment and agree to pay all fees and charges for the person named above. I agree to pay all charges shown by statements, promptly upon their presentation, unless credit arrangements are agreed upon in writing.

I authorize payment directly to POLARIS MEDICAL GROUP of insurance benefits otherwise payable to me. I hereby authorize the release of any medical information necessary in order to process a claim for payment in my behalf.

| Hector M. Valaquez | 6/15/18 |
|---|---|
| (Patient's Signature/Parent or Guardian's Signature) | (Date) |

I plan to make payment of my medical expenses as follows (check one or more):

X Insurance (as above)   X Cash/Check/Credit/Debit Card   ____Medicare   ____Medicaid   ____Workers' Comp.

# ENCOUNTER FORM

| | |
|---|---|
| **6/15/2018**          **9:00am** | **Dr. Robin Crebore** |
| DATE                    TIME | PROVIDER |
| **Hector M. Valaquez** | **VALAQHEO** |
| PATIENT NAME | CHART # |

| OFFICE VISITS - SYMPTOMATIC - NEW | | |
|---|---|---|
| 99201 | OF--New Patient Minimal | X |
| 99202 | OF--New Patient Low | |
| 99203 | OF--New Patient Detailed | |
| 99204 | OF--New Patient Moderate | |
| 99205 | OF--New Patient High | |

| OFFICE VISITS - SYMPTOMATIC - ESTABLISHED | | |
|---|---|---|
| 99211 | OF--Established Patient Minimal | |
| 99212 | OF--Established Patient Low | |
| 99213 | OF--Established Patient Detailed | |
| 99214 | OF--Established Patient Moderate | |
| 99215 | OF--Established Patient High | |

| PREVENTIVE VISITS - NEW | | |
|---|---|---|
| 99381 | Under 1 Year | |
| 99382 | 1 - 4 Years | |
| 99383 | 5 - 11 Years | |
| 99384 | 12 - 17 Years | |
| 99385 | 18 - 39 Years | |
| 99386 | 40 - 64 Years | |
| 99387 | 65 Years & Up | |

| PREVENTIVE VISITS - ESTABLISHED | | |
|---|---|---|
| 99391 | Under 1 Year | |
| 99392 | 1 - 4 Years | |
| 99393 | 5 - 11 Years | |
| 99394 | 12 - 17 Years | |
| 99395 | 18 - 39 Years | |
| 99396 | 40 - 64 Years | |
| 99397 | 65 Years & Up | |

| HOSPITAL/NURSING HOME VISITS | | |
|---|---|---|
| 99221 | Initial hospital care, det. | |
| 99222 | Initial hospital care, comp. | |
| 99223 | Initial hospital care, high | |
| 99281 | ER Visit, min. | |
| 99282 | ER Visit, low | |
| 99283 | ER Visit, det. | |
| 99284 | ER Visit, moderate | |
| 99285 | ER Visit, high | |
| 99307 | Subseq. nursing facility care, pf. | |
| | | |
| | | |

| PROCEDURES | | |
|---|---|---|
| 10060 | Incision/drainage, abscess | |
| 20610 | Aspiration, bursa | |
| 29505 | Splint, long leg | |
| 29515 | Splint, short leg | |
| 36415 | Routine venipuncture | |
| 45330 | Sigmoidoscopy, flex | |
| 46600 | Anoscopy, diagnostic | |
| 71030 | Chest x-ray, complete | |
| 73610 | Radiology, ankle, complete | |
| 93000 | Routine ECG | |
| 93018 | Cardiovascular stress test | |
| 99070 | Supplies and materials | |

| LABORATORY | | |
|---|---|---|
| 80050 | General health panel | |
| 81000 | Urinalysis, complete | |
| 82270 | Blood, occult, feces screening | |
| 82607 | Vitamin B-12 test | |
| 82948 | Glucose, blood reagent | |
| 85027 | CBC, automated | |
| 85651 | Sedimentation rate test, manual | |
| 86360 | Absolute CD4/CD8 ratio | |
| 86592 | Syphilis test | |
| 87070 | Throat culture | |
| 87088 | Urine culture | |
| 88150 | Cytopathology, cervical or vaginal | |

| INJECTIONS | | |
|---|---|---|
| 90471 | Immunization administration | |
| 90472 | Immunization administration, 2nd | |
| 90658 | Influenza injection, ages >3 | |
| 90702 | DT immunization, ages <7 | |
| 90703 | Tetanus immunization | |
| 90707 | MMR immunization | |
| 96372 | Therapeutic injection | |
| 90723 | DTaP - HepB - IPV | |
| 90732 | Pneumococcal immunization | |
| | | |
| | | |

## POLARIS MEDICAL GROUP

| | | NOTES |
|---|---|---|
| REFERRING PHYSICIAN | NPI | |
| AUTHORIZATION # | | |
| DIAGNOSIS **L55.9** | | |
| PAYMENT AMOUNT **$15.00 copay, check #3231** | | |

# ENCOUNTER FORM

| | | |
|---|---|---|
| **6/15/2018** | **9:30am** | **Dr. Robin Crebore** |
| DATE | TIME | PROVIDER |
| **Seymour B. Colbs** | | **COLBSSE0** |
| PATIENT NAME | | CHART # |

| OFFICE VISITS - SYMPTOMATIC - NEW | | |
|---|---|---|
| 99201 | OF--New Patient Minimal | |
| 99202 | OF--New Patient Low | |
| 99203 | OF--New Patient Detailed | |
| 99204 | OF--New Patient Moderate | |
| 99205 | OF--New Patient High | |

| OFFICE VISITS - SYMPTOMATIC - ESTABLISHED | | |
|---|---|---|
| 99211 | OF--Established Patient Minimal | |
| 99212 | OF--Established Patient Low | |
| 99213 | OF--Established Patient Detailed | X |
| 99214 | OF--Established Patient Moderate | |
| 99215 | OF--Established Patient High | |

| PREVENTIVE VISITS - NEW | | |
|---|---|---|
| 99381 | Under 1 Year | |
| 99382 | 1 - 4 Years | |
| 99383 | 5 - 11 Years | |
| 99384 | 12 - 17 Years | |
| 99385 | 18 - 39 Years | |
| 99386 | 40 - 64 Years | |
| 99387 | 65 Years & Up | |

| PREVENTIVE VISITS - ESTABLISHED | | |
|---|---|---|
| 99391 | Under 1 Year | |
| 99392 | 1 - 4 Years | |
| 99393 | 5 - 11 Years | |
| 99394 | 12 - 17 Years | |
| 99395 | 18 - 39 Years | |
| 99396 | 40 - 64 Years | |
| 99397 | 65 Years & Up | |

| HOSPITAL/NURSING HOME VISITS | | |
|---|---|---|
| 99221 | Initial hospital care, det. | |
| 99222 | Initial hospital care, comp. | |
| 99223 | Initial hospital care, high | |
| 99281 | ER Visit, min. | |
| 99282 | ER Visit, low | |
| 99283 | ER Visit, det. | |
| 99284 | ER Visit, moderate | |
| 99285 | ER Visit, high | |
| 99307 | Subseq. nursing facility care, pf. | |

| PROCEDURES | | |
|---|---|---|
| 10060 | Incision/drainage, abscess | |
| 20610 | Aspiration, bursa | |
| 29505 | Splint, long leg | |
| 29515 | Splint, short leg | |
| 36415 | Routine venipuncture | |
| 45330 | Sigmoidoscopy, flex | |
| 46600 | Anoscopy, diagnostic | |
| 71030 | Chest x-ray, complete | |
| 73610 | Radiology, ankle, complete | |
| 93000 | Routine ECG | |
| 93018 | Cardiovascular stress test | |
| 99070 | Supplies and materials | |

| LABORATORY | | |
|---|---|---|
| 80050 | General health panel | |
| 81000 | Urinalysis, complete | |
| 82270 | Blood, occult, feces screening | |
| 82607 | Vitamin B-12 test | |
| 82948 | Glucose, blood reagent | |
| 85027 | CBC, automated | |
| 85651 | Sedimentation rate test, manual | |
| 86360 | Absolute CD4/CD8 ratio | |
| 86592 | Syphilis test | |
| 87070 | Throat culture | |
| 87088 | Urine culture | |
| 88150 | Cytopathology, cervical or vaginal | |

| INJECTIONS | | |
|---|---|---|
| 90471 | Immunization administration | |
| 90472 | Immunization administration, 2nd | |
| 90658 | Influenza injection, ages >3 | |
| 90702 | DT immunization, ages <7 | |
| 90703 | Tetanus immunization | |
| 90707 | MMR immunization | |
| 96372 | Therapeutic injection | |
| 90723 | DTaP - HepB - IPV | |
| 90732 | Pneumococcal immunization | |
| | | |
| | | |

| POLARIS MEDICAL GROUP | | NOTES |
|---|---|---|
| REFERRING PHYSICIAN | NPI | |
| AUTHORIZATION # | | |
| DIAGNOSIS **S61.409A** | | |
| PAYMENT AMOUNT **$8.25 copay, check #839** | | |

# ENCOUNTER FORM

| | | |
|---|---|---|
| **6/15/2018** | **10:00am** | **Dr. Robin Crebore** |
| DATE | TIME | PROVIDER |

| | |
|---|---|
| **David R. Weatherly** | **WEATHDA0** |
| PATIENT NAME | CHART # |

| OFFICE VISITS - SYMPTOMATIC - NEW | | |
|---|---|---|
| 99201 | OF--New Patient Minimal | |
| 99202 | OF--New Patient Low | |
| 99203 | OF--New Patient Detailed | |
| 99204 | OF--New Patient Moderate | |
| 99205 | OF--New Patient High | |

| OFFICE VISITS - SYMPTOMATIC - ESTABLISHED | | |
|---|---|---|
| 99211 | OF--Established Patient Minimal | |
| 99212 | OF--Established Patient Low | |
| 99213 | OF--Established Patient Detailed | |
| 99214 | OF--Established Patient Moderate | X |
| 99215 | OF--Established Patient High | |

| PREVENTIVE VISITS - NEW | | |
|---|---|---|
| 99381 | Under 1 Year | |
| 99382 | 1 - 4 Years | |
| 99383 | 5 - 11 Years | |
| 99384 | 12 - 17 Years | |
| 99385 | 18 - 39 Years | |
| 99386 | 40 - 64 Years | |
| 99387 | 65 Years & Up | |

| PREVENTIVE VISITS - ESTABLISHED | | |
|---|---|---|
| 99391 | Under 1 Year | |
| 99392 | 1 - 4 Years | |
| 99393 | 5 - 11 Years | |
| 99394 | 12 - 17 Years | |
| 99395 | 18 - 39 Years | |
| 99396 | 40 - 64 Years | |
| 99397 | 65 Years & Up | |

| HOSPITAL/NURSING HOME VISITS | | |
|---|---|---|
| 99221 | Initial hospital care, det. | |
| 99222 | Initial hospital care, comp. | |
| 99223 | Initial hospital care, high | |
| 99281 | ER Visit, min. | |
| 99282 | ER Visit, low | |
| 99283 | ER Visit, det. | |
| 99284 | ER Visit, moderate | |
| 99285 | ER Visit, high | |
| 99307 | Subseq. nursing facility care, pf. | |
| | | |
| | | |

| PROCEDURES | | |
|---|---|---|
| 10060 | Incision/drainage, abscess | |
| 20610 | Aspiration, bursa | |
| 29505 | Splint, long leg | |
| 29515 | Splint, short leg | |
| 36415 | Routine venipuncture | |
| 45330 | Sigmoidoscopy, flex | |
| 46600 | Anoscopy, diagnostic | |
| 71030 | Chest x-ray, complete | X |
| 73610 | Radiology, ankle, complete | |
| 93000 | Routine ECG | X |
| 93018 | Cardiovascular stress test | |
| 99070 | Supplies and materials | |

| LABORATORY | | |
|---|---|---|
| 80050 | General health panel | |
| 81000 | Urinalysis, complete | |
| 82270 | Blood, occult, feces screening | |
| 82607 | Vitamin B-12 test | |
| 82948 | Glucose, blood reagent | |
| 85027 | CBC, automated | |
| 85651 | Sedimentation rate test, manual | |
| 86360 | Absolute CD4/CD8 ratio | |
| 86592 | Syphilis test | |
| 87070 | Throat culture | |
| 87088 | Urine culture | |
| 88150 | Cytopathology, cervical or vaginal | |

| INJECTIONS | | |
|---|---|---|
| 90471 | Immunization administration | |
| 90472 | Immunization administration, 2nd | |
| 90658 | Influenza injection, ages >3 | |
| 90702 | DT immunization, ages <7 | |
| 90703 | Tetanus immunization | |
| 90707 | MMR immunization | |
| 96372 | Therapeutic injection | |
| 90723 | DTaP - HepB - IPV | |
| 90732 | Pneumococcal immunization | |
| | | |
| | | |
| | | |

## POLARIS MEDICAL GROUP

| | | NOTES |
|---|---|---|
| REFERRING PHYSICIAN | NPI | |
| AUTHORIZATION # | | |
| DIAGNOSIS | | |
| **J45.20** | | |
| PAYMENT AMOUNT | | |
| **$18.00 copay, check #2312** | | |

# Electronic Claim Audit/Edit Report

Polaris Medical Group
2100 Grace Avenue
Columbus, OH 43214

Transmission Number: 6071298

Insurance Carrier: Medicare

| Patient's Name | Dates of Service From - Thru | POS | Proc | Qty | Status |
|---|---|---|---|---|---|
| Atchely, Rachel | 5/23/18 – 5/23/18 | 31 | 99202 | 1 | Rejected** |

** see reason for rejection below

********* *Incorrect procedure code* *********

# ENCOUNTER FORM

| 6/15/2018 | 10:45am | Dr. Michael Mahabir |
|-----------|---------|---------------------|
| DATE | TIME | PROVIDER |

| Roberta Yange-Sang | YANGEROO |
|--------------------|----------|
| PATIENT NAME | CHART # |

| OFFICE VISITS - SYMPTOMATIC - NEW | | |
|---|---|---|
| 99201 | OF--New Patient Minimal | |
| 99202 | OF--New Patient Low | |
| 99203 | OF--New Patient Detailed | |
| 99204 | OF--New Patient Moderate | |
| 99205 | OF--New Patient High | |
| **OFFICE VISITS - SYMPTOMATIC - ESTABLISHED** | | |
| 99211 | OF--Established Patient Minimal | |
| 99212 | OF--Established Patient Low | X |
| 99213 | OF--Established Patient Detailed | |
| 99214 | OF--Established Patient Moderate | |
| 99215 | OF--Established Patient High | |
| **PREVENTIVE VISITS - NEW** | | |
| 99381 | Under 1 Year | |
| 99382 | 1 - 4 Years | |
| 99383 | 5 - 11 Years | |
| 99384 | 12 - 17 Years | |
| 99385 | 18 - 39 Years | |
| 99386 | 40 - 64 Years | |
| 99387 | 65 Years & Up | |
| **PREVENTIVE VISITS - ESTABLISHED** | | |
| 99391 | Under 1 Year | |
| 99392 | 1 - 4 Years | |
| 99393 | 5 - 11 Years | |
| 99394 | 12 - 17 Years | |
| 99395 | 18 - 39 Years | |
| 99396 | 40 - 64 Years | |
| 99397 | 65 Years & Up | |
| **HOSPITAL/NURSING HOME VISITS** | | |
| 99221 | Initial hospital care, det. | |
| 99222 | Initial hospital care, comp. | |
| 99223 | Initial hospital care, high | |
| 99281 | ER Visit, min. | |
| 99282 | ER Visit, low | |
| 99283 | ER Visit, det. | |
| 99284 | ER Visit, moderate | |
| 99285 | ER Visit, high | |
| 99307 | Subseq. nursing facility care, pf. | |
| | | |

| PROCEDURES | | |
|---|---|---|
| 10060 | Incision/drainage, abscess | |
| 20610 | Aspiration, bursa | |
| 29505 | Splint, long leg | |
| 29515 | Splint, short leg | |
| 36415 | Routine venipuncture | |
| 45330 | Sigmoidoscopy, flex | |
| 46600 | Anoscopy, diagnostic | |
| 71030 | Chest x-ray, complete | |
| 73610 | Radiology, ankle, complete | |
| 93000 | Routine ECG | |
| 93018 | Cardiovascular stress test | |
| 99070 | Supplies and materials | |
| **LABORATORY** | | |
| 80050 | General health panel | |
| 81000 | Urinalysis, complete | |
| 82270 | Blood, occult, feces screening | |
| 82607 | Vitamin B-12 test | |
| 82948 | Glucose, blood reagent | |
| 85027 | CBC, automated | |
| 85651 | Sedimentation rate test, manual | |
| 86360 | Absolute CD4/CD8 ratio | |
| 86592 | Syphilis test | |
| 87070 | Throat culture | |
| 87088 | Urine culture | |
| 88150 | Cytopathology, cervical or vaginal | |
| **INJECTIONS** | | |
| 90471 | Immunization administration | |
| 90472 | Immunization administration, 2nd | |
| 90658 | Influenza injection, ages >3 | |
| 90702 | DT immunization, ages <7 | |
| 90703 | Tetanus immunization | |
| 90707 | MMR immunization | |
| 96372 | Therapeutic injection | |
| 90723 | DTaP - HepB - IPV | |
| 90732 | Pneumococcal immunization | |
| | | |
| | | |

## POLARIS MEDICAL GROUP

| | | NOTES |
|---|---|---|
| REFERRING PHYSICIAN | NPI | |
| AUTHORIZATION # | | |
| DIAGNOSIS<br>**S81.009A** | | |
| PAYMENT AMOUNT<br>**$8.25 copay, check #240** | | |

# ENCOUNTER FORM

| 6/15/2018 | 2:45pm | | Dr. Michael Mahabir |
|---|---|---|---|
| DATE | TIME | | PROVIDER |

| Gloria Berkel-Rees | | BERKEGLO |
|---|---|---|
| PATIENT NAME | | CHART # |

| OFFICE VISITS - SYMPTOMATIC - NEW | | |
|---|---|---|
| 99201 | OF--New Patient Minimal | |
| 99202 | OF--New Patient Low | |
| 99203 | OF--New Patient Detailed | |
| 99204 | OF--New Patient Moderate | |
| 99205 | OF--New Patient High | |
| **OFFICE VISITS - SYMPTOMATIC - ESTABLISHED** | | |
| 99211 | OF--Established Patient Minimal | |
| 99212 | OF--Established Patient Low | |
| 99213 | OF--Established Patient Detailed | X |
| 99214 | OF--Established Patient Moderate | |
| 99215 | OF--Established Patient High | |
| **PREVENTIVE VISITS - NEW** | | |
| 99381 | Under 1 Year | |
| 99382 | 1 - 4 Years | |
| 99383 | 5 - 11 Years | |
| 99384 | 12 - 17 Years | |
| 99385 | 18 - 39 Years | |
| 99386 | 40 - 64 Years | |
| 99387 | 65 Years & Up | |
| **PREVENTIVE VISITS - ESTABLISHED** | | |
| 99391 | Under 1 Year | |
| 99392 | 1 - 4 Years | |
| 99393 | 5 - 11 Years | |
| 99394 | 12 - 17 Years | |
| 99395 | 18 - 39 Years | |
| 99396 | 40 - 64 Years | |
| 99397 | 65 Years & Up | |
| **HOSPITAL/NURSING HOME VISITS** | | |
| 99221 | Initial hospital care, det. | |
| 99222 | Initial hospital care, comp. | |
| 99223 | Initial hospital care, high | |
| 99281 | ER Visit, min. | |
| 99282 | ER Visit, low | |
| 99283 | ER Visit, det. | |
| 99284 | ER Visit, moderate | |
| 99285 | ER Visit, high | |
| 99307 | Subseq. nursing facility care, pf. | |
| | | |

| PROCEDURES | | |
|---|---|---|
| 10060 | Incision/drainage, abscess | |
| 20610 | Aspiration, bursa | |
| 29505 | Splint, long leg | |
| 29515 | Splint, short leg | |
| 36415 | Routine venipuncture | |
| 45330 | Sigmoidoscopy, flex | |
| 46600 | Anoscopy, diagnostic | |
| 71030 | Chest x-ray, complete | |
| 73610 | Radiology, ankle, complete | |
| 93000 | Routine ECG | |
| 93018 | Cardiovascular stress test | |
| 99070 | Supplies and materials | X |
| **LABORATORY** | | |
| 80050 | General health panel | |
| 81000 | Urinalysis, complete | |
| 82270 | Blood, occult, feces screening | |
| 82607 | Vitamin B-12 test | |
| 82948 | Glucose, blood reagent | |
| 85027 | CBC, automated | |
| 85651 | Sedimentation rate test, manual | |
| 86360 | Absolute CD4/CD8 ratio | |
| 86592 | Syphilis test | |
| 87070 | Throat culture | |
| 87088 | Urine culture | |
| 88150 | Cytopathology, cervical or vaginal | |
| **INJECTIONS** | | |
| 90471 | Immunization administration | |
| 90472 | Immunization administration, 2nd | |
| 90658 | Influenza injection, ages >3 | |
| 90702 | DT immunization, ages <7 | |
| 90703 | Tetanus immunization | |
| 90707 | MMR immunization | |
| 96372 | Therapeutic injection | |
| 90723 | DTaP - HepB - IPV | |
| 90732 | Pneumococcal immunization | |
| | | |
| | | |

| POLARIS MEDICAL GROUP | | NOTES |
|---|---|---|
| REFERRING PHYSICIAN | NPI | **99070 supplies and materials $15.00** |
| AUTHORIZATION # | | |
| DIAGNOSIS **J45.20** | | |
| PAYMENT AMOUNT | | |

# ENCOUNTER FORM

| | |
|---|---|
| 6/15/2018  DATE | 4:00pm  TIME |

**Dr. Michael Mahabir**
PROVIDER

**Alan J. Harcar**
PATIENT NAME

**HARCAALO**
CHART #

| OFFICE VISITS - SYMPTOMATIC - NEW | | |
|---|---|---|
| 99201 | OF--New Patient Minimal | |
| 99202 | OF--New Patient Low | |
| 99203 | OF--New Patient Detailed | |
| 99204 | OF--New Patient Moderate | |
| 99205 | OF--New Patient High | |
| **OFFICE VISITS - SYMPTOMATIC - ESTABLISHED** | | |
| 99211 | OF--Established Patient Minimal | |
| 99212 | OF--Established Patient Low | |
| 99213 | OF--Established Patient Detailed | |
| 99214 | OF--Established Patient Moderate | |
| 99215 | OF--Established Patient High | |
| **PREVENTIVE VISITS - NEW** | | |
| 99381 | Under 1 Year | |
| 99382 | 1 - 4 Years | |
| 99383 | 5 - 11 Years | |
| 99384 | 12 - 17 Years | |
| 99385 | 18 - 39 Years | |
| 99386 | 40 - 64 Years | |
| 99387 | 65 Years & Up | |
| **PREVENTIVE VISITS - ESTABLISHED** | | |
| 99391 | Under 1 Year | |
| 99392 | 1 - 4 Years | |
| 99393 | 5 - 11 Years | |
| 99394 | 12 - 17 Years | |
| 99395 | 18 - 39 Years | |
| 99396 | 40 - 64 Years | |
| 99397 | 65 Years & Up | X |
| **HOSPITAL/NURSING HOME VISITS** | | |
| 99221 | Initial hospital care, det. | |
| 99222 | Initial hospital care, comp. | |
| 99223 | Initial hospital care, high | |
| 99281 | ER Visit, min. | |
| 99282 | ER Visit, low | |
| 99283 | ER Visit, det. | |
| 99284 | ER Visit, moderate | |
| 99285 | ER Visit, high | |
| 99307 | Subseq. nursing facility care, pf. | |
| | | |
| | | |

| PROCEDURES | | |
|---|---|---|
| 10060 | Incision/drainage, abscess | |
| 20610 | Aspiration, bursa | |
| 29505 | Splint, long leg | |
| 29515 | Splint, short leg | |
| 36415 | Routine venipuncture | X |
| 45330 | Sigmoidoscopy, flex | |
| 46600 | Anoscopy, diagnostic | |
| 71030 | Chest x-ray, complete | |
| 73610 | Radiology, ankle, complete | |
| 93000 | Routine ECG | X |
| 93018 | Cardiovascular stress test | |
| 99070 | Supplies and materials | |
| **LABORATORY** | | |
| 80050 | General health panel | X |
| 81000 | Urinalysis, complete | X |
| 82270 | Blood, occult, feces screening | |
| 82607 | Vitamin B-12 test | |
| 82948 | Glucose, blood reagent | |
| 85027 | CBC, automated | |
| 85651 | Sedimentation rate test, manual | |
| 86360 | Absolute CD4/CD8 ratio | |
| 86592 | Syphilis test | |
| 87070 | Throat culture | |
| 87088 | Urine culture | |
| 88150 | Cytopathology, cervical or vaginal | |
| **INJECTIONS** | | |
| 90471 | Immunization administration | |
| 90472 | Immunization administration, 2nd | |
| 90658 | Influenza injection, ages >3 | |
| 90702 | DT immunization, ages <7 | |
| 90703 | Tetanus immunization | |
| 90707 | MMR immunization | |
| 96372 | Therapeutic injection | |
| 90723 | DTaP - HepB - IPV | |
| 90732 | Pneumococcal immunization | |
| | | |
| | | |

## POLARIS MEDICAL GROUP

| | | NOTES |
|---|---|---|
| REFERRING PHYSICIAN | NPI | |
| AUTHORIZATION # | | |
| DIAGNOSIS  Z00.00 | | |
| PAYMENT AMOUNT  $18.00 copay, check #1024 | | |

**Diagnosis and Procedure Codes: Hospital Visit**

Patient:    Myrna Beedon

Subject:    Hospital Visit, 6/18/18

ICD:        Q24.9

CPT:        99222

# PATIENT INFORMATION FORM

## THIS SECTION REFERS TO PATIENT ONLY

| | | | |
|---|---|---|---|
| Name:<br>Fran C. Ferrone | Sex:<br>F | Marital Status:<br>☐ S ☐ M ☒ D ☐ W | Birth Date:<br>3/30/58 |

| | |
|---|---|
| Address:<br>1050 Southway | SS#:<br>332-75-9360 |

| | | | | |
|---|---|---|---|---|
| City:<br>Fairview | State:<br>OH | Zip:<br>43773 | Employer:<br>Woodworkers Warehouse (full-time) | Phone:<br>999-555-9001 |

| | |
|---|---|
| Home Phone:<br>999-555-7735 | Employer's Address:<br>301 Valley Plaza |

| | | | |
|---|---|---|---|
| Work Phone: | City:<br>Fairview | State:<br>OH | Zip:<br>43773 |

| | | |
|---|---|---|
| Race:<br><br>__American Indian or Alaska Native   __Other<br>__Asian   __Native Hawaiian or Other Pacific Islander<br>__Black or African American<br>X_White   __Declined | Ethnicity:<br><br>__Hispanic or Latino<br>X_Non-Hispanic or Latino<br>__Declined | Language:<br>English |

| | |
|---|---|
| Spouse's Name: | Spouse's Employer: |

| | | |
|---|---|---|
| Emergency Contact:<br>Ann Ferrone | Relationship:<br>daughter | Phone #:<br>999-555-3237 |

## FILL IN IF PATIENT IS A MINOR

| | | | |
|---|---|---|---|
| Parent/Guardian's Name: | Sex: | Marital Status:<br>☐ S ☐ M ☐ D ☐ W | Birth Date: |

| | |
|---|---|
| Phone: | SS#: |

| | | |
|---|---|---|
| Address: | Employer: | Phone: |

| | |
|---|---|
| City:   State:   Zip: | Employer's Address: |

| | | | |
|---|---|---|---|
| Student Status: | City: | State: | Zip: |

## INSURANCE INFORMATION

| | |
|---|---|
| Primary Insurance Company:<br>Blue Cross/Blue Shield of Ohio | Secondary Insurance Company: |

| | | | |
|---|---|---|---|
| Subscriber's Name:<br>Fran C. Ferrone | Birth Date:<br>3/30/58 | Subscriber's Name: | Birth Date: |

| | | |
|---|---|---|
| Plan:<br>Traditional | SS#:<br>332-75-9360 | Plan: |

| | | | |
|---|---|---|---|
| Policy #:<br>XRS332759360 | Group #: | Policy #: | Group #: |

| | | |
|---|---|---|
| Copayment/Deductible:<br>$500 deductible | Price Code:<br>A | |

## OTHER INFORMATION

| | |
|---|---|
| Reason for visit:<br>cough | Allergy to Medication (list): |

| | |
|---|---|
| Name of referring physician: | If auto accident, list date and state in which it occurred: |

I authorize treatment and agree to pay all fees and charges for the person named above. I agree to pay all charges shown by statements, promptly upon their presentation, unless credit arrangements are agreed upon in writing.

I authorize payment directly to POLARIS MEDICAL GROUP of insurance benefits otherwise payable to me. I hereby authorize the release of any medical information necessary in order to process a claim for payment in my behalf.

| | |
|---|---|
| Fran C. Ferrone | 6/18/18 |
| (Patient's Signature/Parent or Guardian's Signature) | (Date) |

I plan to make payment of my medical expenses as follows (check one or more):

X_Insurance (as above)   X_Cash/Check/Credit/Debit Card   ___Medicare   ___Medicaid   ___Workers' Comp.

# ENCOUNTER FORM

| 6/18/2018 | 9:00am | Dr. Robin Crebore |
|---|---|---|
| DATE | TIME | PROVIDER |

| Fran C. Ferrone | FERROFRO |
|---|---|
| PATIENT NAME | CHART # |

| OFFICE VISITS - SYMPTOMATIC - NEW | | |
|---|---|---|
| 99201 | OF--New Patient Minimal | |
| 99202 | OF--New Patient Low | X |
| 99203 | OF--New Patient Detailed | |
| 99204 | OF--New Patient Moderate | |
| 99205 | OF--New Patient High | |
| **OFFICE VISITS - SYMPTOMATIC - ESTABLISHED** | | |
| 99211 | OF--Established Patient Minimal | |
| 99212 | OF--Established Patient Low | |
| 99213 | OF--Established Patient Detailed | |
| 99214 | OF--Established Patient Moderate | |
| 99215 | OF--Established Patient High | |
| **PREVENTIVE VISITS - NEW** | | |
| 99381 | Under 1 Year | |
| 99382 | 1 - 4 Years | |
| 99383 | 5 - 11 Years | |
| 99384 | 12 - 17 Years | |
| 99385 | 18 - 39 Years | |
| 99386 | 40 - 64 Years | |
| 99387 | 65 Years & Up | |
| **PREVENTIVE VISITS - ESTABLISHED** | | |
| 99391 | Under 1 Year | |
| 99392 | 1 - 4 Years | |
| 99393 | 5 - 11 Years | |
| 99394 | 12 - 17 Years | |
| 99395 | 18 - 39 Years | |
| 99396 | 40 - 64 Years | |
| 99397 | 65 Years & Up | |
| **HOSPITAL/NURSING HOME VISITS** | | |
| 99221 | Initial hospital care, det. | |
| 99222 | Initial hospital care, comp. | |
| 99223 | Initial hospital care, high | |
| 99281 | ER Visit, min. | |
| 99282 | ER Visit, low | |
| 99283 | ER Visit, det. | |
| 99284 | ER Visit, moderate | |
| 99285 | ER Visit, high | |
| 99307 | Subseq. nursing facility care, pf. | |
| | | |

| PROCEDURES | | |
|---|---|---|
| 10060 | Incision/drainage, abscess | |
| 20610 | Aspiration, bursa | |
| 29505 | Splint, long leg | |
| 29515 | Splint, short leg | |
| 36415 | Routine venipuncture | |
| 45330 | Sigmoidoscopy, flex | |
| 46600 | Anoscopy, diagnostic | |
| 71030 | Chest x-ray, complete | |
| 73610 | Radiology, ankle, complete | |
| 93000 | Routine ECG | |
| 93018 | Cardiovascular stress test | |
| 99070 | Supplies and materials | |
| **LABORATORY** | | |
| 80050 | General health panel | |
| 81000 | Urinalysis, complete | |
| 82270 | Blood, occult, feces screening | |
| 82607 | Vitamin B-12 test | |
| 82948 | Glucose, blood reagent | |
| 85027 | CBC, automated | |
| 85651 | Sedimentation rate test, manual | |
| 86360 | Absolute CD4/CD8 ratio | |
| 86592 | Syphilis test | |
| 87070 | Throat culture | |
| 87088 | Urine culture | |
| 88150 | Cytopathology, cervical or vaginal | |
| **INJECTIONS** | | |
| 90471 | Immunization administration | |
| 90472 | Immunization administration, 2nd | |
| 90658 | Influenza injection, ages >3 | |
| 90702 | DT immunization, ages <7 | |
| 90703 | Tetanus immunization | |
| 90707 | MMR immunization | |
| 96372 | Therapeutic injection | |
| 90723 | DTaP - HepB - IPV | |
| 90732 | Pneumococcal immunization | |
| | | |
| | | |

## POLARIS MEDICAL GROUP

| REFERRING PHYSICIAN | NPI | NOTES |
|---|---|---|
| AUTHORIZATION # | | |
| DIAGNOSIS **J40** | | |
| PAYMENT AMOUNT | | |

# ENCOUNTER FORM

| | | | |
|---|---|---|---|
| **6/18/2018** | **9:30am** | **Dr. Michael Mahabir** | |
| DATE | TIME | PROVIDER | |
| **Jimmy R. Hellery** | | **HELLEJIO** | |
| PATIENT NAME | | CHART # | |

| **OFFICE VISITS - SYMPTOMATIC - NEW** | | |
|---|---|---|
| 99201 | OF--New Patient Minimal | |
| 99202 | OF--New Patient Low | |
| 99203 | OF--New Patient Detailed | |
| 99204 | OF--New Patient Moderate | |
| 99205 | OF--New Patient High | |
| **OFFICE VISITS - SYMPTOMATIC - ESTABLISHED** | | |
| 99211 | OF--Established Patient Minimal | |
| 99212 | OF--Established Patient Low | X |
| 99213 | OF--Established Patient Detailed | |
| 99214 | OF--Established Patient Moderate | |
| 99215 | OF--Established Patient High | |
| **PREVENTIVE VISITS - NEW** | | |
| 99381 | Under 1 Year | |
| 99382 | 1 - 4 Years | |
| 99383 | 5 - 11 Years | |
| 99384 | 12 - 17 Years | |
| 99385 | 18 - 39 Years | |
| 99386 | 40 - 64 Years | |
| 99387 | 65 Years & Up | |
| **PREVENTIVE VISITS - ESTABLISHED** | | |
| 99391 | Under 1 Year | |
| 99392 | 1 - 4 Years | |
| 99393 | 5 - 11 Years | |
| 99394 | 12 - 17 Years | |
| 99395 | 18 - 39 Years | |
| 99396 | 40 - 64 Years | |
| 99397 | 65 Years & Up | |
| **HOSPITAL/NURSING HOME VISITS** | | |
| 99221 | Initial hospital care, det. | |
| 99222 | Initial hospital care, comp. | |
| 99223 | Initial hospital care, high | |
| 99281 | ER Visit, min. | |
| 99282 | ER Visit, low | |
| 99283 | ER Visit, det. | |
| 99284 | ER Visit, moderate | |
| 99285 | ER Visit, high | |
| 99307 | Subseq. nursing facility care, pf. | |

| **PROCEDURES** | | |
|---|---|---|
| 10060 | Incision/drainage, abscess | |
| 20610 | Aspiration, bursa | |
| 29505 | Splint, long leg | |
| 29515 | Splint, short leg | |
| 36415 | Routine venipuncture | |
| 45330 | Sigmoidoscopy, flex | |
| 46600 | Anoscopy, diagnostic | |
| 71030 | Chest x-ray, complete | |
| 73610 | Radiology, ankle, complete | |
| 93000 | Routine ECG | |
| 93018 | Cardiovascular stress test | |
| 99070 | Supplies and materials | |
| **LABORATORY** | | |
| 80050 | General health panel | |
| 81000 | Urinalysis, complete | |
| 82270 | Blood, occult, feces screening | |
| 82607 | Vitamin B-12 test | |
| 82948 | Glucose, blood reagent | |
| 85027 | CBC, automated | |
| 85651 | Sedimentation rate test, manual | |
| 86360 | Absolute CD4/CD8 ratio | |
| 86592 | Syphilis test | |
| 87070 | Throat culture | X |
| 87088 | Urine culture | |
| 88150 | Cytopathology, cervical or vaginal | |
| **INJECTIONS** | | |
| 90471 | Immunization administration | |
| 90472 | Immunization administration, 2nd | |
| 90658 | Influenza injection, ages >3 | |
| 90702 | DT immunization, ages <7 | |
| 90703 | Tetanus immunization | |
| 90707 | MMR immunization | |
| 96372 | Therapeutic injection | |
| 90723 | DTaP - HepB - IPV | |
| 90732 | Pneumococcal immunization | |
| | | |
| | | |

## POLARIS MEDICAL GROUP

| | | NOTES |
|---|---|---|
| REFERRING PHYSICIAN | NPI | |
| AUTHORIZATION # | | |
| DIAGNOSIS **J02.2** | | |
| PAYMENT AMOUNT **$8.25 copay, check #1019** | | |

# ENCOUNTER FORM

| | |
|---|---|
| 6/18/2018   10:00am | Dr. Robin Crebore |
| DATE        TIME | PROVIDER |
| Floyd S. Deysenrothe | DEYSEFLO |
| PATIENT NAME | CHART # |

| OFFICE VISITS - SYMPTOMATIC - NEW | | |
|---|---|---|
| 99201 | OF--New Patient Minimal | |
| 99202 | OF--New Patient Low | |
| 99203 | OF--New Patient Detailed | |
| 99204 | OF--New Patient Moderate | |
| 99205 | OF--New Patient High | |

| OFFICE VISITS - SYMPTOMATIC - ESTABLISHED | | |
|---|---|---|
| 99211 | OF--Established Patient Minimal | |
| 99212 | OF--Established Patient Low | |
| 99213 | OF--Established Patient Detailed | |
| 99214 | OF--Established Patient Moderate | |
| 99215 | OF--Established Patient High | |

| PREVENTIVE VISITS - NEW | | |
|---|---|---|
| 99381 | Under 1 Year | |
| 99382 | 1 - 4 Years | |
| 99383 | 5 - 11 Years | |
| 99384 | 12 - 17 Years | |
| 99385 | 18 - 39 Years | |
| 99386 | 40 - 64 Years | |
| 99387 | 65 Years & Up | |

| PREVENTIVE VISITS - ESTABLISHED | | |
|---|---|---|
| 99391 | Under 1 Year | |
| 99392 | 1 - 4 Years | |
| 99393 | 5 - 11 Years | |
| 99394 | 12 - 17 Years | |
| 99395 | 18 - 39 Years | |
| 99396 | 40 - 64 Years | |
| 99397 | 65 Years & Up | |

| HOSPITAL/NURSING HOME VISITS | | |
|---|---|---|
| 99221 | Initial hospital care, det. | |
| 99222 | Initial hospital care, comp. | |
| 99223 | Initial hospital care, high | |
| 99281 | ER Visit, min. | |
| 99282 | ER Visit, low | |
| 99283 | ER Visit, det. | |
| 99284 | ER Visit, moderate | |
| 99285 | ER Visit, high | |
| 99307 | Subseq. nursing facility care, pf. | |
| | | |
| | | |

| PROCEDURES | | |
|---|---|---|
| 10060 | Incision/drainage, abscess | |
| 20610 | Aspiration, bursa | |
| 29505 | Splint, long leg | |
| 29515 | Splint, short leg | |
| 36415 | Routine venipuncture | |
| 45330 | Sigmoidoscopy, flex | |
| 46600 | Anoscopy, diagnostic | |
| 71030 | Chest x-ray, complete | |
| 73610 | Radiology, ankle, complete | |
| 93000 | Routine ECG | |
| 93018 | Cardiovascular stress test | |
| 99070 | Supplies and materials | |

| LABORATORY | | |
|---|---|---|
| 80050 | General health panel | |
| 81000 | Urinalysis, complete | |
| 82270 | Blood, occult, feces screening | |
| 82607 | Vitamin B-12 test | |
| 82948 | Glucose, blood reagent | |
| 85027 | CBC, automated | |
| 85651 | Sedimentation rate test, manual | |
| 86360 | Absolute CD4/CD8 ratio | |
| 86592 | Syphilis test | |
| 87070 | Throat culture | |
| 87088 | Urine culture | |
| 88150 | Cytopathology, cervical or vaginal | |

| INJECTIONS | | |
|---|---|---|
| 90471 | Immunization administration | X |
| 90472 | Immunization administration, 2nd | |
| 90658 | Influenza injection, ages >3 | |
| 90702 | DT immunization, ages <7 | |
| 90703 | Tetanus immunization | X |
| 90707 | MMR immunization | |
| 96372 | Therapeutic injection | |
| 90723 | DTaP - HepB - IPV | |
| 90732 | Pneumococcal immunization | |
| | | |
| | | |

## POLARIS MEDICAL GROUP

| | | NOTES |
|---|---|---|
| REFERRING PHYSICIAN | NPI | |
| AUTHORIZATION # | | |
| DIAGNOSIS | | |
| Z23 | | |
| PAYMENT AMOUNT | | |
| $12.00 copay, check #1117 | | |

Blue Cross Blue Shield of Ohio
5000 First Street
Worthington, OH 43085

Polaris Medical Group
2100 Grace Avenue
Columbus, OH 43214

Practice ID: 04-5678901

Date Prepared: 6/18/18                                              EFT Number: 1238963

| Patient's Name | Dates of Service From - Thru | POS | Proc | Qty | Charge Amount | Allowed Amount | Patient Resp. | Amt. Paid Provider |
|---|---|---|---|---|---|---|---|---|
| Brown, William | 5/4/18 – 5/4/18 | 11 | 99213 | 1 | $72.00 | $72.00 | $21.60 | $50.40 |
| | | | | | | | | |
| Totals | | | | | $72.00 | $72.00 | $21.60 | $50.40 |

* * * * * * *     *EFT transmitted in the amount of $50.40*     * * * * * * *

# ENCOUNTER FORM

| | |
|---|---|
| **6/18/2018**     **4:15pm** | **Dr. Robin Crebore** |
| DATE            TIME | PROVIDER |
| **Elizabeth I. Wu** | **WUELIZA0** |
| PATIENT NAME | CHART # |

| OFFICE VISITS - SYMPTOMATIC - NEW | | |
|---|---|---|
| 99201 | OF--New Patient Minimal | |
| 99202 | OF--New Patient Low | |
| 99203 | OF--New Patient Detailed | |
| 99204 | OF--New Patient Moderate | |
| 99205 | OF--New Patient High | |

| OFFICE VISITS - SYMPTOMATIC - ESTABLISHED | | |
|---|---|---|
| 99211 | OF--Established Patient Minimal | |
| 99212 | OF--Established Patient Low | X |
| 99213 | OF--Established Patient Detailed | |
| 99214 | OF--Established Patient Moderate | |
| 99215 | OF--Established Patient High | |

| PREVENTIVE VISITS - NEW | | |
|---|---|---|
| 99381 | Under 1 Year | |
| 99382 | 1 - 4 Years | |
| 99383 | 5 - 11 Years | |
| 99384 | 12 - 17 Years | |
| 99385 | 18 - 39 Years | |
| 99386 | 40 - 64 Years | |
| 99387 | 65 Years & Up | |

| PREVENTIVE VISITS - ESTABLISHED | | |
|---|---|---|
| 99391 | Under 1 Year | |
| 99392 | 1 - 4 Years | |
| 99393 | 5 - 11 Years | |
| 99394 | 12 - 17 Years | |
| 99395 | 18 - 39 Years | |
| 99396 | 40 - 64 Years | |
| 99397 | 65 Years & Up | |

| HOSPITAL/NURSING HOME VISITS | | |
|---|---|---|
| 99221 | Initial hospital care, det. | |
| 99222 | Initial hospital care, comp. | |
| 99223 | Initial hospital care, high | |
| 99281 | ER Visit, min. | |
| 99282 | ER Visit, low | |
| 99283 | ER Visit, det. | |
| 99284 | ER Visit, moderate | |
| 99285 | ER Visit, high | |
| 99307 | Subseq. nursing facility care, pf. | |

| PROCEDURES | | |
|---|---|---|
| 10060 | Incision/drainage, abscess | |
| 20610 | Aspiration, bursa | |
| 29505 | Splint, long leg | |
| 29515 | Splint, short leg | |
| 36415 | Routine venipuncture | |
| 45330 | Sigmoidoscopy, flex | |
| 46600 | Anoscopy, diagnostic | |
| 71030 | Chest x-ray, complete | |
| 73610 | Radiology, ankle, complete | |
| 93000 | Routine ECG | |
| 93018 | Cardiovascular stress test | |
| 99070 | Supplies and materials | |

| LABORATORY | | |
|---|---|---|
| 80050 | General health panel | |
| 81000 | Urinalysis, complete | |
| 82270 | Blood, occult, feces screening | |
| 82607 | Vitamin B-12 test | |
| 82948 | Glucose, blood reagent | |
| 85027 | CBC, automated | |
| 85651 | Sedimentation rate test, manual | |
| 86360 | Absolute CD4/CD8 ratio | |
| 86592 | Syphilis test | |
| 87070 | Throat culture | |
| 87088 | Urine culture | |
| 88150 | Cytopathology, cervical or vaginal | |

| INJECTIONS | | |
|---|---|---|
| 90471 | Immunization administration | |
| 90472 | Immunization administration, 2nd | |
| 90658 | Influenza injection, ages >3 | |
| 90702 | DT immunization, ages <7 | |
| 90703 | Tetanus immunization | |
| 90707 | MMR immunization | |
| 96372 | Therapeutic injection | |
| 90723 | DTaP - HepB - IPV | |
| 90732 | Pneumococcal immunization | |
| | | |
| | | |

## POLARIS MEDICAL GROUP

| | | NOTES |
|---|---|---|
| REFERRING PHYSICIAN | NPI | |
| AUTHORIZATION # | | |
| DIAGNOSIS **L70.0** | | |
| PAYMENT AMOUNT **$10.00 copay, check #1202** | | |

## Additional ICD Codes

| Code | Description |
|------|-------------|
| Z80.0 | Family history of malignant neoplasm, digestive organs |
| Z39.2 | Routine postpartum follow-up |
| R94.31 | Abnormal ECG |
| I20.9 | Angina pectoris, unspecified |
| I49.9 | Cardiac arrhythmia, unspecified |

# ENCOUNTER FORM

| | |
|---|---|
| **6/19/2018**     **9:45am** | **Dr. Robin Crebore** |
| DATE     TIME | PROVIDER |
| **Flora K. Torres-Gil** | **TORREFLO** |
| PATIENT NAME | CHART # |

| OFFICE VISITS - SYMPTOMATIC - NEW | | |
|---|---|---|
| 99201 | OF--New Patient Minimal | |
| 99202 | OF--New Patient Low | |
| 99203 | OF--New Patient Detailed | |
| 99204 | OF--New Patient Moderate | |
| 99205 | OF--New Patient High | |

| OFFICE VISITS - SYMPTOMATIC - ESTABLISHED | | |
|---|---|---|
| 99211 | OF--Established Patient Minimal | |
| 99212 | OF--Established Patient Low | |
| 99213 | OF--Established Patient Detailed | |
| 99214 | OF--Established Patient Moderate | |
| 99215 | OF--Established Patient High | |

| PREVENTIVE VISITS - NEW | | |
|---|---|---|
| 99381 | Under 1 Year | |
| 99382 | 1 - 4 Years | |
| 99383 | 5 - 11 Years | |
| 99384 | 12 - 17 Years | |
| 99385 | 18 - 39 Years | |
| 99386 | 40 - 64 Years | |
| 99387 | 65 Years & Up | |

| PREVENTIVE VISITS - ESTABLISHED | | |
|---|---|---|
| 99391 | Under 1 Year | |
| 99392 | 1 - 4 Years | |
| 99393 | 5 - 11 Years | |
| 99394 | 12 - 17 Years | |
| 99395 | 18 - 39 Years | |
| 99396 | 40 - 64 Years | |
| 99397 | 65 Years & Up | |

| HOSPITAL/NURSING HOME VISITS | | |
|---|---|---|
| 99221 | Initial hospital care, det. | |
| 99222 | Initial hospital care, comp. | |
| 99223 | Initial hospital care, high | |
| 99281 | ER Visit, min. | |
| 99282 | ER Visit, low | |
| 99283 | ER Visit, det. | |
| 99284 | ER Visit, moderate | |
| 99285 | ER Visit, high | |
| 99307 | Subseq. nursing facility care, pf. | |
| | | |
| | | |

| PROCEDURES | | |
|---|---|---|
| 10060 | Incision/drainage, abscess | |
| 20610 | Aspiration, bursa | X |
| 29505 | Splint, long leg | |
| 29515 | Splint, short leg | |
| 36415 | Routine venipuncture | |
| 45330 | Sigmoidoscopy, flex | |
| 46600 | Anoscopy, diagnostic | |
| 71030 | Chest x-ray, complete | |
| 73610 | Radiology, ankle, complete | |
| 93000 | Routine ECG | |
| 93018 | Cardiovascular stress test | |
| 99070 | Supplies and materials | |

| LABORATORY | | |
|---|---|---|
| 80050 | General health panel | |
| 81000 | Urinalysis, complete | |
| 82270 | Blood, occult, feces screening | |
| 82607 | Vitamin B-12 test | |
| 82948 | Glucose, blood reagent | |
| 85027 | CBC, automated | |
| 85651 | Sedimentation rate test, manual | |
| 86360 | Absolute CD4/CD8 ratio | |
| 86592 | Syphilis test | |
| 87070 | Throat culture | |
| 87088 | Urine culture | |
| 88150 | Cytopathology, cervical or vaginal | |

| INJECTIONS | | |
|---|---|---|
| 90471 | Immunization administration | |
| 90472 | Immunization administration, 2nd | |
| 90658 | Influenza injection, ages >3 | |
| 90702 | DT immunization, ages <7 | |
| 90703 | Tetanus immunization | |
| 90707 | MMR immunization | |
| 96372 | Therapeutic injection | |
| 90723 | DTaP - HepB - IPV | |
| 90732 | Pneumococcal immunization | |
| | | |
| | | |

## POLARIS MEDICAL GROUP

| | | NOTES |
|---|---|---|
| REFERRING PHYSICIAN | NPI | |
| AUTHORIZATION # | | |
| DIAGNOSIS | | |
| **M71.50** | | |
| PAYMENT AMOUNT | | |
| **$5.00 copay, check #1309** | | |

**Information on Ohio Maxcare PPO, 6/19/2018**

**Address Tab**

Ohio Maxcare PPO

4001 Bridgeway Center

Columbus, OH  43214

Office Phone: 800-555-0060

Fax: 999 555-8814

Contact: Sharon Lucas

Plan Name: Maxcare Plus

**Options and Codes Tab**

Procedure Code Set: 1

Diagnosis Code Set: ICD-10

Default Billing Method 1: Electronic

Default Payment Application Codes:

    Payment: PAYMAX

    Adjustment: ADJMAX

    Withhold: WITMAX

    Deductible: DEDMAX

    Take Back: TBKMAX

**EDI/Eligibility Tab**

Primary EDI Receiver: NDCO

Claims Payer ID: 0123

Type: PPO

NDC Record Code: 07

**Allowed Tab**

Allowed Amounts: Refer to SD 48

# POLARIS MEDICAL GROUP
Discounted Fee Schedule: Ohio Maxcare PPO

## OFFICE VISITS - SYMPTOMATIC

### NEW
| | | |
|---|---|---|
| 99201 | OF-New Patient Minimal | 56 |
| 99202 | OF-New Patient Low | 75 |
| 99203 | OF-New Patient Detailed | 103 |
| 99204 | OF-New Patient Moderate | 150 |
| 99205 | OF-New Patient High | 194 |

### ESTABLISHED
| | | |
|---|---|---|
| 99211 | OF-Est. Patient Minimal | 30 |
| 99212 | OF-Est. Patient Low | 46 |
| 99213 | OF-Est. Patient Detailed | 62 |
| 99214 | OF-Est. Patient Moderate | 91 |
| 99215 | OF-Est. Patient High | 140 |

## PREVENTIVE VISITS

### NEW
| | | |
|---|---|---|
| 99381 | Under 1 Year | 140 |
| 99382 | 1 - 4 Years | 146 |
| 99383 | 5 - 11 Years | 143 |
| 99384 | 12 - 17 Years | 178 |
| 99385 | 18 - 39 Years | 166 |
| 99386 | 40 - 64 Years | 180 |
| 99387 | 65 Years & Up | 200 |

### ESTABLISHED
| | | |
|---|---|---|
| 99391 | Under 1 Year | 111 |
| 99392 | 1 - 4 Years | 124 |
| 99393 | 5 - 11 Years | 130 |
| 99394 | 12 - 17 Years | 149 |
| 99395 | 18 - 39 Years | 137 |
| 99396 | 40 - 64 Years | 149 |
| 99397 | 65 Years & Up | 120 |

## HOSPITAL/NURSING HOME VISITS
| | | |
|---|---|---|
| 99221 | Initial hospital care, det. | 160 |
| 99222 | Initial hospital care, comp. | 177 |
| 99223 | Initial hospital care, high | 218 |
| 99281 | ER visit, min. | 87 |
| 99282 | ER visit, low | 109 |
| 99283 | ER visit, det. | 131 |
| 99284 | ER visit, moderate | 153 |
| 99285 | ER visit, high | 175 |
| 99307 | Subseq. nursing facility care, pf. | 54 |

## PROCEDURES
| | | |
|---|---|---|
| 10060 | Incision/drainage, abscess | 98 |
| 20610 | Aspiration, bursa | 91 |
| 29505 | Splint, long leg | 110 |
| 29515 | Splint, short leg | 94 |
| 36415 | Routine venipuncture | 17 |
| 45330 | Sigmoidoscopy, flex | 226 |
| 46600 | Anoscopy, collection | 72 |
| 71030 | Chest x-ray, complete | 128 |
| 73610 | Radiology, ankle, complete | 94 |
| 93000 | Routine ECG | 70 |
| 93018 | Cardiovascular stress test | 162 |
| 99070 | Supplies and materials | 0 |

## LABORATORY
| | | |
|---|---|---|
| 80050 | General health panel | 120 |
| 81000 | Urinalysis, complete | 17 |
| 82270 | Blood, occult, feces screening | 15 |
| 82607 | Vitamin B-12 test | 72 |
| 82948 | Glucose, blood reagent | 15 |
| 85027 | CBC, automated | 27 |
| 85651 | Sedimentation rate test, manual | 20 |
| 86360 | Absolute CD4/CD8 ratio | 195 |
| 86592 | Syphilis test | 20 |
| 87070 | Throat culture | 38 |
| 87088 | Urine culture | 34 |
| 88150 | Cytopathology, cervical or vaginal | 29 |

## INJECTIONS
| | | |
|---|---|---|
| 90471 | Immunization administration | 14 |
| 90472 | Immunization administration, 2nd | 8 |
| 90658 | Influenza injection, ages >3 | 23 |
| 90702 | DT immunization, ages <7 | 27 |
| 90703 | Tetanus immunization | 24 |
| 90707 | MMR immunization | 75 |
| 96372 | Therapeutic injection | 20 |
| 90723 | DTaP - HepB - IPV | 67 |
| 90732 | Pneumococcal immunization | 32 |

| | | |
|---|---|---|
| LABINS | Lab Charges - Inside | 0 |
| LABOUT | Lab Charges - Outside | 0 |
| NSFFEE | Returned Check Fee | 35 |

# ENCOUNTER FORM

| | |
|---|---|
| **6/19/2018**     **10:45am** | **Dr. Robin Crebore** |
| DATE         TIME | PROVIDER |
| **Diana E. O'Keefe** | **OKEEFDIO** |
| PATIENT NAME | CHART # |

| OFFICE VISITS - SYMPTOMATIC - NEW | | |
|---|---|---|
| 99201 | OF--New Patient Minimal | |
| 99202 | OF--New Patient Low | |
| 99203 | OF--New Patient Detailed | |
| 99204 | OF--New Patient Moderate | |
| 99205 | OF--New Patient High | |

| OFFICE VISITS - SYMPTOMATIC - ESTABLISHED | | |
|---|---|---|
| 99211 | OF--Established Patient Minimal | X |
| 99212 | OF--Established Patient Low | |
| 99213 | OF--Established Patient Detailed | |
| 99214 | OF--Established Patient Moderate | |
| 99215 | OF--Established Patient High | |

| PREVENTIVE VISITS - NEW | | |
|---|---|---|
| 99381 | Under 1 Year | |
| 99382 | 1 - 4 Years | |
| 99383 | 5 - 11 Years | |
| 99384 | 12 - 17 Years | |
| 99385 | 18 - 39 Years | |
| 99386 | 40 - 64 Years | |
| 99387 | 65 Years & Up | |

| PREVENTIVE VISITS - ESTABLISHED | | |
|---|---|---|
| 99391 | Under 1 Year | |
| 99392 | 1 - 4 Years | |
| 99393 | 5 - 11 Years | |
| 99394 | 12 - 17 Years | |
| 99395 | 18 - 39 Years | |
| 99396 | 40 - 64 Years | |
| 99397 | 65 Years & Up | |

| HOSPITAL/NURSING HOME VISITS | | |
|---|---|---|
| 99221 | Initial hospital care, det. | |
| 99222 | Initial hospital care, comp. | |
| 99223 | Initial hospital care, high | |
| 99281 | ER Visit, min. | |
| 99282 | ER Visit, low | |
| 99283 | ER Visit, det. | |
| 99284 | ER Visit, moderate | |
| 99285 | ER Visit, high | |
| 99307 | Subseq. nursing facility care, pf. | |

| PROCEDURES | | |
|---|---|---|
| 10060 | Incision/drainage, abscess | |
| 20610 | Aspiration, bursa | |
| 29505 | Splint, long leg | |
| 29515 | Splint, short leg | |
| 36415 | Routine venipuncture | |
| 45330 | Sigmoidoscopy, flex | |
| 46600 | Anoscopy, diagnostic | |
| 71030 | Chest x-ray, complete | |
| 73610 | Radiology, ankle, complete | |
| 93000 | Routine ECG | |
| 93018 | Cardiovascular stress test | |
| 99070 | Supplies and materials | |

| LABORATORY | | |
|---|---|---|
| 80050 | General health panel | |
| 81000 | Urinalysis, complete | |
| 82270 | Blood, occult, feces screening | |
| 82607 | Vitamin B-12 test | |
| 82948 | Glucose, blood reagent | |
| 85027 | CBC, automated | |
| 85651 | Sedimentation rate test, manual | X |
| 86360 | Absolute CD4/CD8 ratio | |
| 86592 | Syphilis test | |
| 87070 | Throat culture | |
| 87088 | Urine culture | |
| 88150 | Cytopathology, cervical or vaginal | |

| INJECTIONS | | |
|---|---|---|
| 90471 | Immunization administration | |
| 90472 | Immunization administration, 2nd | |
| 90658 | Influenza injection, ages >3 | |
| 90702 | DT immunization, ages <7 | |
| 90703 | Tetanus immunization | |
| 90707 | MMR immunization | |
| 96372 | Therapeutic injection | |
| 90723 | DTaP - HepB - IPV | |
| 90732 | Pneumococcal immunization | |

## POLARIS MEDICAL GROUP

| | | NOTES |
|---|---|---|
| REFERRING PHYSICIAN | NPI | |
| AUTHORIZATION # | | |
| DIAGNOSIS **M06.9** | | |
| PAYMENT AMOUNT | | |

# ENCOUNTER FORM

| 6/20/2018 | 9:00am |
|---|---|
| DATE | TIME |

**Felidia E. Jonas**
PATIENT NAME

**Dr. Robin Crebore**
PROVIDER

**JONASFE0**
CHART #

| OFFICE VISITS - SYMPTOMATIC - NEW | | |
|---|---|---|
| 99201 | OF--New Patient Minimal | |
| 99202 | OF--New Patient Low | |
| 99203 | OF--New Patient Detailed | |
| 99204 | OF--New Patient Moderate | |
| 99205 | OF--New Patient High | |
| **OFFICE VISITS - SYMPTOMATIC - ESTABLISHED** | | |
| 99211 | OF--Established Patient Minimal | X |
| 99212 | OF--Established Patient Low | |
| 99213 | OF--Established Patient Detailed | |
| 99214 | OF--Established Patient Moderate | |
| 99215 | OF--Established Patient High | |
| **PREVENTIVE VISITS - NEW** | | |
| 99381 | Under 1 Year | |
| 99382 | 1 - 4 Years | |
| 99383 | 5 - 11 Years | |
| 99384 | 12 - 17 Years | |
| 99385 | 18 - 39 Years | |
| 99386 | 40 - 64 Years | |
| 99387 | 65 Years & Up | |
| **PREVENTIVE VISITS - ESTABLISHED** | | |
| 99391 | Under 1 Year | |
| 99392 | 1 - 4 Years | |
| 99393 | 5 - 11 Years | |
| 99394 | 12 - 17 Years | |
| 99395 | 18 - 39 Years | |
| 99396 | 40 - 64 Years | |
| 99397 | 65 Years & Up | |
| **HOSPITAL/NURSING HOME VISITS** | | |
| 99221 | Initial hospital care, det. | |
| 99222 | Initial hospital care, comp. | |
| 99223 | Initial hospital care, high | |
| 99281 | ER Visit, min. | |
| 99282 | ER Visit, low | |
| 99283 | ER Visit, det. | |
| 99284 | ER Visit, moderate | |
| 99285 | ER Visit, high | |
| 99307 | Subseq. nursing facility care, pf. | |
| | | |
| | | |

| PROCEDURES | | |
|---|---|---|
| 10060 | Incision/drainage, abscess | |
| 20610 | Aspiration, bursa | |
| 29505 | Splint, long leg | |
| 29515 | Splint, short leg | |
| 36415 | Routine venipuncture | |
| 45330 | Sigmoidoscopy, flex | |
| 46600 | Anoscopy, diagnostic | |
| 71030 | Chest x-ray, complete | |
| 73610 | Radiology, ankle, complete | |
| 93000 | Routine ECG | |
| 93018 | Cardiovascular stress test | |
| 99070 | Supplies and materials | |
| **LABORATORY** | | |
| 80050 | General health panel | |
| 81000 | Urinalysis, complete | |
| 82270 | Blood, occult, feces screening | |
| 82607 | Vitamin B-12 test | |
| 82948 | Glucose, blood reagent | |
| 85027 | CBC, automated | |
| 85651 | Sedimentation rate test, manual | |
| 86360 | Absolute CD4/CD8 ratio | |
| 86592 | Syphilis test | |
| 87070 | Throat culture | |
| 87088 | Urine culture | |
| 88150 | Cytopathology, cervical or vaginal | |
| **INJECTIONS** | | |
| 90471 | Immunization administration | |
| 90472 | Immunization administration, 2nd | |
| 90658 | Influenza injection, ages >3 | |
| 90702 | DT immunization, ages <7 | |
| 90703 | Tetanus immunization | |
| 90707 | MMR immunization | |
| 96372 | Therapeutic injection | |
| 90723 | DTaP - HepB - IPV | |
| 90732 | Pneumococcal immunization | |
| | | |
| | | |

## POLARIS MEDICAL GROUP

| REFERRING PHYSICIAN | NPI |
|---|---|
| | |

AUTHORIZATION #

DIAGNOSIS
**L01.00**

PAYMENT AMOUNT
**$15.00 copay, check #2349**

NOTES

# ENCOUNTER FORM

**6/20/2018**          **10:00am**                              **Dr. Robin Crebore**
DATE                         TIME                                       PROVIDER

**Cynthia I. Cashell**                                            **CASHECYO**
PATIENT NAME                                                 CHART #

| OFFICE VISITS - SYMPTOMATIC - NEW | | |
|---|---|---|
| 99201 | OF--New Patient Minimal | |
| 99202 | OF--New Patient Low | |
| 99203 | OF--New Patient Detailed | |
| 99204 | OF--New Patient Moderate | |
| 99205 | OF--New Patient High | |

| OFFICE VISITS - SYMPTOMATIC - ESTABLISHED | | |
|---|---|---|
| 99211 | OF--Established Patient Minimal | |
| 99212 | OF--Established Patient Low | |
| 99213 | OF--Established Patient Detailed | |
| 99214 | OF--Established Patient Moderate | X |
| 99215 | OF--Established Patient High | |

| PREVENTIVE VISITS - NEW | | |
|---|---|---|
| 99381 | Under 1 Year | |
| 99382 | 1 - 4 Years | |
| 99383 | 5 - 11 Years | |
| 99384 | 12 - 17 Years | |
| 99385 | 18 - 39 Years | |
| 99386 | 40 - 64 Years | |
| 99387 | 65 Years & Up | |

| PREVENTIVE VISITS - ESTABLISHED | | |
|---|---|---|
| 99391 | Under 1 Year | |
| 99392 | 1 - 4 Years | |
| 99393 | 5 - 11 Years | |
| 99394 | 12 - 17 Years | |
| 99395 | 18 - 39 Years | |
| 99396 | 40 - 64 Years | |
| 99397 | 65 Years & Up | |

| HOSPITAL/NURSING HOME VISITS | | |
|---|---|---|
| 99221 | Initial hospital care, det. | |
| 99222 | Initial hospital care, comp. | |
| 99223 | Initial hospital care, high | |
| 99281 | ER Visit, min. | |
| 99282 | ER Visit, low | |
| 99283 | ER Visit, det. | |
| 99284 | ER Visit, moderate | |
| 99285 | ER Visit, high | |
| 99307 | Subseq. nursing facility care, pf. | |
| | | |
| | | |

| PROCEDURES | | |
|---|---|---|
| 10060 | Incision/drainage, abscess | |
| 20610 | Aspiration, bursa | |
| 29505 | Splint, long leg | |
| 29515 | Splint, short leg | |
| 36415 | Routine venipuncture | |
| 45330 | Sigmoidoscopy, flex | |
| 46600 | Anoscopy, diagnostic | |
| 71030 | Chest x-ray, complete | |
| 73610 | Radiology, ankle, complete | |
| 93000 | Routine ECG | |
| 93018 | Cardiovascular stress test | |
| 99070 | Supplies and materials | X |

| LABORATORY | | |
|---|---|---|
| 80050 | General health panel | |
| 81000 | Urinalysis, complete | |
| 82270 | Blood, occult, feces screening | |
| 82607 | Vitamin B-12 test | |
| 82948 | Glucose, blood reagent | |
| 85027 | CBC, automated | |
| 85651 | Sedimentation rate test, manual | |
| 86360 | Absolute CD4/CD8 ratio | |
| 86592 | Syphilis test | |
| 87070 | Throat culture | |
| 87088 | Urine culture | |
| 88150 | Cytopathology, cervical or vaginal | |

| INJECTIONS | | |
|---|---|---|
| 90471 | Immunization administration | |
| 90472 | Immunization administration, 2nd | |
| 90658 | Influenza injection, ages >3 | |
| 90702 | DT immunization, ages <7 | |
| 90703 | Tetanus immunization | |
| 90707 | MMR immunization | |
| 96372 | Therapeutic injection | |
| 90723 | DTaP - HepB - IPV | |
| 90732 | Pneumococcal immunization | |
| | | |
| | | |

## POLARIS MEDICAL GROUP

| REFERRING PHYSICIAN | NPI |
|---|---|
| AUTHORIZATION # | |

DIAGNOSIS
**L40.0**

PAYMENT AMOUNT
**$125, check #102**

NOTES
**99070 supplies
and materials $20.00**

Copyright ©2016 McGraw-Hill Education

# PATIENT INFORMATION FORM

## THIS SECTION REFERS TO PATIENT ONLY

| Name: Chantalle E. Usdan | Sex: F | Marital Status: ☒ S ☐ M ☐ D ☐ W | Birth Date: 2/23/62 |
|---|---|---|---|

| Address: 28 Fairview Blvd. | SS#: 234-60-8721 |
|---|---|

| City: Columbus | State: OH | Zip: 43214 | Employer: Argene Interiors (full-time) | Phone: |
|---|---|---|---|---|

| Home Phone: 999-555-4555 | Employer's Address: 1760 Watertown Avenue |
|---|---|

| Work Phone: 999-555-6978 | City: Jackson | State: OH | Zip: 45640 |
|---|---|---|---|

| Race: __American Indian or Alaska Native  __Asian  __Black or African American  X White  __Other  __Native Hawaiian or Other Pacific Islander  __Declined | Ethnicity: __Hispanic or Latino  X Non-Hispanic or Latino  __Declined | Language: English |
|---|---|---|

| Spouse's Name: | Spouse's Employer: |
|---|---|

| Emergency Contact: Laraine Modell | Relationship: sister | Phone #: 999-555-9910 |
|---|---|---|

## FILL IN IF PATIENT IS A MINOR

| Parent/Guardian's Name: | Sex: | Marital Status: ☐ S ☐ M ☐ D ☐ W | Birth Date: |
|---|---|---|---|

| Phone: | SS#: |
|---|---|

| Address: | Employer: | Phone: |
|---|---|---|

| City: | State: | Zip: | Employer's Address: |
|---|---|---|---|

| Student Status: | City: | State: | Zip: |
|---|---|---|---|

## INSURANCE INFORMATION

| Primary Insurance Company: Cigna Healthplan | Secondary Insurance Company: |
|---|---|

| Subscriber's Name: Chantalle E. Usdan | Birth Date: 2/23/62 | Subscriber's Name: | Birth Date: |
|---|---|---|---|

| Plan: HMO, capitated | SS#: 234-60-8721 | Plan: |
|---|---|---|

| Policy #: 723-C48 | Group #: AAA66668 | Policy #: | Group #: |
|---|---|---|---|

| Copayment/Deductible: $18 copay | Price Code: A | |
|---|---|---|

## OTHER INFORMATION

| Reason for visit: flexible sigmoidoscopy | Allergy to Medication (list): |
|---|---|

| Name of referring physician: Dr. Rachel P. Innanni | If auto accident, list date and state in which it occurred: |
|---|---|

I authorize treatment and agree to pay all fees and charges for the person named above. I agree to pay all charges shown by statements, promptly upon their presentation, unless credit arrangements are agreed upon in writing.

I authorize payment directly to POLARIS MEDICAL GROUP of insurance benefits otherwise payable to me. I hereby authorize the release of any medical information necessary in order to process a claim for payment in my behalf.

| Chantalle E. Usdan | 6/20/18 |
|---|---|
| (Patient's Signature/Parent or Guardian's Signature) | (Date) |

I plan to make payment of my medical expenses as follows (check one or more):

X Insurance (as above)     X Cash/Check/Credit/Debit Card     ___ Medicare     ___ Medicaid     ___ Workers' Comp.

# ENCOUNTER FORM

**6/20/2018**          **10:00am**                    **Dr. Michael Mahabir**
DATE                    TIME                          PROVIDER

**Chantalle E. Usdan**                               **USDANCHO**
PATIENT NAME                                         CHART #

| OFFICE VISITS - SYMPTOMATIC - NEW | | |
|---|---|---|
| 99201 | OF--New Patient Minimal | |
| 99202 | OF--New Patient Low | |
| 99203 | OF--New Patient Detailed | |
| 99204 | OF--New Patient Moderate | |
| 99205 | OF--New Patient High | |
| **OFFICE VISITS - SYMPTOMATIC - ESTABLISHED** | | |
| 99211 | OF--Established Patient Minimal | |
| 99212 | OF--Established Patient Low | |
| 99213 | OF--Established Patient Detailed | |
| 99214 | OF--Established Patient Moderate | |
| 99215 | OF--Established Patient High | |
| **PREVENTIVE VISITS - NEW** | | |
| 99381 | Under 1 Year | |
| 99382 | 1 - 4 Years | |
| 99383 | 5 - 11 Years | |
| 99384 | 12 - 17 Years | |
| 99385 | 18 - 39 Years | |
| 99386 | 40 - 64 Years | |
| 99387 | 65 Years & Up | |
| **PREVENTIVE VISITS - ESTABLISHED** | | |
| 99391 | Under 1 Year | |
| 99392 | 1 - 4 Years | |
| 99393 | 5 - 11 Years | |
| 99394 | 12 - 17 Years | |
| 99395 | 18 - 39 Years | |
| 99396 | 40 - 64 Years | |
| 99397 | 65 Years & Up | |
| **HOSPITAL/NURSING HOME VISITS** | | |
| 99221 | Initial hospital care, det. | |
| 99222 | Initial hospital care, comp. | |
| 99223 | Initial hospital care, high | |
| 99281 | ER Visit, min. | |
| 99282 | ER Visit, low | |
| 99283 | ER Visit, det. | |
| 99284 | ER Visit, moderate | |
| 99285 | ER Visit, high | |
| 99307 | Subseq. nursing facility care, pf. | |
| | | |

| PROCEDURES | | |
|---|---|---|
| 10060 | Incision/drainage, abscess | |
| 20610 | Aspiration, bursa | |
| 29505 | Splint, long leg | |
| 29515 | Splint, short leg | |
| 36415 | Routine venipuncture | |
| 45330 | Sigmoidoscopy, flex | X |
| 46600 | Anoscopy, diagnostic | |
| 71030 | Chest x-ray, complete | |
| 73610 | Radiology, ankle, complete | |
| 93000 | Routine ECG | |
| 93018 | Cardiovascular stress test | |
| 99070 | Supplies and materials | |
| **LABORATORY** | | |
| 80050 | General health panel | |
| 81000 | Urinalysis, complete | |
| 82270 | Blood, occult, feces screening | |
| 82607 | Vitamin B-12 test | |
| 82948 | Glucose, blood reagent | |
| 85027 | CBC, automated | |
| 85651 | Sedimentation rate test, manual | |
| 86360 | Absolute CD4/CD8 ratio | |
| 86592 | Syphilis test | |
| 87070 | Throat culture | |
| 87088 | Urine culture | |
| 88150 | Cytopathology, cervical or vaginal | |
| **INJECTIONS** | | |
| 90471 | Immunization administration | |
| 90472 | Immunization administration, 2nd | |
| 90658 | Influenza injection, ages >3 | |
| 90702 | DT immunization, ages <7 | |
| 90703 | Tetanus immunization | |
| 90707 | MMR immunization | |
| 96372 | Therapeutic injection | |
| 90723 | DTaP - HepB - IPV | |
| 90732 | Pneumococcal immunization | |
| | | |

## POLARIS MEDICAL GROUP

NOTES

REFERRING PHYSICIAN                     NPI
**Dr. Rachel Innanni**

AUTHORIZATION #

DIAGNOSIS

PAYMENT AMOUNT
**$18.00 copay, check #409**

# ENCOUNTER FORM

**6/20/2018**           **12:00pm**
DATE                    TIME

**Rachel D. Atchely**
PATIENT NAME

**Dr. Michael Mahabir**
PROVIDER

**ATCHERA0**
CHART #

| OFFICE VISITS - SYMPTOMATIC - NEW | | |
|---|---|---|
| 99201 | OF--New Patient Minimal | |
| 99202 | OF--New Patient Low | |
| 99203 | OF--New Patient Detailed | |
| 99204 | OF--New Patient Moderate | |
| 99205 | OF--New Patient High | |
| **OFFICE VISITS - SYMPTOMATIC - ESTABLISHED** | | |
| 99211 | OF--Established Patient Minimal | |
| 99212 | OF--Established Patient Low | |
| 99213 | OF--Established Patient Detailed | |
| 99214 | OF--Established Patient Moderate | |
| 99215 | OF--Established Patient High | |
| **PREVENTIVE VISITS - NEW** | | |
| 99381 | Under 1 Year | |
| 99382 | 1 - 4 Years | |
| 99383 | 5 - 11 Years | |
| 99384 | 12 - 17 Years | |
| 99385 | 18 - 39 Years | |
| 99386 | 40 - 64 Years | |
| 99387 | 65 Years & Up | |
| **PREVENTIVE VISITS - ESTABLISHED** | | |
| 99391 | Under 1 Year | |
| 99392 | 1 - 4 Years | |
| 99393 | 5 - 11 Years | |
| 99394 | 12 - 17 Years | |
| 99395 | 18 - 39 Years | |
| 99396 | 40 - 64 Years | |
| 99397 | 65 Years & Up | |
| **HOSPITAL/NURSING HOME VISITS** | | |
| 99221 | Initial hospital care, det. | |
| 99222 | Initial hospital care, comp. | |
| 99223 | Initial hospital care, high | |
| 99281 | ER Visit, min. | |
| 99282 | ER Visit, low | |
| 99283 | ER Visit, det. | |
| 99284 | ER Visit, moderate | |
| 99285 | ER Visit, high | |
| 99307 | Subseq. nursing facility care, pf. | X |
| | | |
| | | |

| PROCEDURES | | |
|---|---|---|
| 10060 | Incision/drainage, abscess | |
| 20610 | Aspiration, bursa | |
| 29505 | Splint, long leg | |
| 29515 | Splint, short leg | |
| 36415 | Routine venipuncture | |
| 45330 | Sigmoidoscopy, flex | |
| 46600 | Anoscopy, diagnostic | |
| 71030 | Chest x-ray, complete | |
| 73610 | Radiology, ankle, complete | |
| 93000 | Routine ECG | |
| 93018 | Cardiovascular stress test | |
| 99070 | Supplies and materials | |
| **LABORATORY** | | |
| 80050 | General health panel | |
| 81000 | Urinalysis, complete | |
| 82270 | Blood, occult, feces screening | |
| 82607 | Vitamin B-12 test | |
| 82948 | Glucose, blood reagent | |
| 85027 | CBC, automated | |
| 85651 | Sedimentation rate test, manual | |
| 86360 | Absolute CD4/CD8 ratio | |
| 86592 | Syphilis test | |
| 87070 | Throat culture | |
| 87088 | Urine culture | |
| 88150 | Cytopathology, cervical or vaginal | |
| **INJECTIONS** | | |
| 90471 | Immunization administration | |
| 90472 | Immunization administration, 2nd | |
| 90658 | Influenza injection, ages >3 | |
| 90702 | DT immunization, ages <7 | |
| 90703 | Tetanus immunization | |
| 90707 | MMR immunization | |
| 96372 | Therapeutic injection | |
| 90723 | DTaP - HepB - IPV | |
| 90732 | Pneumococcal immunization | |
| | | |
| | | |
| | | |

## POLARIS MEDICAL GROUP

| REFERRING PHYSICIAN | NPI |
|---|---|
| | |

AUTHORIZATION #

DIAGNOSIS
**L03.031**

PAYMENT AMOUNT
**$5.00 copay, check #1078**

NOTES

# ENCOUNTER FORM

| 6/20/2018 | 2:15pm | Dr. Michael Mahabir |
|---|---|---|
| DATE | TIME | PROVIDER |

| Mae J. Deysenrothe | DEYSEMA0 |
|---|---|
| PATIENT NAME | CHART # |

| OFFICE VISITS - SYMPTOMATIC - NEW | | |
|---|---|---|
| 99201 | OF--New Patient Minimal | |
| 99202 | OF--New Patient Low | |
| 99203 | OF--New Patient Detailed | |
| 99204 | OF--New Patient Moderate | |
| 99205 | OF--New Patient High | |
| **OFFICE VISITS - SYMPTOMATIC - ESTABLISHED** | | |
| 99211 | OF--Established Patient Minimal | |
| 99212 | OF--Established Patient Low | |
| 99213 | OF--Established Patient Detailed | |
| 99214 | OF--Established Patient Moderate | |
| 99215 | OF--Established Patient High | |
| **PREVENTIVE VISITS - NEW** | | |
| 99381 | Under 1 Year | |
| 99382 | 1 - 4 Years | |
| 99383 | 5 - 11 Years | |
| 99384 | 12 - 17 Years | |
| 99385 | 18 - 39 Years | |
| 99386 | 40 - 64 Years | |
| 99387 | 65 Years & Up | |
| **PREVENTIVE VISITS - ESTABLISHED** | | |
| 99391 | Under 1 Year | |
| 99392 | 1 - 4 Years | |
| 99393 | 5 - 11 Years | |
| 99394 | 12 - 17 Years | |
| 99395 | 18 - 39 Years | X |
| 99396 | 40 - 64 Years | |
| 99397 | 65 Years & Up | |
| **HOSPITAL/NURSING HOME VISITS** | | |
| 99221 | Initial hospital care, det. | |
| 99222 | Initial hospital care, comp. | |
| 99223 | Initial hospital care, high | |
| 99281 | ER Visit, min. | |
| 99282 | ER Visit, low | |
| 99283 | ER Visit, det. | |
| 99284 | ER Visit, moderate | |
| 99285 | ER Visit, high | |
| 99307 | Subseq. nursing facility care, pf. | |
| | | |

| PROCEDURES | | |
|---|---|---|
| 10060 | Incision/drainage, abscess | |
| 20610 | Aspiration, bursa | |
| 29505 | Splint, long leg | |
| 29515 | Splint, short leg | |
| 36415 | Routine venipuncture | X |
| 45330 | Sigmoidoscopy, flex | |
| 46600 | Anoscopy, diagnostic | |
| 71030 | Chest x-ray, complete | |
| 73610 | Radiology, ankle, complete | |
| 93000 | Routine ECG | X |
| 93018 | Cardiovascular stress test | |
| 99070 | Supplies and materials | |
| **LABORATORY** | | |
| 80050 | General health panel | X |
| 81000 | Urinalysis, complete | X |
| 82270 | Blood, occult, feces screening | |
| 82607 | Vitamin B-12 test | |
| 82948 | Glucose, blood reagent | |
| 85027 | CBC, automated | |
| 85651 | Sedimentation rate test, manual | |
| 86360 | Absolute CD4/CD8 ratio | |
| 86592 | Syphilis test | |
| 87070 | Throat culture | |
| 87088 | Urine culture | |
| 88150 | Cytopathology, cervical or vaginal | X |
| **INJECTIONS** | | |
| 90471 | Immunization administration | |
| 90472 | Immunization administration, 2nd | |
| 90658 | Influenza injection, ages >3 | |
| 90702 | DT immunization, ages <7 | |
| 90703 | Tetanus immunization | |
| 90707 | MMR immunization | |
| 96372 | Therapeutic injection | |
| 90723 | DTaP - HepB - IPV | |
| 90732 | Pneumococcal immunization | |
| | | |

## POLARIS MEDICAL GROUP

| REFERRING PHYSICIAN | NPI |
|---|---|
| | |

NOTES

AUTHORIZATION #

DIAGNOSIS
**Z00.00**

PAYMENT AMOUNT
**$12.00 copay, check #2043**

# ENCOUNTER FORM

| | |
|---|---|
| **6/20/2018** DATE | **4:30pm** TIME |

**Dr. Michael Mahabir**
PROVIDER

**Ann R. LeConey**
PATIENT NAME

**LECONANO**
CHART #

| OFFICE VISITS - SYMPTOMATIC - NEW | | |
|---|---|---|
| 99201 | OF--New Patient Minimal | |
| 99202 | OF--New Patient Low | |
| 99203 | OF--New Patient Detailed | |
| 99204 | OF--New Patient Moderate | |
| 99205 | OF--New Patient High | |
| **OFFICE VISITS - SYMPTOMATIC - ESTABLISHED** | | |
| 99211 | OF--Established Patient Minimal | |
| 99212 | OF--Established Patient Low | X |
| 99213 | OF--Established Patient Detailed | |
| 99214 | OF--Established Patient Moderate | |
| 99215 | OF--Established Patient High | |
| **PREVENTIVE VISITS - NEW** | | |
| 99381 | Under 1 Year | |
| 99382 | 1 - 4 Years | |
| 99383 | 5 - 11 Years | |
| 99384 | 12 - 17 Years | |
| 99385 | 18 - 39 Years | |
| 99386 | 40 - 64 Years | |
| 99387 | 65 Years & Up | |
| **PREVENTIVE VISITS - ESTABLISHED** | | |
| 99391 | Under 1 Year | |
| 99392 | 1 - 4 Years | |
| 99393 | 5 - 11 Years | |
| 99394 | 12 - 17 Years | |
| 99395 | 18 - 39 Years | |
| 99396 | 40 - 64 Years | |
| 99397 | 65 Years & Up | |
| **HOSPITAL/NURSING HOME VISITS** | | |
| 99221 | Initial hospital care, det. | |
| 99222 | Initial hospital care, comp. | |
| 99223 | Initial hospital care, high | |
| 99281 | ER Visit, min. | |
| 99282 | ER Visit, low | |
| 99283 | ER Visit, det. | |
| 99284 | ER Visit, moderate | |
| 99285 | ER Visit, high | |
| 99307 | Subseq. nursing facility care, pf. | |

| PROCEDURES | | |
|---|---|---|
| 10060 | Incision/drainage, abscess | |
| 20610 | Aspiration, bursa | |
| 29505 | Splint, long leg | |
| 29515 | Splint, short leg | |
| 36415 | Routine venipuncture | |
| 45330 | Sigmoidoscopy, flex | |
| 46600 | Anoscopy, diagnostic | |
| 71030 | Chest x-ray, complete | |
| 73610 | Radiology, ankle, complete | |
| 93000 | Routine ECG | |
| 93018 | Cardiovascular stress test | |
| 99070 | Supplies and materials | |
| **LABORATORY** | | |
| 80050 | General health panel | |
| 81000 | Urinalysis, complete | |
| 82270 | Blood, occult, feces screening | |
| 82607 | Vitamin B-12 test | |
| 82948 | Glucose, blood reagent | |
| 85027 | CBC, automated | |
| 85651 | Sedimentation rate test, manual | |
| 86360 | Absolute CD4/CD8 ratio | |
| 86592 | Syphilis test | |
| 87070 | Throat culture | |
| 87088 | Urine culture | |
| 88150 | Cytopathology, cervical or vaginal | |
| **INJECTIONS** | | |
| 90471 | Immunization administration | |
| 90472 | Immunization administration, 2nd | |
| 90658 | Influenza injection, ages >3 | |
| 90702 | DT immunization, ages <7 | |
| 90703 | Tetanus immunization | |
| 90707 | MMR immunization | |
| 96372 | Therapeutic injection | |
| 90723 | DTaP - HepB - IPV | |
| 90732 | Pneumococcal immunization | |
| | | |

## POLARIS MEDICAL GROUP

| | | NOTES |
|---|---|---|
| REFERRING PHYSICIAN | NPI | |
| AUTHORIZATION # | | |
| DIAGNOSIS **L91.9** | | |
| PAYMENT AMOUNT **$15.00 copay, check #1834** | | |

# PATIENT INFORMATION FORM

## THIS SECTION REFERS TO PATIENT ONLY

| Name:<br>Hanna Z. Wong | Sex:<br>F | Marital Status:<br>☐ S  ☐ M  ☐ D  ☒ W | Birth Date:<br>11/5/45 |
|---|---|---|---|

| Address:<br>22-B 22nd Avenue | SS#:<br>015-98-2139 | | |
|---|---|---|---|

| City:<br>Highland | State:<br>OH | Zip:<br>45132 | Employer:<br>retired | Phone: |
|---|---|---|---|---|

| Home Phone:<br>999-555-1122 | Employer's Address: |
|---|---|

| Work Phone: | City: | State: | Zip: |
|---|---|---|---|

| Race:<br>__American Indian or Alaska Native  __Other<br>X Asian  __Native Hawaiian or<br>__Black or African American  Other Pacific Islander<br>__White  __Declined | Ethnicity:<br>__Hispanic or Latino<br>X Non-Hispanic or Latino<br>__Declined | Language:<br>English |
|---|---|---|

| Spouse's Name: | Spouse's Employer: |
|---|---|

| Emergency Contact:<br>John Wong | Relationship:<br>son | Phone #:<br>999-555-0364 |
|---|---|---|

## FILL IN IF PATIENT IS A MINOR

| Parent/Guardian's Name: | Sex: | Marital Status:<br>☐ S  ☐ M  ☐ D  ☐ W | Birth Date: |
|---|---|---|---|

| Phone: | SS#: | | |
|---|---|---|---|

| Address: | Employer: | Phone: |
|---|---|---|

| City: | State: | Zip: | Employer's Address: |
|---|---|---|---|

| Student Status: | City: | State: | Zip: |
|---|---|---|---|

## INSURANCE INFORMATION

| Primary Insurance Company:<br>Nationwide Medicare HMO | Secondary Insurance Company: |
|---|---|

| Subscriber's Name:<br>Hanna Z. Wong | Birth Date:<br>11/5/45 | Subscriber's Name: | Birth Date: |
|---|---|---|---|

| Plan:<br>HMO | SS#:<br>015-98-2139 | Plan: |
|---|---|---|

| Policy #:<br>015-98-2139A | Group #: | Policy #: | Group #: |
|---|---|---|---|

| Copayment/Deductible:<br>$5 copay | Price Code:<br>A | |
|---|---|---|

## OTHER INFORMATION

| Reason for visit:<br>chest pain | Allergy to Medication (list): |
|---|---|

| Name of referring physician: | If auto accident, list date and state in which<br>it occurred: |
|---|---|

I authorize treatment and agree to pay all fees and charges for the person named above. I agree to pay all charges shown by statements, promptly upon their presentation, unless credit arrangements are agreed upon in writing.

I authorize payment directly to POLARIS MEDICAL GROUP of insurance benefits otherwise payable to me. I hereby authorize the release of any medical information necessary in order to process a claim for payment in my behalf.

| Hanna Z. Wong | 6/21/18 |
|---|---|
| (Patient's Signature/Parent or Guardian's Signature) | (Date) |

I plan to make payment of my medical expenses as follows (check one or more):

_____Insurance (as above)  __X__Cash/Check/Credit/Debit Card  __X__Medicare  _____Medicaid  _____Workers' Comp.

# ENCOUNTER FORM

| | | |
|---|---|---|
| **6/21/2018** | **10:00am** | **Dr. Michael Mahabir** |
| DATE | TIME | PROVIDER |
| **Hanna Z. Wong** | | **WONGHAN0** |
| PATIENT NAME | | CHART # |

| OFFICE VISITS - SYMPTOMATIC - NEW | | |
|---|---|---|
| 99201 | OF--New Patient Minimal | |
| 99202 | OF--New Patient Low | |
| 99203 | OF--New Patient Detailed | |
| 99204 | OF--New Patient Moderate | |
| 99205 | OF--New Patient High | X |

| OFFICE VISITS - SYMPTOMATIC - ESTABLISHED | | |
|---|---|---|
| 99211 | OF--Established Patient Minimal | |
| 99212 | OF--Established Patient Low | |
| 99213 | OF--Established Patient Detailed | |
| 99214 | OF--Established Patient Moderate | |
| 99215 | OF--Established Patient High | |

| PREVENTIVE VISITS - NEW | | |
|---|---|---|
| 99381 | Under 1 Year | |
| 99382 | 1 - 4 Years | |
| 99383 | 5 - 11 Years | |
| 99384 | 12 - 17 Years | |
| 99385 | 18 - 39 Years | |
| 99386 | 40 - 64 Years | |
| 99387 | 65 Years & Up | |

| PREVENTIVE VISITS - ESTABLISHED | | |
|---|---|---|
| 99391 | Under 1 Year | |
| 99392 | 1 - 4 Years | |
| 99393 | 5 - 11 Years | |
| 99394 | 12 - 17 Years | |
| 99395 | 18 - 39 Years | |
| 99396 | 40 - 64 Years | |
| 99397 | 65 Years & Up | |

| HOSPITAL/NURSING HOME VISITS | | |
|---|---|---|
| 99221 | Initial hospital care, det. | |
| 99222 | Initial hospital care, comp. | |
| 99223 | Initial hospital care, high | |
| 99281 | ER Visit, min. | |
| 99282 | ER Visit, low | |
| 99283 | ER Visit, det. | |
| 99284 | ER Visit, moderate | |
| 99285 | ER Visit, high | |
| 99307 | Subseq. nursing facility care, pf. | |

| PROCEDURES | | |
|---|---|---|
| 10060 | Incision/drainage, abscess | |
| 20610 | Aspiration, bursa | |
| 29505 | Splint, long leg | |
| 29515 | Splint, short leg | |
| 36415 | Routine venipuncture | |
| 45330 | Sigmoidoscopy, flex | |
| 46600 | Anoscopy, diagnostic | |
| 71030 | Chest x-ray, complete | |
| 73610 | Radiology, ankle, complete | |
| 93000 | Routine ECG | X |
| 93018 | Cardiovascular stress test | |
| 99070 | Supplies and materials | |

| LABORATORY | | |
|---|---|---|
| 80050 | General health panel | |
| 81000 | Urinalysis, complete | |
| 82270 | Blood, occult, feces screening | |
| 82607 | Vitamin B-12 test | |
| 82948 | Glucose, blood reagent | |
| 85027 | CBC, automated | |
| 85651 | Sedimentation rate test, manual | |
| 86360 | Absolute CD4/CD8 ratio | |
| 86592 | Syphilis test | |
| 87070 | Throat culture | |
| 87088 | Urine culture | |
| 88150 | Cytopathology, cervical or vaginal | |

| INJECTIONS | | |
|---|---|---|
| 90471 | Immunization administration | |
| 90472 | Immunization administration, 2nd | |
| 90658 | Influenza injection, ages >3 | |
| 90702 | DT immunization, ages <7 | |
| 90703 | Tetanus immunization | |
| 90707 | MMR immunization | |
| 96372 | Therapeutic injection | |
| 90723 | DTaP - HepB - IPV | |
| 90732 | Pneumococcal immunization | |

## POLARIS MEDICAL GROUP

| REFERRING PHYSICIAN | NPI |
|---|---|
| | |

AUTHORIZATION #

DIAGNOSIS
**R07.9**

PAYMENT AMOUNT
**$5.00 copay, check #840**

NOTES

# Electronic Claim Audit/Edit Report

Polaris Medical Group
2100 Grace Avenue
Columbus, OH 43214

Transmission Number: 6084998

Insurance Carrier: Medicare

| Patient's Name | Dates of Service From - Thru | POS | Proc | Qty | Status |
|---|---|---|---|---|---|
| Connolly, Daniel | 5/31/18 – 5/31/18 | 11 | 99397 | 1 | Rejected**A |
| Connolly, Daniel | 5/31/18 – 5/31/18 | 11 | 80050 | 1 | Rejected**A |

** see reason for rejection below

*\*\*A Procedure not covered*

**Additional CPT Codes**

| Code | Description | POS | Charge A |
|------|-------------|-----|----------|
| 74240** | X-ray exam, upper GI tract | 11 | $88.00 |
| 74290** | Contrast X-ray, gallbladder | 11 | $130.00 |

** Require modifier 26, interpretation only

**Insurance Company Allowed Amounts:**

| Insurance Name | Code 74240 | Code 74290 |
|----------------|-----------|-----------|
| Aetna Health Plans | $ 74.00 | $ 108.00 |
| BCBS of Ohio - Workers' Comp. | 88.00 | 130.00 |
| Blue Cross/Blue Shield of Ohio | 88.00 | 130.00 |
| CIGNA Healthplan | 74.00 | 108.00 |
| Columbus Medical Care | 74.00 | 108.00 |
| Nationwide Medicare (HMO) | 36.00 | 68.00 |
| Nationwide Medicare (Trad) | 36.00 | 68.00 |
| Ohio Depart. of Human Services | 36.00 | 68.00 |
| Ohio Insurance Company | 88.00 | 130.00 |
| Ohio Maxcare PPO | 74.00 | 108.00 |
| Standard Health Care, Inc. | 74.00 | 108.00 |
| TRICARE | 36.00 | 68.00 |

## PATIENT INFORMATION FORM

### THIS SECTION REFERS TO PATIENT ONLY

| Name: Jorge Z. Martinez | Sex: M | Marital Status: ☐ S ☒ M ☐ D ☐ W | Birth Date: 9/16/50 |
|---|---|---|---|

| Address: 900 Andover Circle | SS#: 198-22-8463 | | |
|---|---|---|---|

| City: Fairview | State: OH | Zip: 43773 | Employer: COSTINC (full-time) | Phone: |
|---|---|---|---|---|

| Home Phone: 999-555-4009 | Employer's Address: 3504 Overland Avenue |
|---|---|

| Work Phone: 999-555-4300 | City: Columbus | State: OH | Zip: 43214 |
|---|---|---|---|

| Race:<br>__American Indian or Alaska Native<br>__Asian<br>__Black or African American<br>X White<br>__Other<br>__Native Hawaiian or Other Pacific Islander<br>__Declined | Ethnicity:<br>X Hispanic or Latino<br>__Non-Hispanic or Latino<br>__Declined | Language: English |
|---|---|---|

| Spouse's Name: Janis Martinez | Spouse's Employer: Computer Consultants |
|---|---|

| Emergency Contact: Janis Martinez | Relationship: wife | Phone #: 999-555-4009 |
|---|---|---|

### FILL IN IF PATIENT IS A MINOR

| Parent/Guardian's Name: | Sex: | Marital Status: ☐ S ☐ M ☐ D ☐ W | Birth Date: |
|---|---|---|---|

| Phone: | SS#: | | |
|---|---|---|---|

| Address: | Employer: | Phone: |
|---|---|---|

| City: | State: | Zip: | Employer's Address: |
|---|---|---|---|

| Student Status: | City: | State: | Zip: |
|---|---|---|---|

### INSURANCE INFORMATION

| Primary Insurance Company: Aetna Health Plans | Secondary Insurance Company: |
|---|---|

| Subscriber's Name: Jorge Z. Martinez | Birth Date: 9/16/50 | Subscriber's Name: | Birth Date: |
|---|---|---|---|

| Plan: HMO, capitated | SS#: 198-22-8463 | Plan: |
|---|---|---|

| Policy #: 777JM | Group #: COS-41 | Policy #: | Group #: |
|---|---|---|---|

| Copayment/Deductible: $15 copay | Price Code: A | |
|---|---|---|

### OTHER INFORMATION

| Reason for visit: burning upon urination | Allergy to Medication (list): |
|---|---|

| Name of referring physician: | If auto accident, list date and state in which it occurred: |
|---|---|

I authorize treatment and agree to pay all fees and charges for the person named above. I agree to pay all charges shown by statements, promptly upon their presentation, unless credit arrangements are agreed upon in writing.

I authorize payment directly to POLARIS MEDICAL GROUP of insurance benefits otherwise payable to me. I hereby authorize the release of any medical information necessary in order to process a claim for payment in my behalf.

| Jorge Z. Martinez | 6/21/18 |
|---|---|
| (Patient's Signature/Parent or Guardian's Signature) | (Date) |

I plan to make payment of my medical expenses as follows (check one or more):

X Insurance (as above)   X Cash/Check/Credit/Debit Card   ____ Medicare   ____ Medicaid   ____ Workers' Comp.

# ENCOUNTER FORM

| 6/21/2018 | 4:00pm | Dr. Michael Mahabir |
|-----------|--------|---------------------|
| DATE | TIME | PROVIDER |

| Jorge Z. Martinez | MARTIJO0 |
|-------------------|----------|
| PATIENT NAME | CHART # |

### OFFICE VISITS - SYMPTOMATIC - NEW

| | | |
|---|---|---|
| 99201 | OF--New Patient Minimal | |
| 99202 | OF--New Patient Low | |
| 99203 | OF--New Patient Detailed | X |
| 99204 | OF--New Patient Moderate | |
| 99205 | OF--New Patient High | |

### OFFICE VISITS - SYMPTOMATIC - ESTABLISHED

| | | |
|---|---|---|
| 99211 | OF--Established Patient Minimal | |
| 99212 | OF--Established Patient Low | |
| 99213 | OF--Established Patient Detailed | |
| 99214 | OF--Established Patient Moderate | |
| 99215 | OF--Established Patient High | |

### PREVENTIVE VISITS - NEW

| | | |
|---|---|---|
| 99381 | Under 1 Year | |
| 99382 | 1 - 4 Years | |
| 99383 | 5 - 11 Years | |
| 99384 | 12 - 17 Years | |
| 99385 | 18 - 39 Years | |
| 99386 | 40 - 64 Years | |
| 99387 | 65 Years & Up | |

### PREVENTIVE VISITS - ESTABLISHED

| | | |
|---|---|---|
| 99391 | Under 1 Year | |
| 99392 | 1 - 4 Years | |
| 99393 | 5 - 11 Years | |
| 99394 | 12 - 17 Years | |
| 99395 | 18 - 39 Years | |
| 99396 | 40 - 64 Years | |
| 99397 | 65 Years & Up | |

### HOSPITAL/NURSING HOME VISITS

| | | |
|---|---|---|
| 99221 | Initial hospital care, det. | |
| 99222 | Initial hospital care, comp. | |
| 99223 | Initial hospital care, high | |
| 99281 | ER Visit, min. | |
| 99282 | ER Visit, low | |
| 99283 | ER Visit, det. | |
| 99284 | ER Visit, moderate | |
| 99285 | ER Visit, high | |
| 99307 | Subseq. nursing facility care, pf. | |
| | | |
| | | |

### PROCEDURES

| | | |
|---|---|---|
| 10060 | Incision/drainage, abscess | |
| 20610 | Aspiration, bursa | |
| 29505 | Splint, long leg | |
| 29515 | Splint, short leg | |
| 36415 | Routine venipuncture | |
| 45330 | Sigmoidoscopy, flex | |
| 46600 | Anoscopy, diagnostic | |
| 71030 | Chest x-ray, complete | |
| 73610 | Radiology, ankle, complete | |
| 93000 | Routine ECG | |
| 93018 | Cardiovascular stress test | |
| 99070 | Supplies and materials | |

### LABORATORY

| | | |
|---|---|---|
| 80050 | General health panel | |
| 81000 | Urinalysis, complete | X |
| 82270 | Blood, occult, feces screening | |
| 82607 | Vitamin B-12 test | |
| 82948 | Glucose, blood reagent | |
| 85027 | CBC, automated | |
| 85651 | Sedimentation rate test, manual | |
| 86360 | Absolute CD4/CD8 ratio | |
| 86592 | Syphilis test | |
| 87070 | Throat culture | |
| 87088 | Urine culture | X |
| 88150 | Cytopathology, cervical or vaginal | |

### INJECTIONS

| | | |
|---|---|---|
| 90471 | Immunization administration | |
| 90472 | Immunization administration, 2nd | |
| 90658 | Influenza injection, ages >3 | |
| 90702 | DT immunization, ages <7 | |
| 90703 | Tetanus immunization | |
| 90707 | MMR immunization | |
| 96372 | Therapeutic injection | |
| 90723 | DTaP - HepB - IPV | |
| 90732 | Pneumococcal immunization | |
| | | |
| | | |

## POLARIS MEDICAL GROUP

| REFERRING PHYSICIAN | NPI | NOTES |
|---------------------|-----|-------|
| AUTHORIZATION # | | |
| DIAGNOSIS N39.0 | | |
| PAYMENT AMOUNT $15.00 copay, check #1819 | | |

# ENCOUNTER FORM

| 6/21/2018 | 4:30pm | Dr. Robin Crebore |
|-----------|--------|-------------------|
| DATE | TIME | PROVIDER |

| Susan R. Jonas | JONASSU0 |
|----------------|----------|
| PATIENT NAME | CHART # |

| OFFICE VISITS - SYMPTOMATIC - NEW | | |
|---|---|---|
| 99201 | OF--New Patient Minimal | |
| 99202 | OF--New Patient Low | |
| 99203 | OF--New Patient Detailed | |
| 99204 | OF--New Patient Moderate | |
| 99205 | OF--New Patient High | |
| **OFFICE VISITS - SYMPTOMATIC - ESTABLISHED** | | |
| 99211 | OF--Established Patient Minimal | |
| 99212 | OF--Established Patient Low | X |
| 99213 | OF--Established Patient Detailed | |
| 99214 | OF--Established Patient Moderate | |
| 99215 | OF--Established Patient High | |
| **PREVENTIVE VISITS - NEW** | | |
| 99381 | Under 1 Year | |
| 99382 | 1 - 4 Years | |
| 99383 | 5 - 11 Years | |
| 99384 | 12 - 17 Years | |
| 99385 | 18 - 39 Years | |
| 99386 | 40 - 64 Years | |
| 99387 | 65 Years & Up | |
| **PREVENTIVE VISITS - ESTABLISHED** | | |
| 99391 | Under 1 Year | |
| 99392 | 1 - 4 Years | |
| 99393 | 5 - 11 Years | |
| 99394 | 12 - 17 Years | |
| 99395 | 18 - 39 Years | |
| 99396 | 40 - 64 Years | |
| 99397 | 65 Years & Up | |
| **HOSPITAL/NURSING HOME VISITS** | | |
| 99221 | Initial hospital care, det. | |
| 99222 | Initial hospital care, comp. | |
| 99223 | Initial hospital care, high | |
| 99281 | ER Visit, min. | |
| 99282 | ER Visit, low | |
| 99283 | ER Visit, det. | |
| 99284 | ER Visit, moderate | |
| 99285 | ER Visit, high | |
| 99307 | Subseq. nursing facility care, pf. | |

| PROCEDURES | | |
|---|---|---|
| 10060 | Incision/drainage, abscess | |
| 20610 | Aspiration, bursa | |
| 29505 | Splint, long leg | |
| 29515 | Splint, short leg | |
| 36415 | Routine venipuncture | |
| 45330 | Sigmoidoscopy, flex | |
| 46600 | Anoscopy, diagnostic | |
| 71030 | Chest x-ray, complete | |
| 73610 | Radiology, ankle, complete | |
| 93000 | Routine ECG | |
| 93018 | Cardiovascular stress test | |
| 99070 | Supplies and materials | |
| **LABORATORY** | | |
| 80050 | General health panel | |
| 81000 | Urinalysis, complete | |
| 82270 | Blood, occult, feces screening | |
| 82607 | Vitamin B-12 test | |
| 82948 | Glucose, blood reagent | |
| 85027 | CBC, automated | |
| 85651 | Sedimentation rate test, manual | |
| 86360 | Absolute CD4/CD8 ratio | |
| 86592 | Syphilis test | |
| 87070 | Throat culture | |
| 87088 | Urine culture | |
| 88150 | Cytopathology, cervical or vaginal | |
| **INJECTIONS** | | |
| 90471 | Immunization administration | |
| 90472 | Immunization administration, 2nd | |
| 90658 | Influenza injection, ages >3 | |
| 90702 | DT immunization, ages <7 | |
| 90703 | Tetanus immunization | |
| 90707 | MMR immunization | |
| 96372 | Therapeutic injection | |
| 90723 | DTaP - HepB - IPV | |
| 90732 | Pneumococcal immunization | |
| | | |
| | | |

| POLARIS MEDICAL GROUP | | NOTES |
|---|---|---|
| REFERRING PHYSICIAN | NPI | |
| AUTHORIZATION # | | |
| DIAGNOSIS | | |
| PAYMENT AMOUNT **$15.00 copay, check #349** | | |

**Polaris Medical Group**

**Name:** Susan R. Jonas     **Telephone:** 614-555-9908

**Date of Birth:** 4/4/79     **Age:** 39

| | | |
|---|---|---|
| 6/23/16 | **PROBLEM 1:** | Dermatitis, contact, NOS |
| | **CHIEF COMPLAINT:** | Rash |

**S:**     Rash on leg, itching; reports probable exposure to poison ivy.
**O:**     Swelling, blistering, some scaling of area.
**A:**     Contact dermatitis, mild.
**P:**     Topical application of Benadryl® cream.


Robin Crebore, M.D.

# ENCOUNTER FORM

**6/22/2018**          **9:15am**
DATE                    TIME

**Dr. Robin Crebore**
PROVIDER

**Martin G. Szinovacz**
PATIENT NAME

**SZINOMA0**
CHART #

| OFFICE VISITS - SYMPTOMATIC - NEW | | |
|---|---|---|
| 99201 | OF--New Patient Minimal | |
| 99202 | OF--New Patient Low | |
| 99203 | OF--New Patient Detailed | |
| 99204 | OF--New Patient Moderate | |
| 99205 | OF--New Patient High | |
| **OFFICE VISITS - SYMPTOMATIC - ESTABLISHED** | | |
| 99211 | OF--Established Patient Minimal | |
| 99212 | OF--Established Patient Low | |
| 99213 | OF--Established Patient Detailed | X |
| 99214 | OF--Established Patient Moderate | |
| 99215 | OF--Established Patient High | |
| **PREVENTIVE VISITS - NEW** | | |
| 99381 | Under 1 Year | |
| 99382 | 1 - 4 Years | |
| 99383 | 5 - 11 Years | |
| 99384 | 12 - 17 Years | |
| 99385 | 18 - 39 Years | |
| 99386 | 40 - 64 Years | |
| 99387 | 65 Years & Up | |
| **PREVENTIVE VISITS - ESTABLISHED** | | |
| 99391 | Under 1 Year | |
| 99392 | 1 - 4 Years | |
| 99393 | 5 - 11 Years | |
| 99394 | 12 - 17 Years | |
| 99395 | 18 - 39 Years | |
| 99396 | 40 - 64 Years | |
| 99397 | 65 Years & Up | |
| **HOSPITAL/NURSING HOME VISITS** | | |
| 99221 | Initial hospital care, det. | |
| 99222 | Initial hospital care, comp. | |
| 99223 | Initial hospital care, high | |
| 99281 | ER Visit, min. | |
| 99282 | ER Visit, low | |
| 99283 | ER Visit, det. | |
| 99284 | ER Visit, moderate | |
| 99285 | ER Visit, high | |
| 99307 | Subseq. nursing facility care, pf. | |

| PROCEDURES | | |
|---|---|---|
| 10060 | Incision/drainage, abscess | |
| 20610 | Aspiration, bursa | |
| 29505 | Splint, long leg | |
| 29515 | Splint, short leg | |
| 36415 | Routine venipuncture | |
| 45330 | Sigmoidoscopy, flex | |
| 46600 | Anoscopy, diagnostic | |
| 71030 | Chest x-ray, complete | |
| 73610 | Radiology, ankle, complete | |
| 93000 | Routine ECG | |
| 93018 | Cardiovascular stress test | |
| 99070 | Supplies and materials | |
| **LABORATORY** | | |
| 80050 | General health panel | |
| 81000 | Urinalysis, complete | |
| 82270 | Blood, occult, feces screening | |
| 82607 | Vitamin B-12 test | |
| 82948 | Glucose, blood reagent | |
| 85027 | CBC, automated | |
| 85651 | Sedimentation rate test, manual | |
| 86360 | Absolute CD4/CD8 ratio | |
| 86592 | Syphilis test | |
| 87070 | Throat culture | |
| 87088 | Urine culture | |
| 88150 | Cytopathology, cervical or vaginal | |
| **INJECTIONS** | | |
| 90471 | Immunization administration | |
| 90472 | Immunization administration, 2nd | |
| 90658 | Influenza injection, ages >3 | |
| 90702 | DT immunization, ages <7 | |
| 90703 | Tetanus immunization | |
| 90707 | MMR immunization | |
| 96372 | Therapeutic injection | |
| 90723 | DTaP - HepB - IPV | |
| 90732 | Pneumococcal immunization | |
| | | |
| | | |
| | | |

## POLARIS MEDICAL GROUP

REFERRING PHYSICIAN

NPI

AUTHORIZATION #

DIAGNOSIS
I10

PAYMENT AMOUNT
**$15.00 copay, check #3404**

NOTES

# PATIENT INFORMATION FORM

## THIS SECTION REFERS TO PATIENT ONLY

| | | |
|---|---|---|
| Name: Eugene S. Kadar | Sex: M | Marital Status: ☒ S ☐ M ☐ D ☐ W | Birth Date: 6/1/85 |

| | |
|---|---|
| Address: 8003 Oxford Lane | SS#: 499-09-7453 |

| | | | | |
|---|---|---|---|---|
| City: Highland | State: OH | Zip: 45132 | Employer: Columbus Insurance Company (full-time) | Phone: |

| | |
|---|---|
| Home Phone: 999-555-5858 | Employer's Address: 9800 Overland Avenue |

| | | | |
|---|---|---|---|
| Work Phone: 999-555-1212 | City: Columbus | State: OH | Zip: 43214 |

**Race:**

__American Indian or Alaska Native
__Asian
__Black or African American
X White

__Other
__Native Hawaiian or Other Pacific Islander
__Declined

**Ethnicity:**

__Hispanic or Latino
X Non-Hispanic or Latino
__Declined

**Language:** English

| | |
|---|---|
| Spouse's Name: | Spouse's Employer: |

| | | |
|---|---|---|
| Emergency Contact: Roger Kadar | Relationship: brother | Phone #: 999-555-4443 |

## FILL IN IF PATIENT IS A MINOR

| | | | |
|---|---|---|---|
| Parent/Guardian's Name: | Sex: | Marital Status: ☐ S ☐ M ☐ D ☐ W | Birth Date: |

| | |
|---|---|
| Phone: | SS#: |

| | | |
|---|---|---|
| Address: | Employer: | Phone: |

| | | | |
|---|---|---|---|
| City: | State: | Zip: | Employer's Address: |

| | | | |
|---|---|---|---|
| Student Status: | City: | State: | Zip: |

## INSURANCE INFORMATION

| | |
|---|---|
| Primary Insurance Company: Cigna Healthplan | Secondary Insurance Company: |

| | | | |
|---|---|---|---|
| Subscriber's Name: Eugene S. Kadar | Birth Date: 6/1/85 | Subscriber's Name: | Birth Date: |

| | | |
|---|---|---|
| Plan: HMO, capitated | SS#: 499-09-7453 | Plan: |

| | | | |
|---|---|---|---|
| Policy #: 762-TTY | Group #: BBA998534 | Policy #: | Group #: |

| | |
|---|---|
| Copayment/Deductible: $18 copay | Price Code: A |

## OTHER INFORMATION

| | |
|---|---|
| Reason for visit: sores on lip | Allergy to Medication (list): |

| | |
|---|---|
| Name of referring physician: | If auto accident, list date and state in which it occurred: |

I authorize treatment and agree to pay all fees and charges for the person named above. I agree to pay all charges shown by statements, promptly upon their presentation, unless credit arrangements are agreed upon in writing.

I authorize payment directly to POLARIS MEDICAL GROUP of insurance benefits otherwise payable to me. I hereby authorize the release of any medical information necessary in order to process a claim for payment in my behalf.

| | |
|---|---|
| Eugene S. Kadar | 6/22/18 |
| (Patient's Signature/Parent or Guardian's Signature) | (Date) |

I plan to make payment of my medical expenses as follows (check one or more):

X Insurance (as above)     X Cash/Check/Credit/Debit Card     ____Medicare     ____Medicaid     ____Workers' Comp.

# ENCOUNTER FORM

**6/22/2018**      **10:15am**

DATE            TIME

**Eugene S. Kadar**

PATIENT NAME

**Dr. Robin Crebore**

PROVIDER

**KADAREU0**

CHART #

| OFFICE VISITS - SYMPTOMATIC - NEW | | |
|---|---|---|
| 99201 | OF--New Patient Minimal | |
| 99202 | OF--New Patient Low | X |
| 99203 | OF--New Patient Detailed | |
| 99204 | OF--New Patient Moderate | |
| 99205 | OF--New Patient High | |
| **OFFICE VISITS - SYMPTOMATIC - ESTABLISHED** | | |
| 99211 | OF--Established Patient Minimal | |
| 99212 | OF--Established Patient Low | |
| 99213 | OF--Established Patient Detailed | |
| 99214 | OF--Established Patient Moderate | |
| 99215 | OF--Established Patient High | |
| **PREVENTIVE VISITS - NEW** | | |
| 99381 | Under 1 Year | |
| 99382 | 1 - 4 Years | |
| 99383 | 5 - 11 Years | |
| 99384 | 12 - 17 Years | |
| 99385 | 18 - 39 Years | |
| 99386 | 40 - 64 Years | |
| 99387 | 65 Years & Up | |
| **PREVENTIVE VISITS - ESTABLISHED** | | |
| 99391 | Under 1 Year | |
| 99392 | 1 - 4 Years | |
| 99393 | 5 - 11 Years | |
| 99394 | 12 - 17 Years | |
| 99395 | 18 - 39 Years | |
| 99396 | 40 - 64 Years | |
| 99397 | 65 Years & Up | |
| **HOSPITAL/NURSING HOME VISITS** | | |
| 99221 | Initial hospital care, det. | |
| 99222 | Initial hospital care, comp. | |
| 99223 | Initial hospital care, high | |
| 99281 | ER Visit, min. | |
| 99282 | ER Visit, low | |
| 99283 | ER Visit, det. | |
| 99284 | ER Visit, moderate | |
| 99285 | ER Visit, high | |
| 99307 | Subseq. nursing facility care, pf. | |
| | | |
| | | |

| PROCEDURES | | |
|---|---|---|
| 10060 | Incision/drainage, abscess | |
| 20610 | Aspiration, bursa | |
| 29505 | Splint, long leg | |
| 29515 | Splint, short leg | |
| 36415 | Routine venipuncture | |
| 45330 | Sigmoidoscopy, flex | |
| 46600 | Anoscopy, diagnostic | |
| 71030 | Chest x-ray, complete | |
| 73610 | Radiology, ankle, complete | |
| 93000 | Routine ECG | |
| 93018 | Cardiovascular stress test | |
| 99070 | Supplies and materials | |
| **LABORATORY** | | |
| 80050 | General health panel | |
| 81000 | Urinalysis, complete | |
| 82270 | Blood, occult, feces screening | |
| 82607 | Vitamin B-12 test | |
| 82948 | Glucose, blood reagent | |
| 85027 | CBC, automated | |
| 85651 | Sedimentation rate test, manual | |
| 86360 | Absolute CD4/CD8 ratio | |
| 86592 | Syphilis test | |
| 87070 | Throat culture | |
| 87088 | Urine culture | |
| 88150 | Cytopathology, cervical or vaginal | |
| **INJECTIONS** | | |
| 90471 | Immunization administration | |
| 90472 | Immunization administration, 2nd | |
| 90658 | Influenza injection, ages >3 | |
| 90702 | DT immunization, ages <7 | |
| 90703 | Tetanus immunization | |
| 90707 | MMR immunization | |
| 96372 | Therapeutic injection | |
| 90723 | DTaP - HepB - IPV | |
| 90732 | Pneumococcal immunization | |
| | | |
| | | |

## POLARIS MEDICAL GROUP

NOTES

| REFERRING PHYSICIAN | NPI |
|---|---|

AUTHORIZATION #

DIAGNOSIS

**herpes simplex**

PAYMENT AMOUNT

**$18.00 copay, check #2039**

# PATIENT INFORMATION FORM

### THIS SECTION REFERS TO PATIENT ONLY

| Name: William R. Nisinson | Sex: M | Marital Status: ☐ S ☐ M ☒ D ☐ W | Birth Date: 6/12/72 |
|---|---|---|---|

| Address: 459 Radford Street | SS#: 336-97-9162 | |
|---|---|---|

| City: Homeworth | State: OH | Zip: 43909 | Employer: Dan's Hardware (full-time) | Phone: |
|---|---|---|---|---|

| Home Phone: 999-555-5757 | Employer's Address: 3778 Old Turnpike | |
|---|---|---|

| Work Phone: 999-555-4433 | City: Cincinnati | State: OH | Zip: 43999 |
|---|---|---|---|

Race:
__American Indian or Alaska Native  __Other
__Asian  __Native Hawaiian or Other Pacific Islander
__Black or African American
X White  __Declined

Ethnicity:
__Hispanic or Latino
X Non-Hispanic or Latino
__Declined

Language: English

| Spouse's Name: | Spouse's Employer: |
|---|---|

| Emergency Contact: John Nisinson | Relationship: brother | Phone #: 999-555-0321 |
|---|---|---|

### FILL IN IF PATIENT IS A MINOR

| Parent/Guardian's Name: | Sex: | Marital Status: ☐ S ☐ M ☐ D ☐ W | Birth Date: |
|---|---|---|---|

| Phone: | SS#: | |
|---|---|---|

| Address: | Employer: | Phone: |
|---|---|---|

| City: | State: | Zip: | Employer's Address: |
|---|---|---|---|

| Student Status: | City: | State: | Zip: |
|---|---|---|---|

### INSURANCE INFORMATION

| Primary Insurance Company: Workers' Compensation - BCBS of Ohio | Secondary Insurance Company: |
|---|---|

| Subscriber's Name: | Birth Date: | Subscriber's Name: | Birth Date: |
|---|---|---|---|

| Plan: | SS#: | Plan: |
|---|---|---|

| Policy #: | Group #: | Policy #: | Group #: |
|---|---|---|---|

| Copayment/Deductible: | Price Code: A | |
|---|---|---|

### OTHER INFORMATION

| Reason for visit: fall while on the job (WC) | Allergy to Medication (list): |
|---|---|

| Name of referring physician: | If auto accident, list date and state in which it occurred: |
|---|---|

I authorize treatment and agree to pay all fees and charges for the person named above. I agree to pay all charges shown by statements, promptly upon their presentation, unless credit arrangements are agreed upon in writing.

I authorize payment directly to POLARIS MEDICAL GROUP of insurance benefits otherwise payable to me. I hereby authorize the release of any medical information necessary in order to process a claim for payment in my behalf.

William R. Nisinson  6/22/18

(Patient's Signature/Parent or Guardian's Signature)  (Date)

I plan to make payment of my medical expenses as follows (check one or more):

___ Insurance (as above)  ___ Cash/Check/Credit/Debit Card  ___ Medicare  ___ Medicaid  X Workers' Comp.

# ENCOUNTER FORM

**6/22/2018**          **12:00pm**
DATE                  TIME

**Dr. Michael Mahabir**
PROVIDER

**William R. Nisinson**
PATIENT NAME

**NISINWIO**
CHART #

### OFFICE VISITS - SYMPTOMATIC - NEW

|  |  | |
|---|---|---|
| 99201 | OF--New Patient Minimal | |
| 99202 | OF--New Patient Low | X |
| 99203 | OF--New Patient Detailed | |
| 99204 | OF--New Patient Moderate | |
| 99205 | OF--New Patient High | |

### OFFICE VISITS - SYMPTOMATIC - ESTABLISHED

|  |  | |
|---|---|---|
| 99211 | OF--Established Patient Minimal | |
| 99212 | OF--Established Patient Low | |
| 99213 | OF--Established Patient Detailed | |
| 99214 | OF--Established Patient Moderate | |
| 99215 | OF--Established Patient High | |

### PREVENTIVE VISITS - NEW

|  |  | |
|---|---|---|
| 99381 | Under 1 Year | |
| 99382 | 1 - 4 Years | |
| 99383 | 5 - 11 Years | |
| 99384 | 12 - 17 Years | |
| 99385 | 18 - 39 Years | |
| 99386 | 40 - 64 Years | |
| 99387 | 65 Years & Up | |

### PREVENTIVE VISITS - ESTABLISHED

|  |  | |
|---|---|---|
| 99391 | Under 1 Year | |
| 99392 | 1 - 4 Years | |
| 99393 | 5 - 11 Years | |
| 99394 | 12 - 17 Years | |
| 99395 | 18 - 39 Years | |
| 99396 | 40 - 64 Years | |
| 99397 | 65 Years & Up | |

### HOSPITAL/NURSING HOME VISITS

|  |  | |
|---|---|---|
| 99221 | Initial hospital care, det. | |
| 99222 | Initial hospital care, comp. | |
| 99223 | Initial hospital care, high | |
| 99281 | ER Visit, min. | |
| 99282 | ER Visit, low | |
| 99283 | ER Visit, det. | |
| 99284 | ER Visit, moderate | |
| 99285 | ER Visit, high | |
| 99307 | Subseq. nursing facility care, pf. | |
| | | |

### PROCEDURES

|  |  | |
|---|---|---|
| 10060 | Incision/drainage, abscess | |
| 20610 | Aspiration, bursa | |
| 29505 | Splint, long leg | |
| 29515 | Splint, short leg | X |
| 36415 | Routine venipuncture | |
| 45330 | Sigmoidoscopy, flex | |
| 46600 | Anoscopy, diagnostic | |
| 71030 | Chest x-ray, complete | |
| 73610 | Radiology, ankle, complete | X |
| 93000 | Routine ECG | |
| 93018 | Cardiovascular stress test | |
| 99070 | Supplies and materials | |

### LABORATORY

|  |  | |
|---|---|---|
| 80050 | General health panel | |
| 81000 | Urinalysis, complete | |
| 82270 | Blood, occult, feces screening | |
| 82607 | Vitamin B-12 test | |
| 82948 | Glucose, blood reagent | |
| 85027 | CBC, automated | |
| 85651 | Sedimentation rate test, manual | |
| 86360 | Absolute CD4/CD8 ratio | |
| 86592 | Syphilis test | |
| 87070 | Throat culture | |
| 87088 | Urine culture | |
| 88150 | Cytopathology, cervical or vaginal | |

### INJECTIONS

|  |  | |
|---|---|---|
| 90471 | Immunization administration | |
| 90472 | Immunization administration, 2nd | |
| 90658 | Influenza injection, ages >3 | |
| 90702 | DT immunization, ages <7 | |
| 90703 | Tetanus immunization | |
| 90707 | MMR immunization | |
| 96372 | Therapeutic injection | |
| 90723 | DTaP - HepB - IPV | |
| 90732 | Pneumococcal immunization | |

## POLARIS MEDICAL GROUP

NOTES

REFERRING PHYSICIAN

NPI

AUTHORIZATION #

DIAGNOSIS
**S82.899A**

PAYMENT AMOUNT

# ENCOUNTER FORM

| 6/22/2018 | 2:45pm | | Dr. Michael Mahabir |
|-----------|--------|---|---------------------|
| DATE | TIME | | PROVIDER |
| **Daniel Connolly** | | | **CONNODA0** |
| PATIENT NAME | | | CHART # |

| OFFICE VISITS - SYMPTOMATIC - NEW | | |
|---|---|---|
| 99201 | OF--New Patient Minimal | |
| 99202 | OF--New Patient Low | |
| 99203 | OF--New Patient Detailed | |
| 99204 | OF--New Patient Moderate | |
| 99205 | OF--New Patient High | |
| **OFFICE VISITS - SYMPTOMATIC - ESTABLISHED** | | |
| 99211 | OF--Established Patient Minimal | |
| 99212 | OF--Established Patient Low | X |
| 99213 | OF--Established Patient Detailed | |
| 99214 | OF--Established Patient Moderate | |
| 99215 | OF--Established Patient High | |
| **PREVENTIVE VISITS - NEW** | | |
| 99381 | Under 1 Year | |
| 99382 | 1 - 4 Years | |
| 99383 | 5 - 11 Years | |
| 99384 | 12 - 17 Years | |
| 99385 | 18 - 39 Years | |
| 99386 | 40 - 64 Years | |
| 99387 | 65 Years & Up | |
| **PREVENTIVE VISITS - ESTABLISHED** | | |
| 99391 | Under 1 Year | |
| 99392 | 1 - 4 Years | |
| 99393 | 5 - 11 Years | |
| 99394 | 12 - 17 Years | |
| 99395 | 18 - 39 Years | |
| 99396 | 40 - 64 Years | |
| 99397 | 65 Years & Up | |
| **HOSPITAL/NURSING HOME VISITS** | | |
| 99221 | Initial hospital care, det. | |
| 99222 | Initial hospital care, comp. | |
| 99223 | Initial hospital care, high | |
| 99281 | ER Visit, min. | |
| 99282 | ER Visit, low | |
| 99283 | ER Visit, det. | |
| 99284 | ER Visit, moderate | |
| 99285 | ER Visit, high | |
| 99307 | Subseq. nursing facility care, pf. | |
| | | |
| | | |

| PROCEDURES | | |
|---|---|---|
| 10060 | Incision/drainage, abscess | |
| 20610 | Aspiration, bursa | |
| 29505 | Splint, long leg | |
| 29515 | Splint, short leg | |
| 36415 | Routine venipuncture | |
| 45330 | Sigmoidoscopy, flex | |
| 46600 | Anoscopy, diagnostic | |
| 71030 | Chest x-ray, complete | |
| 73610 | Radiology, ankle, complete | |
| 93000 | Routine ECG | |
| 93018 | Cardiovascular stress test | |
| 99070 | Supplies and materials | |
| **LABORATORY** | | |
| 80050 | General health panel | |
| 81000 | Urinalysis, complete | |
| 82270 | Blood, occult, feces screening | |
| 82607 | Vitamin B-12 test | |
| 82948 | Glucose, blood reagent | |
| 85027 | CBC, automated | |
| 85651 | Sedimentation rate test, manual | |
| 86360 | Absolute CD4/CD8 ratio | |
| 86592 | Syphilis test | |
| 87070 | Throat culture | |
| 87088 | Urine culture | |
| 88150 | Cytopathology, cervical or vaginal | |
| **INJECTIONS** | | |
| 90471 | Immunization administration | |
| 90472 | Immunization administration, 2nd | |
| 90658 | Influenza injection, ages >3 | |
| 90702 | DT immunization, ages <7 | |
| 90703 | Tetanus immunization | |
| 90707 | MMR immunization | |
| 96372 | Therapeutic injection | |
| 90723 | DTaP - HepB - IPV | |
| 90732 | Pneumococcal immunization | |
| | | |
| | | |

| POLARIS MEDICAL GROUP | | NOTES |
|---|---|---|
| REFERRING PHYSICIAN | NPI | |
| AUTHORIZATION # | | |
| DIAGNOSIS **M25.559** | | |
| PAYMENT AMOUNT | | |

**Diagnosis and Procedure Codes: Hospital Visit**

Patient:        Yomo Hirosha

Subject:        Hospital Visit, Emergency Dept., 6/22/18

ICD:            I25.9

CPT:            99283

# PATIENT INFORMATION FORM

## THIS SECTION REFERS TO PATIENT ONLY

| | | | |
|---|---|---|---|
| Name: Marilyn K. Rennagel | Sex: F | Marital Status: ☐ S ☒ M ☐ D ☐ W | Birth Date: 6/12/67 |

| | |
|---|---|
| Address: 46 Brossard Avenue | SS#: 445-98-2415 |

| City: Columbus | State: OH | Zip: 43214 | Employer: The Columbus World Press (full-time) | Phone: |
|---|---|---|---|---|

| | |
|---|---|
| Home Phone: 999-555-8574 | Employer's Address: 2399 Overland Way |

| Work Phone: | City: Columbus | State: OH | Zip: 43214 |
|---|---|---|---|

**Race:**
__American Indian or Alaska Native   __Other
__Asian   __Native Hawaiian or Other Pacific Islander
__Black or African American
X White   __Declined

**Ethnicity:**
__Hispanic or Latino
X Non-Hispanic or Latino
__Declined

**Language:** English

| | |
|---|---|
| Spouse's Name: | Spouse's Employer: |

| | | |
|---|---|---|
| Emergency Contact: | Relationship: | Phone #: |

## FILL IN IF PATIENT IS A MINOR

| Parent/Guardian's Name: | Sex: | Marital Status: ☐ S ☐ M ☐ D ☐ W | Birth Date: |
|---|---|---|---|

| | |
|---|---|
| Phone: | SS#: |

| | | |
|---|---|---|
| Address: | Employer: | Phone: |

| City: | State: | Zip: | Employer's Address: |
|---|---|---|---|

| Student Status: | City: | State: | Zip: |
|---|---|---|---|

## INSURANCE INFORMATION

| | |
|---|---|
| Primary Insurance Company: Blue Cross Blue Shield of Ohio | Secondary Insurance Company: |

| Subscriber's Name: Marilyn K. Rennagel | Birth Date: 6/12/67 | Subscriber's Name: | Birth Date: |
|---|---|---|---|

| Plan: Standard | SS#: 445-98-2415 | Plan: |
|---|---|---|

| Policy #: XGS0007613045 | Group #: 067544-000 | Policy #: | Group #: |
|---|---|---|---|

| Copayment/Deductible: $500 deductible | Price Code: A | |
|---|---|---|

## OTHER INFORMATION

| | |
|---|---|
| Reason for visit: diabetes | Allergy to Medication (list): |
| Name of referring physician: | If auto accident, list date and state in which it occurred: |

I authorize treatment and agree to pay all fees and charges for the person named above. I agree to pay all charges shown by statements, promptly upon their presentation, unless credit arrangements are agreed upon in writing.

I authorize payment directly to POLARIS MEDICAL GROUP of insurance benefits otherwise payable to me. I hereby authorize the release of any medical information necessary in order to process a claim for payment in my behalf.

| Marilyn K. Rennagel | 6/22/18 |
|---|---|
| (Patient's Signature/Parent or Guardian's Signature) | (Date) |

I plan to make payment of my medical expenses as follows (check one or more):

X Insurance (as above)   X Cash/Check/Credit/Debit Card   ____Medicare   ____Medicaid   ____Workers' Comp.

# ENCOUNTER FORM

**6/22/2018**          **3:00pm**                    **Dr. Robin Crebore**
DATE                  TIME                          PROVIDER

**Marilyn K. Rennagel**                            **RENNAMAO**
PATIENT NAME                                       CHART #

| OFFICE VISITS - SYMPTOMATIC - NEW | | |
|---|---|---|
| 99201 | OF--New Patient Minimal | |
| 99202 | OF--New Patient Low | |
| 99203 | OF--New Patient Detailed | |
| 99204 | OF--New Patient Moderate | |
| 99205 | OF--New Patient High | |
| **OFFICE VISITS - SYMPTOMATIC - ESTABLISHED** | | |
| 99211 | OF--Established Patient Minimal | |
| 99212 | OF--Established Patient Low | |
| 99213 | OF--Established Patient Detailed | X |
| 99214 | OF--Established Patient Moderate | |
| 99215 | OF--Established Patient High | |
| **PREVENTIVE VISITS - NEW** | | |
| 99381 | Under 1 Year | |
| 99382 | 1 - 4 Years | |
| 99383 | 5 - 11 Years | |
| 99384 | 12 - 17 Years | |
| 99385 | 18 - 39 Years | |
| 99386 | 40 - 64 Years | |
| 99387 | 65 Years & Up | |
| **PREVENTIVE VISITS - ESTABLISHED** | | |
| 99391 | Under 1 Year | |
| 99392 | 1 - 4 Years | |
| 99393 | 5 - 11 Years | |
| 99394 | 12 - 17 Years | |
| 99395 | 18 - 39 Years | |
| 99396 | 40 - 64 Years | |
| 99397 | 65 Years & Up | |
| **HOSPITAL/NURSING HOME VISITS** | | |
| 99221 | Initial hospital care, det. | |
| 99222 | Initial hospital care, comp. | |
| 99223 | Initial hospital care, high | |
| 99281 | ER Visit, min. | |
| 99282 | ER Visit, low | |
| 99283 | ER Visit, det. | |
| 99284 | ER Visit, moderate | |
| 99285 | ER Visit, high | |
| 99307 | Subseq. nursing facility care, pf. | |
| | | |
| | | |

| PROCEDURES | | |
|---|---|---|
| 10060 | Incision/drainage, abscess | |
| 20610 | Aspiration, bursa | |
| 29505 | Splint, long leg | |
| 29515 | Splint, short leg | |
| 36415 | Routine venipuncture | |
| 45330 | Sigmoidoscopy, flex | |
| 46600 | Anoscopy, diagnostic | |
| 71030 | Chest x-ray, complete | |
| 73610 | Radiology, ankle, complete | |
| 93000 | Routine ECG | |
| 93018 | Cardiovascular stress test | |
| 99070 | Supplies and materials | |
| **LABORATORY** | | |
| 80050 | General health panel | |
| 81000 | Urinalysis, complete | X |
| 82270 | Blood, occult, feces screening | |
| 82607 | Vitamin B-12 test | |
| 82948 | Glucose, blood reagent | X |
| 85027 | CBC, automated | |
| 85651 | Sedimentation rate test, manual | |
| 86360 | Absolute CD4/CD8 ratio | |
| 86592 | Syphilis test | |
| 87070 | Throat culture | |
| 87088 | Urine culture | |
| 88150 | Cytopathology, cervical or vaginal | |
| **INJECTIONS** | | |
| 90471 | Immunization administration | |
| 90472 | Immunization administration, 2nd | |
| 90658 | Influenza injection, ages >3 | |
| 90702 | DT immunization, ages <7 | |
| 90703 | Tetanus immunization | |
| 90707 | MMR immunization | |
| 96372 | Therapeutic injection | |
| 90723 | DTaP - HepB - IPV | |
| 90732 | Pneumococcal immunization | |
| | | |
| | | |

## POLARIS MEDICAL GROUP

NOTES

REFERRING PHYSICIAN                    NPI

AUTHORIZATION #

DIAGNOSIS
**E11.9, I25.10**

PAYMENT AMOUNT

# ENCOUNTER FORM

| | |
|---|---|
| **6/22/2018**      **3:15pm** | **Dr. Robin Crebore** |
| DATE      TIME | PROVIDER |
| **William A. Brown** | **BROWNWI0** |
| PATIENT NAME | CHART # |

| OFFICE VISITS - SYMPTOMATIC - NEW | | |
|---|---|---|
| 99201 | OF--New Patient Minimal | |
| 99202 | OF--New Patient Low | |
| 99203 | OF--New Patient Detailed | |
| 99204 | OF--New Patient Moderate | |
| 99205 | OF--New Patient High | |

| OFFICE VISITS - SYMPTOMATIC - ESTABLISHED | | |
|---|---|---|
| 99211 | OF--Established Patient Minimal | |
| 99212 | OF--Established Patient Low | X |
| 99213 | OF--Established Patient Detailed | |
| 99214 | OF--Established Patient Moderate | |
| 99215 | OF--Established Patient High | |

| PREVENTIVE VISITS - NEW | | |
|---|---|---|
| 99381 | Under 1 Year | |
| 99382 | 1 - 4 Years | |
| 99383 | 5 - 11 Years | |
| 99384 | 12 - 17 Years | |
| 99385 | 18 - 39 Years | |
| 99386 | 40 - 64 Years | |
| 99387 | 65 Years & Up | |

| PREVENTIVE VISITS - ESTABLISHED | | |
|---|---|---|
| 99391 | Under 1 Year | |
| 99392 | 1 - 4 Years | |
| 99393 | 5 - 11 Years | |
| 99394 | 12 - 17 Years | |
| 99395 | 18 - 39 Years | |
| 99396 | 40 - 64 Years | |
| 99397 | 65 Years & Up | |

| HOSPITAL/NURSING HOME VISITS | | |
|---|---|---|
| 99221 | Initial hospital care, det. | |
| 99222 | Initial hospital care, comp. | |
| 99223 | Initial hospital care, high | |
| 99281 | ER Visit, min. | |
| 99282 | ER Visit, low | |
| 99283 | ER Visit, det. | |
| 99284 | ER Visit, moderate | |
| 99285 | ER Visit, high | |
| 99307 | Subseq. nursing facility care, pf. | |
| | | |

| PROCEDURES | | |
|---|---|---|
| 10060 | Incision/drainage, abscess | |
| 20610 | Aspiration, bursa | |
| 29505 | Splint, long leg | |
| 29515 | Splint, short leg | |
| 36415 | Routine venipuncture | |
| 45330 | Sigmoidoscopy, flex | |
| 46600 | Anoscopy, diagnostic | |
| 71030 | Chest x-ray, complete | |
| 73610 | Radiology, ankle, complete | |
| 93000 | Routine ECG | |
| 93018 | Cardiovascular stress test | |
| 99070 | Supplies and materials | |

| LABORATORY | | |
|---|---|---|
| 80050 | General health panel | |
| 81000 | Urinalysis, complete | |
| 82270 | Blood, occult, feces screening | |
| 82607 | Vitamin B-12 test | |
| 82948 | Glucose, blood reagent | |
| 85027 | CBC, automated | |
| 85651 | Sedimentation rate test, manual | |
| 86360 | Absolute CD4/CD8 ratio | |
| 86592 | Syphilis test | |
| 87070 | Throat culture | |
| 87088 | Urine culture | |
| 88150 | Cytopathology, cervical or vaginal | |

| INJECTIONS | | |
|---|---|---|
| 90471 | Immunization administration | |
| 90472 | Immunization administration, 2nd | |
| 90658 | Influenza injection, ages >3 | |
| 90702 | DT immunization, ages <7 | |
| 90703 | Tetanus immunization | |
| 90707 | MMR immunization | |
| 96372 | Therapeutic injection | |
| 90723 | DTaP - HepB - IPV | |
| 90732 | Pneumococcal immunization | |
| | | |
| | | |

## POLARIS MEDICAL GROUP

| | | NOTES |
|---|---|---|
| REFERRING PHYSICIAN | NPI | |
| AUTHORIZATION # | | |
| DIAGNOSIS<br>**K64.4** | | |
| PAYMENT AMOUNT | | |

Standard Health Care
1500 Summit Avenue, Suite 500
Cincinnati, OH 45000

Polaris Medical Group
2100 Grace Avenue
Columbus, OH 43214

Practice ID: 01-234567

Date Prepared: 6/19/18                                      EFT Number: 0347914

| Patient's Name | Dates of Service From - Thru | POS | Proc | Qty | Charge Amount | Allowed Amount | Patient Resp. | Amt. Paid Provider |
|---|---|---|---|---|---|---|---|---|
| Daiute, Angelo X | 6/14/18 – 6/14/18 | 11 | 99386 | 1 | $233.00 | $180.00 | $15.00 | $165.00 |
| Daiute, Angelo X | 6/14/18 – 6/14/18 | 11 | 36415 | 1 | $22.00 | $17.00 | $0.00 | $17.00 |
| Daiute, Angelo X | 6/14/18 – 6/14/18 | 11 | 93000 | 1 | $84.00 | $70.00 | $0.00 | $70.00 |
| Daiute, Angelo X | 6/14/18 – 6/14/18 | 11 | 80050 | 1 | $143.00 | $120.00 | $0.00 | $120.00 |
| Daiute, Angelo X | 6/14/18 – 6/14/18 | 11 | 81000 | 1 | $22.00 | $17.00 | $0.00 | $17.00 |
| Totals | | | | | $504.00 | $404.00 | $15.00 | $389.00 |

* * * * * * *    *EFT transmitted in the amount of $389.00*    * * * * * * *

Ohio Insurance Company
1600 Galleria Way
Cleveland, OH 44000

Polaris Medical Group
2100 Grace Avenue
Columbus, OH 43214

Practice ID: 09-012345

Date Prepared: 6/28/18                                  EFT Number: 115896

| Patient's Name | Dates of Service From - Thru | POS | Proc | Qty | Charge Amount | Allowed Amount | Patient Resp. | Amt. Paid Provider |
|----------------|------------------------------|-----|------|-----|---------------|----------------|---------------|--------------------|
| Ferrara, Victoria | 6/13/18 – 6/13/18 | 11 | 99212 | 1 | $54.00 | $54.00 | $5.40 | $48.60 |
| Totals | | | | | $54.00 | $54.00 | $5.40 | $48.60 |

*  *  *  *  *  *  *  *    *EFT transmitted in the amount of $48.60*    *  *  *  *  *  *  *  *

Standard Health Care
1500 Summit Avenue, Suite 500
Cincinnati, OH 45000

Polaris Medical Group
2100 Grace Avenue
Columbus, OH 43214

Practice ID: 01-234567

Date Prepared: 6/28/18                                        EFT Number: 65891372

| Patient's Name | Dates of Service From - Thru | POS | Proc | Qty | Charge Amount | Allowed Amount | Patient Resp. | Amt. Paid Provider |
|---|---|---|---|---|---|---|---|---|
| Kavanaugh, Gregory | 6/11/18 – 6/11/18 | 11 | 99212 | 1 | $54.00 | $46.00 | $15.00 | $31.00 |
| Kavanaugh, Gregory | 6/11/18 – 6/11/18 | 11 | 36415 | 1 | $22.00 | $17.00 | $0.00 | $17.00 |
| Kavanaugh, Gregory | 6/11/18 – 6/11/18 | 11 | 86360 | 1 | $263.00 | $195.00 | $0.00 | $195.00 |
| Szinovacz, Martin G | 6/22/18 – 6/22/18 | 11 | 99213 | 1 | $72.00 | $62.00 | $15.00 | $47.00 |
| Totals | | | | | $411.00 | $320.00 | $30.00 | $290.00 |

\* \* \* \* \* \* \*   *EFT transmitted in the amount of $290.00*   \* \* \* \* \* \* \*

Blue Cross Blue Shield of Ohio
5000 First Street
Worthington, OH 43085

Polaris Medical Group
2100 Grace Avenue
Columbus, OH 43214

Practice ID: 04-5678901

Date Prepared: 6/28/18

EFT Number: 9928674

| Patient's Name | Dates of Service From - Thru | POS | Proc | Qty | Charge Amount | Allowed Amount | Patient Resp. | Amt. Paid Provider |
|---|---|---|---|---|---|---|---|---|
| Berkel-Rees, Gloria | 6/15/18 – 6/15/18 | 11 | 99213 | 1 | $72.00 | $72.00 | $21.60 | $50.40 |
| Berkel-Rees, Gloria | 6/15/18 – 6/15/18 | 11 | 99070 | 1 | $15.00 | $15.00 | $4.50 | $10.50 |
| | | | | | | | | |
| Brown, William A | 6/12/18 – 6/12/18 | 11 | 99214 | 1 | $105.00 | $105.00 | $31.50 | $73.50 |
| Brown, William A | 6/12/18 – 6/12/18 | 11 | 82270 | 1 | $19.00 | $19.00 | $5.70 | $13.30 |
| Brown, William A | 6/12/18 – 6/12/18 | 11 | 46600 | 1 | $89.00 | $89.00 | $26.70 | $62.30 |
| Brown, William A | 6/12/18 – 6/12/18 | 11 | 99212 | 1 | $54.00 | $54.00 | $16.20 | $37.80 |
| | | | | | | | | |
| Ferrone, Fran C | 6/18/18 – 6/18/18 | 11 | 99202 | 1 | $88.00 | $88.00 | $26.40 | $61.60 |
| | | | | | | | | |
| LeConey, James I | 6/12/18 – 6/12/18 | 11 | 99214 | 1 | $105.00 | $105.00 | $31.50 | $73.50 |
| | | | | | | | | |
| O'Keefe, Diana E | 6/19/18 – 6/19/18 | 11 | 99211 | 1 | $36.00 | $36.00 | $10.80 | $25.20 |
| O'Keefe, Diana E | 6/19/18 – 6/19/18 | 11 | 85651 | 1 | $24.00 | $24.00 | $7.20 | $16.80 |
| | | | | | | | | |
| Rennagel, Marilyn K | 6/22/18 – 6/22/18 | 11 | 99213 | 1 | $72.00 | $72.00 | $21.60 | $50.40 |
| Rennagel, Marilyn K | 6/22/18 – 6/22/18 | 11 | 81000 | 1 | $22.00 | $22.00 | $6.60 | $15.40 |
| Rennagel, Marilyn K | 6/22/18 – 6/22/18 | 11 | 82948 | 1 | $18.00 | $18.00 | $5.40 | $12.60 |

| | | | | | | | | |
|---|---|---|---|---|---|---|---|---|
| Totals | | | | | $719.00 | $719.00 | $215.70 | $503.30 |

******* *EFT transmitted in the amount of $503.30* *******

Blue Cross Blue Shield of Ohio - Workers' Compensation
5000 First Street
Worthington, OH 43085

Polaris Medical Group
2100 Grace Avenue
Columbus, OH 43214

Practice ID: 02-3456789

Date Prepared: 6/28/18                     EFT Number: 88415629

| Patient's Name | Dates of Service From - Thru | POS | Proc | Qty | Charge Amount | Allowed Amount | Patient Resp. | Amt. Paid Provider |
|---|---|---|---|---|---|---|---|---|
| Nisinson, William R | 6/22/18 – 6/22/18 | 11 | 99202 | 1 | $88.00 | $88.00 | $0.00 | $88.00 |
| Nisinson, William R | 6/22/18 – 6/22/18 | 11 | 29515 | 1 | $114.00 | $114.00 | $0.00 | $114.00 |
| Nisinson, William R | 6/22/18 – 6/22/18 | 11 | 73610 | 1 | $113.00 | $113.00 | $0.00 | $113.00 |

| Totals | | | | | $315.00 | $315.00 | $0.00 | $315.00 |

\* \* \* \* \* \* \*    *EFT transmitted in the amount of $315.00*    \* \* \* \* \* \* \*

Nationwide Medicare HMO
P.O. Box 7000
Columbus, OH 43214

Polaris Medical Group
2100 Grace Avenue
Columbus, OH 43214

Practice ID: 10-123456

Date Prepared: 6/28/18

EFT Number: 378214

| Patient's Name | Dates of Service From - Thru | POS | Proc | Qty | Charge Amount | Allowed Amount | Patient Resp. | Amt. Paid Provider |
|---|---|---|---|---|---|---|---|---|
| Atchely, Rachel D | 5/23/18 – 5/23/18 | 31 | 99307 | 1 | $63.00 | $34.00 | $5.00 | $29.00 |
| Atchely, Rachel D | 6/20/18 – 6/20/18 | 31 | 99307 | 1 | $63.00 | $34.00 | $5.00 | $29.00 |
| | | | | | | | | |
| Beedon, Myrna E | 5/28/18 – 5/28/18 | 11 | 99211 | 1 | $36.00 | $14.00 | $5.00 | $9.00 |
| Beedon, Myrna E | 5/28/18 – 5/28/18 | 11 | 93000 | 1 | $84.00 | $29.00 | $0.00 | $29.00 |
| Beedon, Myrna E | 6/18/18 – 6/18/18 | 21 | 99222 | 1 | $205.00 | $113.00 | $0.00 | $113.00 |
| | | | | | | | | |
| Estephan, Wilma T | 6/12/18 – 6/12/18 | 11 | 99202 | 1 | $88.00 | $50.00 | $5.00 | $45.00 |
| Estephan, Wilma T | 6/12/18 – 6/12/18 | 11 | 81000 | 1 | $22.00 | $10.00 | $0.00 | $10.00 |
| Estephan, Wilma T | 6/12/18 – 6/12/18 | 11 | 87088 | 1 | $42.00 | $18.00 | $0.00 | $18.00 |
| | | | | | | | | |
| McAniff, Nora B | 6/13/18 – 6/13/18 | 11 | 99202 | 1 | $88.00 | $50.00 | $5.00 | $45.00 |
| | | | | | | | | |
| Torres-Gil, Flora K | 6/19/18 – 6/19/18 | 11 | 20610 | 1 | $112.00 | $45.00 | $5.00 | $40.00 |
| | | | | | | | | |
| Wong, Hanna Z | 6/21/18 – 6/21/18 | 11 | 99205 | 1 | $229.00 | $128.00 | $5.00 | $123.00 |
| Wong, Hanna Z | 6/21/18 – 6/21/18 | 11 | 93000 | 1 | $84.00 | $29.00 | $0.00 | $29.00 |

| Totals | | | | | $1116.00 | $554.00 | $35.00 | $519.00 |
|---|---|---|---|---|---|---|---|---|

* * * * * * *  *EFT transmitted in the amount of $519.00*  * * * * * * *

TRICARE
PO Box 1000
Columbus, OH 43214

Polaris Medical Group
2100 Grace Avenue
Columbus, OH 43214

Practice ID: 05-678901

Date Prepared: 6/28/18                     EFT Number: 69876542

| Patient's Name | Dates of Service From - Thru | POS | Proc | Qty | Charge Amount | Allowed Amount | Patient Resp. | Amt. Paid Provider |
|---|---|---|---|---|---|---|---|---|
| Kopelman, Mary A. | 6/11/18 – 6/11/18 | 11 | 99202 | 1 | $88.00 | $50.00 | $10.00 | $40.00 |
| Kopelman, Mary A. | 6/11/18 – 6/11/18 | 11 | 80050 | 1 | $143.00 | $70.00 | $0.00 | $70.00 |
| Kopelman, Mary A. | 6/11/18 – 6/11/18 | 11 | 36415 | 1 | $22.00 | $8.00 | $0.00 | $8.00 |
| Wu, Elizabeth I | 6/18/18 – 6/18/18 | 11 | 99212 | 1 | $54.00 | $28.00 | $10.00 | $18.00 |
| Totals | | | | | $307.00 | $156.00 | $20.00 | $136.00 |

******* *EFT transmitted in the amount of $136.00* *******

Nationwide Medicare
P.O. Box 7001
Columbus, OH 43214

Polaris Medical Group
2100 Grace Avenue
Columbus, OH 43214

Practice ID: 10-123456

Date Prepared: 6/28/18

EFT Number: 3642988

| Patient's Name | Dates of Service From - Thru | POS | Proc | Qty | Charge Amount | Allowed Amount | Patient Resp. | Amt. Paid Provider |
|---|---|---|---|---|---|---|---|---|
| Ahmadian, George | 5/23/18 – 5/23/18 | 11 | 99213 | 1 | $72.00 | $39.00 | $7.80 | $31.20 |
| Ahmadian, George | 6/14/18 – 6/14/18 | 11 | 99215 | 1 | $163.00 | $94.00 | $18.80 | $75.20 |
| | | | | | | | | |
| Connolly, Daniel | 5/31/18 – 5/31/18 | 11 | 99397 | 1 | $155.00 | $118.00 | B | $0.00 |
| Connolly, Daniel | 5/31/18 – 5/31/18 | 11 | 80050 | 1 | $143.00 | $70.00 | B | $0.00 |
| Connolly, Daniel | 6/11/18 – 6/11/18 | 11 | 99214 | 1 | $105.00 | $59.00 | B | $47.20 |
| Connolly, Daniel | 6/22/18 – 6/22/18 | 11 | 99212 | 1 | $54.00 | $28.00 | B | $22.40 |
| | | | | | | | | |
| Stephanos, Lydia | 6/11/18 – 6/11/18 | 11 | 99213 | 1 | $72.00 | $39.00 | $7.80 | $31.20 |
| Stephanos, Lydia | 6/11/18 – 6/11/18 | 11 | 10060 | 1 | $117.00 | $57.00 | $11.40 | $45.60 |

B  Claim submitted to secondary payer.

| Totals | | | | | $881.00 | $504.00 | $45.80 | $252.80 |
|---|---|---|---|---|---|---|---|---|

\* \* \* \* \* \* \*  *EFT transmitted in the amount of $252.80*  \* \* \* \* \* \* \*

Ohio Dept. of Human Resources - Medicaid
PO Box 4000
Columbus OH 43214

Polaris Medical Group
2100 Grace Avenue
Columbus, OH 43214

Practice ID: 11-123456

Date Prepared: 6/28/18

EFT Number: 3968452

| Patient's Name | Dates of Service From - Thru | POS | Proc | Qty | Charge Amount | Allowed Amount | Patient Resp. | Amt. Paid Provider |
|---|---|---|---|---|---|---|---|---|
| Colbs, Seymour | 6/15/18 – 6/15/18 | 11 | 99213 | 1 | $72.00 | $39.00 | $8.25 | $30.75 |
| Connolly, Daniel | 6/11/18 – 6/11/18 | 11 | 99214 | 1 | $105.00 | $59.00A | $0.00 | $11.80 |
| Connolly, Daniel | 6/22/18 – 6/22/18 | 11 | 99212 | 1 | $54.00 | $28.00A | $0.00 | $5.60 |
| Hellery, Jimmy | 5/25/18 – 5/25/18 | 11 | 99211 | 1 | $36.00 | $14.00 | $8.25 | $5.75 |
| Hellery, Jimmy | 6/18/18 – 6/18/18 | 11 | 99212 | 1 | $54.00 | $28.00 | $8.25 | $19.75 |
| Hellery, Jimmy | 6/18/18 – 6/18/18 | 11 | 87070 | 1 | $48.00 | $20.00 | $0.00 | $20.00 |
| Yange-Sang, Roberta | 6/15/18 – 6/15/18 | 11 | 99212 | 1 | $54.00 | $28.00 | $8.25 | $19.75 |

A - Claim forwarded from primary payer.

| Totals | | | | | $423.00 | $216.00 | $33.00 | $113.40 |
|---|---|---|---|---|---|---|---|---|

* * * * * * *   *EFT transmitted in the amount of $113.40*   * * * * * * *

Columbus Medical Care
3000 Arkady Street
Columbus OH 43214


Polaris Medical Group
2100 Grace Avenue
Columbus, OH 43214

Practice ID: 06-789012

Date Prepared: 6/28/18

EFT Number: 00679522

| Patient's Name | Dates of Service From - Thru | POS | Proc | Qty | Charge Amount | Allowed Amount | Patient Resp. | Amt. Paid Provider |
|---|---|---|---|---|---|---|---|---|
| Deysenrothe, Floyd | 6/18/18 – 6/18/18 | 11 | 90471 | 1 | $18.00 | $14.00 | $12.00 | $2.00 |
| Deysenrothe, Floyd | 6/18/18 – 6/18/18 | 11 | 90703 | 1 | $29.00 | $24.00 | $0.00 | $24.00 |
| | | | | | | | | |
| Deysenrothe, Mae J | 6/20/18 – 6/20/18 | 11 | 99395 | 1 | $178.00 | $137.00 | $12.00 | $125.00 |
| Deysenrothe, Mae J | 6/20/18 – 6/20/18 | 11 | 80050 | 1 | $143.00 | $120.00 | $0.00 | $120.00 |
| Deysenrothe, Mae J | 6/20/18 – 6/20/18 | 11 | 81000 | 1 | $22.00 | $17.00 | $0.00 | $17.00 |
| Deysenrothe, Mae J | 6/20/18 – 6/20/18 | 11 | 88150 | 1 | $35.00 | $29.00 | $0.00 | $29.00 |
| Deysenrothe, Mae J | 6/20/18 – 6/20/18 | 11 | 36415 | 1 | $22.00 | $17.00 | $0.00 | $17.00 |
| Deysenrothe, Mae J | 6/20/18 – 6/20/18 | 11 | 93000 | 1 | $84.00 | $70.00 | $0.00 | $70.00 |
| | | | | | | | | |
| Deysenrothe, Roger | 4/30/18 – 4/30/18 | 11 | 99395 | 1 | $178.00 | $137.00 | $12.00 | $125.00 |
| Deysenrothe, Roger | 4/30/18 – 4/30/18 | 11 | 36415 | 1 | $22.00 | $17.00 | $0.00 | $17.00 |
| Deysenrothe, Roger | 4/30/18 – 4/30/18 | 11 | 80050 | 1 | $143.00 | $120.00 | $0.00 | $120.00 |
| Deysenrothe, Roger | 4/30/18 – 4/30/18 | 11 | 81000 | 1 | $22.00 | $17.00 | $0.00 | $17.00 |
| Deysenrothe, Roger | 4/30/18 – 4/30/18 | 11 | 93000 | 1 | $84.00 | $70.00 | $0.00 | $70.00 |
| | | | | | | | | |
| Hirosha, Yomo C | 4/12/18 – 4/12/18 | 11 | 99214 | 1 | $105.00 | $91.00 | $12.00 | $79.00 |
| Hirosha, Yomo C | 4/12/18 – 4/12/18 | 11 | 93000 | 1 | $84.00 | $70.00 | $0.00 | $70.00 |
| Hirosha, Yomo C | 4/12/18 – 4/12/18 | 11 | 93018 | 1 | $202.00 | $162.00 | $0.00 | $162.00 |
| Hirosha, Yomo C | 6/22/18 – 6/22/18 | 23 | 99283 | 1 | $150.00 | $131.00 | $0.00 | $131.00 |
| | | | | | | | | |
| Weintraub, Stewart | 6/13/18 – 6/13/18 | 23 | 99283 | 1 | $150.00 | $131.00 | $0.00 | $131.00 |

| Totals | | | | | $1671.00 | $1374.00 | $48.00 | $1326.00 |
|---|---|---|---|---|---|---|---|---|

\* \* \* \* \* \* \*   *EFT transmitted in the amount of $1326.00*   \* \* \* \* \* \* \*

Aetna Health Plans
5777 Royal Boulevard
Columbus, OH 43214

Polaris Medical Group
2100 Grace Avenue
Columbus, OH 43214

Practice ID: 08-901234

Date Prepared: 6/30/18                                    EFT Number: 00059876521

Capitation payment for May 2018                   $1500.00
Dr. Robin Crebore
Dr. Michael Mahabir

Capitation payment for June 2018                  $1500.00
Dr. Robin Crebore
Dr. Michael Mahabir

* * * * * * *    *EFT transmitted in the amount of $3000.00*    * * * * * * *

CIGNA Healthplan
1200 Green Avenue
Cincinnati, OH 45000

Polaris Medical Group
2100 Grace Avenue
Columbus, OH 43214

Practice ID: 07-890123

Date Prepared: 6/30/18                                     EFT Number: 794620

| | |
|---|---|
| Capitation payment for May 2018<br>Dr. Robin Crebore<br>Dr. Michael Mahabir | $2000.00 |
| Capitation payment for June 2018<br>Dr. Robin Crebore<br>Dr. Michael Mahabir | $2000.00 |

\* \* \* \* \* \* \*     *EFT transmitted in the amount of $4000.00*     \* \* \* \* \* \* \*

# Glossary

**accept assignment** A physician's agreement to accept an allowed charge as payment in full.

**Acknowledgment of Receipt of Notice of Privacy Practices** Form accompanying a covered entity's Notice of Privacy Practices; under HIPAA, medical practices and other covered entities must make a good-faith effort to have patients sign the acknowledgment.

**allowed amount/allowed charge** The amount an insurance carrier or governmental program covers for each service.

**American Recovery and Reinvestment Act of 2009 (ARRA)** A $787 billion economic stimulus bill passed in 2009 that allocates $19.2 billion to promote the use of health information technology.

**assignment of benefits** Authorization by a policyholder that allows an insurance carrier to pay benefits directly to a healthcare provider.

**audit** A third-party examination of a physician's accounting records or patient records relating to claims.

**audit trail** A technical safeguard on a computer that keeps track of who has accessed information and when, which is regularly checked by a manager for errors or irregularities in data entry.

**authorized signature form** A one-time authorization for payment to be made to a physician for services rendered and for the release of medical information to insurance carriers or medical professionals; also called *release of information*.

**benefits** (1) The amount of money an insurance carrier pays for services covered by an insurance policy. (2) Nonmonetary employee compensation, such as a paid vacation.

**billing compliance program** A set of procedures and policies that helps medical office employees comply with applicable laws and regulations and avoid misconduct.

**Blue Cross and Blue Shield Association** The national licensing agency of Blue Cross and Blue Shield plans.

**breach of confidentiality** A party's disclosing to a third party information that was confidential between two original parties.

**breach of contract** A party's failure to comply with the terms of a legal contract.

**capitation** A method of insurance reimbursement to physicians based on the number of patients seen rather than the services performed.

**case** A Medisoft term that refers to a grouping of transactions for visits to a physician's office organized around a condition.

**Centers for Medicare and Medicaid Services (CMS)** The governmental department that runs Medicare and other governmental health programs (formerly HCFA).

**CHAMPUS** Now the TRICARE program; formerly the Civilian Health and Medical Program of the Uniformed Services for spouses and children of active-duty service members, military retirees and their families, some former spouses, and survivors of deceased military members.

**CHAMPVA** The Civilian Health and Medical Program of the Veterans Administration (Department of Veterans Affairs), which shares healthcare costs for families of veterans with 100 percent service-related disabilities and for the surviving spouses and children of veterans who died from service-related disabilities.

**chief complaint (CC)** A description of the symptoms or other reasons a patient seeks medical care on a particular visit to a physician.

**claim appeal** A written request for a review of a payment that the provider feels is inadequate or incorrect.

**clearinghouse** A centralized service bureau that for a fee offers providers the service of receiving electronic media/paper claims, checking and preparing them for processing, and transmitting them in proper data format to the correct carriers.

**COBRA** A federal law requiring employers with 20 or more workers who sponsor a group health benefit plan to continue health insurance plan coverage for up to 18 months for terminated or laid-off employees.

**coding** In medical terminology, the process of assigning numerical codes to diagnoses and treatments.

**coinsurance** The portion of charges under an indemnity plan that the insured must pay for services, based on insurance coverage and payment of a deductible amount.

**consultation** The service performed by one physician for the purpose of advising an attending physician about a patient's condition and care.

**continuity of care** The coordination of care received by a patient over time and across multiple healthcare providers.

**coordination of benefits** A clause in an insurance policy that explains how the policy will pay if more than one insurance policy applies to the claim.

**copayment** The portion or amount of charges that the insured must pay at the time of services, based on insurance coverage and payment of any deductible amounts.

**covered entity** Under HIPAA, a health plan, clearinghouse, or provider that transmits any health information in electronic form in connection with a HIPAA transaction.

**CPT** The abbreviation that refers to *Current Procedural Terminology*.

**Current Procedural Terminology (CPT)** A publication of the American Medical Association containing a standardized system of codes for medical procedures and diagnostic services.

**day sheet** In a medical office, a report that summarizes the business day's charges and payments, drawn from all the patient ledgers for the day.

**deductible** The part of medical charges the insured must pay before insurance payment begins.

**default** The instruction or value a computer is programmed to use unless other instructions or values are entered.

**dependent** A person related to a policyholder, such as a spouse or child.

**diagnosis** A physician's opinion of the nature of a patient's illness or injury.

**diagnostic code** The number assigned to a physician's diagnosis in the International Classification of Diseases (ICD).

**dialog box** A computer screen display with which a user interacts by providing instructions or selecting from among options.

**documentation** The chronological recording of facts and observations about a patient's health status in a logical sequence.

**Dx** An abbreviation for a physician's diagnosis.

**electronic data interchange (EDI)** The electronic exchange of healthcare claims, remittance, and eligibility and claim status inquiries.

**electronic health record (EHR)** Electronic collection and management of health data.

**electronic protected health information (ePHI)** Any protected health information (PHI) that is created, stored, transmitted, or received electronically.

**encounter form** The part of a patient's medical record that contains the diagnosis, services, and fees for a patient's visit.

**established patient** A patient who has been seen by a provider in the practice in the same specialty or subspecialty within three years.

**ethics** Standards of conduct based on moral principles.

**excluded illness** A condition or circumstance specified in a medical insurance contract as not covered.

**explanation of Medicare benefits (EOMB)** Remittance advice that explains how payment for a Medicare claim was determined.

**family practitioner** A physician with a general practice rather than a specialty; also called a *general practitioner*.

**fee-for-service** A way of charging patients for medical services based on the service performed.

**fee schedule** A list of charges for services and procedures performed by a physician.

**fixed fee schedule** A payment method based on a list of maximum fees allowed for specific services.

**fraud** The intentional misrepresentation of information to obtain a benefit.

**grievance** Job-related problem that an employee feels should be corrected.

**guardian** An adult responsible for the care and custody of a minor. The guardian can make decisions regarding the minor's health, care, and maintenance.

**Health Insurance Claim Form (CMS-1500)** The universal form approved by the American Medical Association and CMS for use in requesting benefits from medical insurance carriers and government health programs.

**health maintenance organization (HMO)** A managed care healthcare system under which patients pay fixed periodic rates and receive medical services from an approved list of healthcare providers specified in their contract.

**HIPAA (Health Insurance Portability and Accountability Act of 1996)** A federal law governing many aspects of healthcare, such as electronic transmission standards and the security of healthcare records.

**HIPAA Electronic Health Care Transactions and Code Sets (TCS)** HIPAA standards governing the electronic exchange of health information using standard formats and standard code sets.

**HIPAA Privacy Rule** Legislation that protects individually identifiable health information.

**HIPAA Security Rule** Legislation that outlines the administrative, technical, and physical safeguards required to prevent unauthorized access to protected healthcare information.

**HITECH Act** The Health Information Technology for Economic and Clinical Health Act, part of the American Recovery and Reinvestment Act of 2009, which provides financial incentives to physicians and hospitals to adopt EHRs and strengthens HIPAA privacy and security regulations.

**ICD code** A system of diagnostic codes based on the International Classification of Diseases.

**indemnity plan** An agreement to reimburse a policyholder for healthcare costs due to illness or accidents.

**informed consent** A written document in which the physician notifies the patient of a procedure and the accompanying hazards, complications, alternatives, and risks.

**inpatient** A person admitted to a hospital who generally stays overnight and incurs the hospital's room and board fees.

**insurance carrier** A company or agency that offers financial protection as a result of a specified event.

**insurance claim form** A document filed with an insurance carrier to receive benefits.

**insurance log** A medical office's list of insurance claim forms that have been filed and/or paid.

**insured** The policyholder, or subscriber, to a medical insurance policy or plan.

**International Classification of Diseases (ICD)** A publication known as the ICD that lists diagnostic codes assigned by the World Health Organization and used by the U.S. government, American medical insurance carriers, and others.

**internist** A physician who specializes in the care of adults.

**liable** Legally responsible.

**libel** A harmful, written statement about someone.

**malfeasance** Wrongdoing or misconduct, often by someone who is legally bound to proper actions.

**managed care** A way of supervising medical care to be sure patients get services they need in the most appropriate, cost-effective setting.

**Medicaid** A federal and state assistance program that pays for healthcare services for people with incomes below the national poverty level.

**medical insurance** A financial plan that covers the cost of hospital and/or medical care due to illness or injury.

**medical malpractice** The failure to use an acceptable level of professional skill when giving medical services that results in injury or harm to a patient.

**medical necessity** Payment criterion of third-party payers that requires medical treatments to be appropriate for a patient's diagnosis and to be provided in accordance with generally accepted standards of medical practice.

**medical professional liability policy** An insurance policy that covers a medical office's personnel for unintentional errors in the medical treatment of patients.

**medical record** A file that includes the patient information form, the patient's medical history, record of care, progress notes, insurance correspondence, and other correspondence.

**Medicare** The federal health insurance program for people aged 65 and older and for those with some disabilities and end-stage renal disease.

**Medicare beneficiary** A person covered by Medicare.

**Medicare carrier** A private insurance organization under contract with the federal government to administer Medicare Part B claims.

**Medicare Fee Schedule (MFS)** A list of the allowed fees that are reimbursable to Medicare-participating physicians; based on the RBRVS system.

**Medicare Part A** The part of the Medicare program that pays for hospitalization, care in a skilled nursing facility, home healthcare, and hospice care.

**Medicare Part B** The part of the Medicare program that pays for physician services, outpatient hospital services, durable medical equipment, and other services and supplies.

**Medicare-participating agreement** A document signed by physicians and other providers of medical services who have agreed to accept assignment on all Medicare claims.

**Medigap insurance** An insurance plan offered by a federally approved private insurance carrier designed to supplement Medicare coverage.

**Medi-Medi beneficiary** A person who is eligible for both Medicare and Medicaid benefits.

**menu** A list of choices appearing on a computer screen for selection by a user.

**modem** A device that converts electronic data from computers into signals that can be transmitted over telephone lines.

**modifier** ICD A nonessential word or phrase that helps to define a diagnostic code; CPT: a number indicating a special circumstance that affects a medical procedure in some way, such as surgery being more difficult than usual for some reason.

**multiple modifiers** More than a single two-digit code used to augment a procedure code.

**National Provider Identifier (NPI)** A unique identifier assigned to a healthcare provider that is used in standard transactions, such as healthcare claims.

**new patient** A patient who has not received services from the same provider or a provider of the same specialty or subspecialty within the same practice for a period of three years.

**nonavailability statement** A form required for preauthorization when a TRICARE member seeks medical services in other than a military facility.

**nonparticipating (nonPAR) physician** A physician or other healthcare provider who chooses not to join a particular governmental program or insurance carrier's plan.

**Notice of Privacy Practices (NPP)** A HIPAA-mandated description of a covered entity's principles and procedures related to the protection of patients' health information.

**NSF (nonsufficient funds) check** A check that is not honored by a bank because the account it was written on does not have sufficient funds to cover it.

**outpatient** A patient who receives healthcare in a hospital without admission; the length of stay is generally 23 hours or less.

**participating (PAR) physician** A physician who participates in a governmental program or an insurance carrier's plan.

**patient chart** See *medical record.*

**patient day sheet** A report that summarizes the business day's charges and payments, organized by patient.

**patient information form** A form that includes a patient's personal, employment, and insurance company data needed to complete an insurance claim form; also known as a *registration form.*

**patient ledger** In a medical office, a record of all charges and payments made to a particular patient's account.

**patient update form** A form that is used to update information about a patient's personal, employment, and insurance company data.

**place of service (POS) code** Code that describes a location where medical services are performed.

**policyholder** A person who buys an insurance plan; the insured.

**preauthorization** Prior authorization from an insurance carrier that must be received before a procedure is covered; also known as *precertification.*

**preexisting condition** An illness or disorder that existed before the insured's medical insurance contract went into effect.

**preferred provider organization (PPO)** A managed care network of healthcare providers who agree to perform services for member patients at discounted fees.

**premium** The amount of money paid to an insurance carrier to buy an insurance plan.

**primary care physician** The physician in a health maintenance organization who directs all aspects of a patient's care, including routine services, referrals to specialists within the system, and supervision of hospital admissions; also known as a *gatekeeper.*

**primary diagnosis** The diagnosis that represents the patient's major health problem for a particular insurance claim.

**primary insurance** The insurance plan that pays benefits first when a patient is covered by more than one medical insurance plan.

**primary payer** The insurance plan that pays first when a patient is covered by more than one insurance plan or governmental program.

**prior authorization number** An identifying code assigned by a governmental program or insurance carrier when preauthorization is granted; also called a *preauthorization number.*

**privileged communication** Confidential conversation between physician and patient.

**procedure code** A code that identifies medical or diagnostic services.

**procedure day sheet** A report that summarizes the business day's charges and payments, organized by procedure code.

**prognosis** The physician's prediction of the outcome of a disease or injury and the likelihood of recovery.

**protected health information (PHI)** Individually identifiable health information that is transmitted or maintained in any form or medium.

**provider** In medical insurance, a professional member of the healthcare team, such as a physician, who provides services or supplies to the insured.

**real-time claims adjudication (RTCA)** Electronic health insurance claim processed at patient checkout; allows practice to know what the patient will owe for the visit.

**referral** The transfer of patient care from one physician to another.

**release of information** A statement that authorizes the provider to give the insurance carrier information needed to process an insurance claim.

**remittance advice (RA)** A document from an insurance carrier that reports claim activity and shows how the amount of benefit was determined.

**schedule of benefits** A list of benefits for which an insurance policy will pay.

**secondary insurance** The insurance plan that pays benefits after the primary carrier when a patient is covered by more than one medical insurance plan.

**SOAP format** The documentation of medical records according to the S (subjective data), O (objective data), A (assessment), and P (plan of treatment).

**sponsor** The uniformed service member in a family qualified for TRICARE or CHAMPVA.

**subscriber** An individual who has a contract with an insurance plan for healthcare coverage.

**superbill** A custom-made form used by physicians to note diagnosis and treatment; also known as an *encounter form* or *charge ticket*.

**supplemental insurance** An insurance plan, such as Medigap, that provides benefits for services that are not normally covered by a primary plan.

**third-party liability** An obligation of an insurance plan or governmental program to pay all or part of a patient's medical costs.

**third-party payer** A payer of one entity for another, as an insurance company paying a physician for services received by a patient.

**traditional plan** See *indemnity plan*.

**transaction** In a computerized billing system, a financial exchange, such as a deposit of funds into a provider's bank account.

**TRICARE** A governmental health program offering managed care to dependents of active-duty service members, military retirees and their families, some former spouses, and survivors of deceased military members; formerly called CHAMPUS.

**type of service code** A code that describes the kind of service performed.

**Universal Precautions** Techniques issued by the Centers for Disease Control and Prevention to protect healthcare workers from infection.

**walkout receipt** In a medical office, a completed form a patient receives after a visit. The walkout receipt contains the details of the resulting diagnosis, services provided, fees, and payments received and due.

**workers' compensation insurance** A state or federal plan that covers medical care and other benefits for employees who suffer accidental injury or become ill as a result of employment.

**write off** To discount a patient's fee in accordance with contractual agreements.

**X12 837 Health Care Claim, or 837P** The electronic claim format that is used to bill for a physician's services.

# Index

HIPAA Electronic Health Care Transactions and Code Sets (TCS), 15–17
HIPAA Omnibus Rule, 15
HIPAA Privacy Rule
    authorization to release patient information and, 12–13
    defined, 9–10
    Notice of Privacy Practices and, 11–12, 20
    protected health information and, 10, 52
HIPAA Security Rule, 13–15

ICD-9-CM, 16. *See also* Codes/code sets
ICD-10-CM, 16, 24, 67. *See also* Codes/code sets
ICD-10-PCS, 16. *See also* Codes/code sets
Identification badges, employee, 42
Identifiers, 16–17
Inclement weather, 42
Incoming referrals, 60
Information technology, 54–56
Insurance Carrier List dialog box, 141, 142, 145, 170
Insurance Coverage Percents boxes, 100
*International Classification of Diseases* (ICD), 24
Internists, 3

Laptop computers, 55
Lateness, 47
Leaving early, 47

Managed care plans
    Medicare, 73–74
    visit authorization numbers for, 152
Medicaid, 74
Medical ethics, 46
Medically unnecessary services, 71
Medical necessity, 65
Medical records
    defined, 4
    HIPAA Privacy Rule and, 9–13
    HIPAA Security Rule and, 13–15
    information in, 5–7
    patient privacy and confidentiality issues related to, 8–9 (*See also* Privacy)
    problem-oriented, 7–8
    recording and maintaining patient information in, 19–20
    security issues related to, 13–15 (*See also* Security)
    standards for, 7
Medicare
    allowed amount for procedures covered by, 163
    coverage percent of, 100
    excluded services in, 71
    managed care plans, 73–74
    medically unnecessary services in, 71
    Medigap insurance for, 71–73
    overview of, 70–71
    provider agreement to accept, 115
Medigap insurance, 71–73
Medi-Medi beneficiary, 74
Medisoft
    adding new insurance carrier in, 141–145
    adding new provider, 115–118
    Allowed Amounts feature in, 95–97
    changing insurance carrier code set on, 170
    Claim Rejection Message List in, 98–99
    closing cases in, 152–153
    creating Patient by Insurance Carrier report, 107–109

Diagnosis report, 107
    entering additional diagnosis codes in, 141
    entering additional procedure codes in, 159–164
    entering prior authorization in, 136
    entering referrals in, 151–152
    entering visit authorization numbers in, 152
    printing copayment report in, 135
    printing Patient Face Sheet report, 123
    Quick Balance feature, 129
    Reports menu, 107
    using Final Draft on, 169–170
Messages, telephone, 49–50

National drug code, 162
National Provider Identifier (NPI), 17, 117
New Provider ID dialog box, 117–118
Nonexempt employees, time records for, 38–39
Nonsufficient funds (NSF) checks, 23
Notice of Privacy Practices, 11–12, 20
NSF (nonsufficient funds) checks, 23

Office for Civil Rights (OCR), 15
Office hours, 46–47
Office Hours Lists menu, 119
Office Hours program
    default date in, 101
    locating appointment in, 119
    provider selection in, 103
Office visit procedures
    to check preauthorized requirements, 60
    to check referral requirements, 60
    to conclude patient visits, 61
    to gather patient information, 57–58
    for receptioning, 57
    to schedule appointments, 61–62
    to verify insurance coverage, 59–60
Operations, 10
Oral communication, 52–53. *See also* Telephone procedures
Outgoing referrals, 60
Overtime compensation, 38

Password protection, 54
Patient by Diagnosis report, 107
Patient by Insurance Carrier report, 107–109
Patient day sheets, 67, 68
Patient Face Sheet report, 123
Patient flow, 61–62
Patient information, 52–53. *See also* Medical records
Patient information forms, 5, 6, 182, 186, 190, 192, 197, 206, 211, 220, 233, 238, 242, 247, 249, 253
Patients
    authorization to disclose information about, 12–13
    collecting and recording payments from, 21–22
    educating, 21
    responding to inquiries of, 21
Patient services specialists (PSSs)
    collecting overdue payments from patients by, 23–24
    function of, 8, 17–18
    general responsibilities of, 18
    generating healthcare claims by, 22
    generating patient statements and financial reports by, 23
    maintaining third-party payer information by, 20

monitoring third-party payments by, 22–23
    patient education role of, 21
    recording and maintaining patient information by, 19–20
    recording payments, charges, and adjustments by, 21–22
    responding to patient inquiries by, 21
    scheduling patients for appointments by, 19
    updating CPT and ICD-10-CM codes in database by, 24
Patient statements, 23
Pay dates, 38
Payment for services
    billing cycle and, 63–64
    billing guidelines and, 65–66
    collecting overdue, 23–24
    collections policy and, 62–63
    copayments, 135
    for insurance claims, 64–65
    patient billing disputes and, 67
    Quick Balance feature, 129
    recording, 21–22
    review of remittance advice and, 66–67
    from third-party payers, 22–23
Pay rates, 38
PDF files, 108–109
Performance evaluations, 39
Personal telephone calls, 44
Personal visitors, 44
Personnel conduct, 42–46
PHI. *See* Protected health information (PHI)
Photocopy machines, 53
Physical safeguards, 14
Physicians
    family practice, 3
    internists, 3
    primary care, 4
Place of service (POS) codes, 64, 161
Polaris Medical Group
    discount fee schedule for, 229
    HIPAA Compliance Program and, 17
    HIPAA Privacy Rule and, 9–13
    HIPAA Security Rule and, 13–15
    legislation addressing patient privacy and security and, 8–17
    medical records procedures in, 4–7
    organization and staff of, 2–4
    patient services team in, 2–4
    role of patient services specialist in, 17–24
    SOAP format for, 7–8
    source documents for, 176–267
    statement of purpose for, 2
    typical day at, 19–24
Polaris Medical Group Policy and Procedure Manual (PPM)
    attendance requirements, 47–48
    COBRA benefits, 41
    conduct issues, 42–46
    daily reports, 67–70
    employee benefits, 39–40
    employee conduct issues, 42–46
    employee discharge, 41
    employee grievances, 40
    employee time records, 38–39
    employment levels, 37
    equal employment opportunity, nondiscrimination, and affirmative action statements, 36–37
    ethics, 46
    fee schedule, 76
    health plan information, 77–78
    Medicaid guidelines, 74–75

# NOTES

# NOTES

# NOTES

# NOTES

# NOTES

# NOTES

# NOTES

# NOTES

# NOTES